# Communication Perspectives on HIV/AIDS for the 21st Century

## LEA'S COMMUNICATION SERIES
### Jennings Bryant/Dolf Zillmann, General Editors

# Communication
# Perspectives
# on HIV/AIDS
# for the
# 21st Century

Edited by

Timothy Edgar • Seth M. Noar • Vicki S. Freimuth

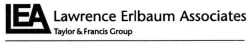

**LEA** Lawrence Erlbaum Associates
Taylor & Francis Group

New York   London

Lawrence Erlbaum Associates
Taylor & Francis Group
270 Madison Avenue
New York, NY 10016

Lawrence Erlbaum Associates
Taylor & Francis Group
2 Park Square
Milton Park, Abingdon
Oxon OX14 4RN

Transferred to Digital Printing 2008

International Standard Book Number-13: 978-0-8058-5827-3 (Softcover) 978-0-8058-5826-6 (Hardcover)

### Library of Congress Cataloging-in-Publication Data

Communication perspectives on HIV/AIDS for the 21st century / editor(s), Timothy
   M. Edgar, Seth M. Noar, Vicki S. Freimuth.
      p. ; cm. -- (LEA's communication series)
   Includes bibliographical references and index.
   ISBN-13: 978-0-8058-5826-6 (hardcover : alk. paper)
   ISBN-10: 0-8058-5826-1 (hardcover : alk. paper)
   ISBN-13: 978-0-8058-5827-3 (softcover : alk. paper)
   ISBN-10: 0-8058-5827-X (softcover : alk. paper)
   1. AIDS (Disease)--Prevention. 2. AIDS (Disease) in mass media. 3. Mass media in
health education. 4. Communication in public health. I. Edgar, Timothy. II. Noar, Seth
M. III. Freimuth, Vicki S. IV. Series.
   [DNLM: 1. Acquired Immunodeficiency Syndrome--prevention & control.
   2. HIV Infections--prevention & control. 3. Health Education. WC
   503.6 C7346 2008]

RA643.8.C64 2008
362.196'9792--dc22                                                    2007023816

**Visit the Taylor & Francis Web site at**
**http://www.taylorandfrancis.com**

# Dedication

*To Wendy and Linda for all of your love,
support, constant friendship, and for proving
that 13 can be a very lucky number*

**Tim Edgar**

*To Elisa, for your love and support. To Jonah,
for coming into our lives and for all the laughs. And
to Sadie, for being the best communicator I know.*

**Seth M. Noar**

*For my grandchildren with the hope that their
generation will be free of HIV/AIDS*

**Vicki S. Freimuth**

# Contents

## Intervention Exemplar Chapters

# Preface

In 1981, the Centers for Disease Control and Prevention (CDC) published a report of cases of a rare pneumonia found in five previously healthy gay men, later determined to be the first five reported AIDS cases in the United States. More than twenty-five years later we are faced with a domestic epidemic that has claimed more than 500,000 lives. Currently, more than 1 million people are living with HIV in the United States and nearly one third of these individuals are unaware of their serostatus. Furthermore, each year approximately 40,000 people become newly infected with HIV, with the epidemic increasingly affecting racial minorities, women, and heterosexuals (CDC, 2006b). Recent data also indicate a resurgence in new infections among men who have sex with men (MSM) (CDC, 2006a, 2006b). Worldwide, the global AIDS epidemic has grown to so-called "pandemic" proportions. In 2005 alone, an estimated 2.8 million people lost their lives to AIDS and 4.1 million people became newly infected with HIV. To date, more than 25 million deaths have been attributed to AIDS and approximately 38.6 million people are currently living with HIV (UNAIDS, 2006).

As the epidemiology and course of HIV/AIDS have changed, so have the salient issues before us. Early in the epidemic (i.e., 1980s) the major focus in the United States was on informing the public about the disease and developing primary prevention efforts to contain the spread of the virus. In that early period, AIDS was essentially a death sentence, as the medical profession had little to offer patients with AIDS. Perhaps the most dramatic shift came in the mid-1990s when highly active antiretroviral therapy (HAART) became available and transformed AIDS from an automatic death sentence to a chronic disease. The medicines that became available have extended individuals' lives and allowed many to cope with the disease, and such medicines have been continually improving since first coming on the market. Although the introduction of HAART brought hope to those with HIV/AIDS and was a significant step forward for those suffering with the disease, there are still many issues related to access to these medicines. In fact, it is estimated that of those currently in need of HIV treatment, only 55% of those in the United States and 20% in low- and middle-income countries have access to HAART (CDC, 2006a). ← *So we must focus on prevention*

Moreover, the post-HAART era of AIDS has brought new challenges with it, and has expanded AIDS issues to include medication adherence and health literacy, social support, and prevention with HIV-positive individuals. In addition, there has been new interest in novel HIV prevention messages and programs given recent reports of AIDS complacency and renewed high-risk sexual behavior among certain at-risk groups such as MSM (CDC, 2006a; Elford & Hart, 2003). In addition, as AIDS has become a global issue and priority, there has been an increased focus and discussion of issues related to technology transfer, dissemination, and cultural adaptation and sensitivity of prevention programs; stigma and denial surrounding HIV; gender inequality, human rights, poverty, and social change; and the politics of funding HIV-related initiatives (e.g., UNAIDS, 2006).

How have communication scholars and practitioners responded to the HIV/AIDS epidemic? Many of those interested in communication issues have, in fact, long been involved in the fight against AIDS. For example, from early on, a number of communication scholars were engaged in various research projects in this area, and one culmination of this work was the publication of *AIDS: A Communication Perspective* in 1992. The volume, edited by Edgar, Fitzpatrick, and Freimuth, focused on many of the key issues of the epidemic throughout the 1980s and early 1990s. Such topics included development and evaluation of HIV prevention media campaigns, examination of HIV/AIDS news coverage, and prevention of HIV through understanding communication patterns and optimizing safer-sex messages. In the preface of that volume, the editors wrote:

> As the number of AIDS cases multiplied throughout the early and mid-1980s, it became apparent that no cure or vaccine was on the horizon. Prevention through appropriate behavior was, and still is, the best weapon to fight further spread of HIV infection. However, individuals take necessary actions to prevent a disease such as AIDS only when (a) they are properly informed and (b) they feel motivated to respond to the information they possess. In order to achieve a clearer understanding of these facets of the prevention process, we must examine the interplay

of the messages individuals receive about AIDS at the public level and
the messages exchanged between individuals at the interpersonal level.
(Edgar, Fitzpatrick, & Freimuth, 1992, p. xi)

Although that passage was written more than 15 years ago (in
1991 when finishing the book), the point is still valid. The only factor
that we might add, based on what we have learned over these many
years, is that individuals need not only to be informed and motivated, but to have the behavioral skills and control over the situation
in order to carry out their intended actions. Clearly, an understanding of effective communication through both mediated and interpersonal channels is *still* essential to winning the continued battle
against AIDS. Although at the time the original book went to press
we thought that the battle against AIDS would be in its last stages
within a decade or so, that clearly has not been the case.

In addition, communication scholars have kept pace with the
changing course of the disease. Researchers have been exploring
some of the same research questions with new methods and insights,
whereas others have conducted research projects in many of the
newer and diverse areas that are now central in understanding and
responding to HIV/AIDS. Thus, we decided that the time had come
to pull together this work and assemble it in a new book, given that
the face of HIV/AIDS has changed so much since 1992. An early decision made regarding the scope of the current book was that it would
focus primarily on domestic HIV/AIDS issues and research. Why
focus on domestic research? Although international work is very
important, particularly given the global impact of AIDS, recently
published volumes have begun to pull together and disseminate key
communication perspectives on responding to the global HIV/AIDS
epidemic (e.g., see McKee, Bertrand, & Becker-Benton, 2004; Singhal & Rogers, 2003). On the other hand, as best we could tell a major
volume pulling together domestic health communication perspectives on HIV/AIDS had not been published since our previous 1992
volume. In addition, focusing primarily on U.S.-based research gives
us an opportunity to focus on a broad spectrum of issues and topics
within a single volume. Such a broad but representative cross section
of topics is much more difficult to accomplish with international volumes, given the massive scope of global HIV/AIDS. Thus, our goal
was to pull together a volume that was primarily focused on domestic
research and featured many different (but central) issues and themes
under study by health communication scholars. Despite this focus,

we encouraged contributors to touch on international issues if possible, and many contributors took us up on this proposition. Furthermore, we should note that approaches developed in the United States or in the West are sometimes adapted to developing countries in the fight against AIDS. Thus, much of the work contained in this volume should have relevance for those pursuing work in other countries.

In addition, some further background on and description of the structure of the book is in order. When we originally conceptualized the book, we first discussed, and subsequently decided on a number of topics that we felt had to be included in the book. The ultimate result of these conversations is the 13 major chapters that reside in the current volume. Many of the topics are as relevant now as they were in 1992. However, the major difference is that we have much more data from which to evaluate the topic/issue now than we did then. In addition, other topics are reflective of the way in which the AIDS epidemic has changed. In chapter 1, Noar and Edgar review the literature on partner communication about safer sex and examine how such communication is related to the enactment of safer sexual behavior. Although few studies of partner communication existed in the 1980s, this review demonstrates that this literature and our subsequent knowledge about this area blossomed greatly in the 1990s through today. In a related chapter, Edgar, Noar, and Murphy (chap. 2) review approaches to communication skills training within the vast HIV prevention intervention literature, and reveal that great diversity exists in the training approaches that have been utilized. In fact, in the original volume, Edgar (1992) reviewed that same literature and was able to locate only three studies on the topic, but in the last 15 years, scores of intervention studies with a communication skills component have been published.

Moreover, now that 25 years of HIV/AIDS have passed and many more people are living with HIV, how has the social stigma associated with the disease changed? What is the current state of research in the area of HIV/AIDS stigma? Rintamaki and Weaver review the literature in the area of stigma and provide answers to these important questions in chapter 3. In addition, given the many challenges that those living with HIV face including the social stigma and uncertainty about the course of their illness, understanding how individuals cope with the disease is very important. In chapter 4, Goldsmith, Brashers, Kosenko, and O'Keefe examine the growing research on social support and those living with HIV/AIDS.

Since the beginning of the epidemic, HIV counseling and testing have been central activities for identifying those who are HIV-positive and counseling individuals with regard to behavior change. What is the state of HIV testing currently and are there ways in which this practice could be improved? Mattson and Basnyat provide an overview of this topic in chapter 5 and suggest ways in which such counseling might be enhanced. Next, chapter 6 by DiIorio, McCarty, and Pluhar features a review of literature on parent–child discussions surrounding HIV/AIDS and safer sexual behavior. This literature has blossomed greatly in the past two decades as evidenced by the more than 100 studies appearing on this topic, and researchers are beginning to better understand how parent–child communication patterns may relate to safer or risky decision making on the part of adolescents. Furthermore, a growing area of concern surrounding HIV/AIDS is the disproportionate impact of HIV on racial minorities such as African Americans. In chapter 7, Resnicow, DiIorio, and Davis examine the issue of cultural sensitivity as it relates to developing HIV prevention and sex education programs, including discussion of cultural targeting and tailoring of programs.

Early in the epidemic the mass media were major tools used to raise awareness about AIDS in the United States and elsewhere. Today, the mass media have become key tools used by numerous countries around the world to transmit HIV/AIDS prevention messages. Are such campaigns capable, however, of effectively impacting not only knowledge levels but also attitudes, norms, and ultimately behavior change? In chapter 8, Palmgreen, Noar, and Zimmerman report on a number of studies that have now been undertaken to examine this important question. In a related chapter, Kennedy, Beck, and Freimuth (chap. 9) report on the current state of entertainment education and its ability to contribute to HIV prevention in both the United States and abroad. Finally, the news media coverage of HIV/AIDS is responsible for bringing HIV/AIDS into our living rooms (or failing to do so). How has the news media coverage of HIV/AIDS changed over time and how does the agenda-setting function of news impact public opinion and policy making? These important issues are considered by Dearing and Kim in chapter 10.

U.S. policy surrounding HIV/AIDS is another very important area and one that has often been controversial. In responding to the AIDS epidemic, are our policies based on science, politics, or some blend of the two? In chapter 11, Scott uses rhetorical analysis to examine the issues surrounding the science versus politics debate and U.S. policy making. Furthermore, in the post-HAART era of AIDS, those living with HIV often have very complex medication regimens that they need to understand and carefully adhere to in order to keep the disease at bay, something that requires significant health literacy skills. In chapter 12, Kalichman gives an overview of research on health literacy and its importance to the health and well-being of those undergoing HIV treatment. And finally, in chapter 13, Bull introduces us to a 21st-century world in which numerous technological innovations, most notably the Internet, are being used every day for both prevention interventions as well as risky behavior (i.e., seeking sex partners online). Although this is still a relatively new area of HIV prevention research, it is rapidly growing and has major implications for public health.

In addition, along the way in the development of the overall volume the editors had a discussion about the number of exciting intervention projects around HIV/AIDS in which health communication researchers were engaged. Thus, we came up with the idea of having a section that included short exemplars of such projects, to be able to provide a collection of such projects in one book and to showcase the varying approaches to health communication that have been used to combat the HIV/AIDS epidemic. Rather than invite every health communication scholar engaged in HIV prevention work to contribute to this section, our goal instead was to carefully select projects so that the patchwork of interventions that resulted demonstrated the diversity of approaches that are being utilized and studied in health communication. To be sure that we were capturing important health communication approaches beyond those developed by individuals working in academic settings, we also invited one foundation (Kaiser Family Foundation) and one community-based group (STOP AIDS Project) to contribute.

In order to have some similarity in structure across the exemplars and to encourage contributors to focus on what we viewed as key issues, we asked each contributor to consider the following when crafting their chapter:

1. What were the goals of your intervention?
2. How was communication used to effect change?
3. Briefly discuss how theory was used (if at all).
4. Does evidence exist that the approach made a difference?
5. What were the most important lessons learned?

ask this of
Vancouver
based organizations.

The result of our efforts and the efforts of the contributors can be found in the latter part of the book. The set of approaches within this part range from interpersonal to mass communication mediums, those that use traditional as well as new media and technology, those conducted by academics as well as practitioners, individual as well as community-based approaches, those based in the United States as well as international projects, and those directed at at-risk, HIV-positive, and general populations.

Thus, given so many new topics, a variety of new contributors, and the broadened scope of the current volume, this book is not simply a revision of the 1992 volume but rather is a whole new book altogether. Moreover, the current book is designed for a variety of audiences—including academics, researchers, practitioners, and graduate and undergraduate students. It is our belief and hope that a variety of readers from a variety of disciplines and backgrounds will find the book accessible and enlightening. We hope that the current volume adds to the growing knowledge base with regard to communication approaches to HIV/AIDS, and that this work ultimately influences those affected by and infected with HIV/AIDS.

## Acknowledgments

We would like to thank all of the contributors to the current volume for their efforts and for being responsive to our suggestions and ideas regarding their chapter contributions. We would also like to thank Linda Bathgate at Lawrence Erlbaum Associates (now part of the Routledge imprint) for her guidance through the early stages of the project and Marsha Hecht from the Taylor & Francis Group for her patience and attention to detail during the production process. Bryan Murphy deserves special recognition for his many hours of painstaking editorial assistance. We greatly appreciate the personal pride Bryan took and the dedication he showed in helping to ensure a high-quality final product. And Katey Dyall, Kelly George, and Georgette Petraglia deserve thanks for their help with the index. Finally, we would like to acknowledge Mary Anne Fitzpatrick, who was a coeditor of the 1992 volume and the one who first had the idea to do the original book. Because Mary Anne's new career as a dean of a large college of arts and sciences occupies all of her professional life, she was not able to participate in the project this time, but we appreciate the encouragement she has provided in the development of the second book.

**Timothy Edgar**
**Seth M. Noar**
**Vicki S. Freimuth**

## References

Centers for Disease Control and Prevention. (2006a). The global HIV/AIDS pandemic. *Morbidity and Mortality Weekly Report, 55*(31), 841–844.

Centers for Disease Control and Prevention. (2006b). Twenty-five years of HIV/AIDS—United States, 1981–2006. *Morbidity and Mortality Weekly Report, 55*(21), 585–589.

Edgar, T. (1992). A compliance-based approach to the study of condom use. In T. Edgar, M. A. Fitzpatrick, & V. S. Freimuth (Eds.), *AIDS: A communication perspective* (pp. 47–67). Hillsdale, NJ: Lawrence Erlbaum Associates.

Edgar, T., Fitzpatrick, M. A., & Freimuth, V. S. (Eds). (1992). *AIDS: A communication perspective.* Hillsdale, NJ: Lawrence Erlbaum Associates.

Elford, J., & Hart, G. (2003). If HIV prevention works, why are rates of high-risk sexual behaviour increasing among MSM? *AIDS Education & Prevention, 15,* 294–308.

McKee, N., Bertrand, J. T., & Becker-Benton, A. (2004). *Strategic communication in the HIV/AIDS epidemic.* Thousand Oaks, CA: Sage.

Singhal, A., & Rogers, E. M. (2003). *Combating AIDS: Communication strategies in action.* Thousand Oaks, CA: Sage.

UNAIDS. (2006). *Report on the global AIDS epidemic: Executive summary.* Geneva, Switzerland: Joint United Nations Program on HIV/AIDS.

# Editors

**Timothy Edgar** (PhD, Purdue University) is an associate professor and director of the Graduate Program in Health Communication at Emerson College, where he teaches behavioral and communication theory, social marketing, and research methods. He also has a secondary appointment as an associate adjunct clinical professor in the Department of Public Health and Family Medicine at the Tufts University School of Medicine. His career has been devoted to conducting research on the use of communication strategies to motivate changes in health-related risk behaviors. Prior to joining the Emerson faculty, Dr. Edgar was a senior study director at Westat in Rockville, Maryland for 9 years. While at Westat, he was the project director for dozens of health communication evaluation studies, primarily for the Centers for Disease Control and Prevention (CDC). Dr. Edgar also led the team that developed the *CDCynergy* training tool for CDC, which is the agency's standard for instruction on health communication planning, implementation, and evaluation. Prior to his career as a professional evaluator, Dr. Edgar was on the health communication faculty at the University of Maryland for 7 years where he primarily conducted HIV/AIDS-related research. His work culminated in the publication of a book titled *AIDS: A Communication Perspective*. Dr. Edgar has been the recipient of numerous academic honors and awards, and he has published widely in professional journals and texts and has been a presenter at various conferences. He is also on the editorial boards of both *Health Communication* and the *Journal of Health Communication*.

**Seth M. Noar** (PhD, University of Rhode Island) is an assistant professor and associate member of the graduate faculty in the Department of Communication at the University of Kentucky. Before joining the University of Kentucky, he was a postdoctoral scholar at the Institute for HIV Prevention Research for 2 years, also located at the University of Kentucky. His research interests focus on health promotion and disease prevention from a health communication perspective, and are mostly concentrated in the area of HIV prevention and safer sexual behavior. His research articles address health behavior theories, sexual communication, safer-sex messages and media campaigns, and methodological topics including meta-analysis, and have appeared in a wide range of journals including *Health Communication, Journal of Health Communication, Health Education Research: Theory & Practice, Health Education & Behavior, AIDS Education and Prevention, AIDS Care, Archives of Sexual Behavior,* and *Psychological Bulletin.* Dr. Noar is currently a co-investigator on HIV prevention projects funded by both the National Institutes of Health and the Centers for Disease Control and Prevention. He also is on the editorial boards of *Health Communication* and *Communication Monographs.*

**Vicki S. Freimuth** (PhD, Florida State University) is director of the Center for Health and Risk Communication and a professor in the Department of Speech Communication and the Grady School of Journalism at the University of Georgia. Her major research interests center on health communication, specifically studying the role of communication in health promotion. Before joining the faculty at the University of Georgia, she served as director of communication at the CDC for 7 years. Prior to that position, she was professor and director of the Health Communication Program at the University of Maryland. She is author of *Searching for Health Information,* coeditor of *AIDS: A Communication Perspective,* and author of chapters in several major books in health communication. Her research has appeared in journals such as *Human Communication Research, Journal of Communication, Journal of Health Communication, American Journal of Public Health, Social Science and Medicine,* and *Journal of Emerging Infectious Diseases.* She is the recipient of several grants including ones from the National Cancer Institute and the CDC. She has served on the editorial boards of several journals including the *Journal of Communication, Human Communication Research,* and the *Journal of Health Communication.* She won a Distinguished Career Award from the American Association of Public Health in 2003. She was selected as the first Outstanding Health Communication Scholar by the International Communication Association and the National Communication Association and was selected as the Woman of the Year at the University of Maryland in 1990. She has provided consultation to many organizations including the U.S. Agency for International Development, the World Health Organization, the World Bank, the National Cancer Institute, the National Eye Institute, and the Robert Wood Johnson Foundation.

# Contributors

**Paul Robert Appleby, PhD**
Department of Psychology
University of Southern California
Los Angeles, California

**Iccha Basnyat, MPH**
Department of Communication
Purdue University
West Lafayette, Indiana

**Vicki Beck, MS**
Hollywood, Health & Society at the Annenberg Norman Lear
    Center
University of Southern California
Beverly Hills, California

**Anne Bowen, PhD**
Department of Psychology
University of Wyoming
Laramie, Wyoming

**Dale E. Brashers, PhD**
Department of Speech Communication
University of Illinois at Urbana-Champaign
Urbana, Illinois

**Nikia D. Braxton, MPH**
Rollins School of Public Health
Emory University
Atlanta, Georgia

**Sheana Bull, PhD, MPH**
Colorado Health Outcomes Program and Department
    of Family Medicine
University of Colorado at Denver and Health Sciences Center
Aurora, Colorado

**Kellie E. Carlyle, MA**
School of Communication
The Ohio State University
Columbus, Ohio

**Sara Clayton, MS**
Department of Psychology
University of Wyoming
Laramie, Wyoming

**Candice M. Daniel, MS**
Department of Psychology
University of Wyoming
Laramie, Wyoming

**Julia L. Davis, BA**
Benjamin N. Cardozo School of Law
Yeshiva University
New York, New York

**Rachel Davis, MPH**
Health Behavior & Health Education
School of Public Health
University of Michigan
Ann Arbor, Michigan

**James W. Dearing, PhD**
Clinical Research Unit
Kaiser Permanente Colorado
Denver, Colorado

**Ralph J. DiClemente, PhD**
Rollins School of Public Health
Emory University
Atlanta, Georgia

**Colleen K. DiIorio, PhD, RN, FAAN**
Department of Behavioral Sciences and Health Education
Rollins School of Public Health
Emory University
Atlanta, Georgia

**Timothy Edgar, PhD**
Department of Marketing Communication
Emerson College
Boston, Massachusetts

**Lilia Espinoza, MPH**
Department of Preventive Medicine
Keck School of Medicine
University of Southern California
Los Angeles, California

**Vicki S. Freimuth, PhD**
Department of Speech Communication and Grady College
   of Journalism and Mass Communication
University of Georgia
Athens, Georgia

**Carlos Godoy, MA**
Annenberg School for Communication
University of Southern California
Los Angeles, California

**Daena J. Goldsmith, PhD**
Department of Communication
Lewis and Clark College
Portland, Oregon

**Jennifer Hecht, MPH**
STOP AIDS Project
San Francisco, California

**Tina Hoff, BS**
Entertainment Media Partnerships
Henry J. Kaiser Family Foundation
Menlo Park, California

**John Howson, MSc**
Health Communication Partnership/International HIV/AIDS
    Alliance
Center for Communication Programs
Johns Hopkins University Bloomberg School of Public Health
Baltimore, Maryland

**Matt James, BA**
Media & Pubic Education
Henry J. Kaiser Family Foundation
Menlo Park, California

**Seth C. Kalichman, PhD**
Department of Psychology
University of Connecticut
Storrs, Connecticut

**May G. Kennedy, PhD**
Department of Behavioral Science and Health Promotion
Virginia Commonwealth University
Richmond, Virginia

**Do Kyun Kim, MA**
School of Communication Studies
Ohio University
Athens, Ohio

**Amy R. Knowlton, ScD, MPH**
Department of Health, Behavior, and Society
Johns Hopkins School of Public Health
Baltimore, Maryland

**Kami Kosenko, MA**
Department of Speech Communication
University of Illinois at Urbana-Champaign
Urbana, Illinois

**Carl A. Latkin, PhD**
Department of Health, Behavior, and Society
Johns Hopkins School of Public Health
Baltimore, Maryland

**Marifran Mattson, PhD**
Department of Communication
Purdue University
West Lafayette, Indiana

**Frances McCarty, PhD**
Department of Behavioral Sciences and Health Education
Rollins School of Public Health
Emory University
Atlanta, Georgia

**Kathryn S. Meier, MPH**
Cancer Prevention Research Center
University of Rhode Island
Kingston, Rhode Island

**Joel Milam, PhD**
Department of Preventive Medicine
Keck School of Medicine
University of Southern California
Los Angeles, California

**Ann Neville Miller, PhD**
Daystar University
Nairobi, Kenya

**Lynn Carol Miller, PhD**
Annenberg School for Communication
University of Southern California
Los Angeles, California

**Patricia J. Morokoff, PhD**
Department of Psychology
University of Rhode Island
Kingston, Rhode Island

**Bryan Murphy, MA**
Emerson College
Boston, Massachusetts

**Seth M. Noar, PhD**
Department of Communication
University of Kentucky
Lexington, Kentucky

**Daniel J. O'Keefe, PhD**
Department of Communication Studies
Northwestern University
Evanston, Illinois

**Philip Palmgreen, PhD**
Department of Communication
University of Kentucky
Lexington, Kentucky

**Erika Pluhar, PhD**
Department of Behavioral Sciences and Health Education
Rollins School of Public Health
Emory University
Atlanta, Georgia

**Stephen J. Read, PhD**
Department of Psychology
University of Southern California
Los Angeles, California

**Colleen A. Redding, PhD**
Cancer Prevention Research Center
University of Rhode Island
Kingston, Rhode Island

**Ken Resnicow, PhD**
Health Behavior & Health Education School of Public Health
University of Michigan
Ann Arbor, Michigan

**Jean L. Richardson, PhD**
Department of Preventive Medicine
Keck School of Medicine
Los Angeles, California

**Lance S. Rintamaki, PhD**
State University of New York at Buffalo
Buffalo, New York

**Anthony J. Roberto, PhD**
School of Communication
The Ohio State University
Columbus, Ohio

**Joseph S. Rossi, PhD**
Cancer Prevention Research Center
University of Rhode Island
Kingston, Rhode Island

**Jessica McDermott Sales, PhD**
Rollins School of Public Health
Emory University
Atlanta, Georgia

**J. Blake Scott, PhD**
Department of English
University of Central Florida
Orlando, Florida

**Frances M. Weaver, PhD**
Department of Veteran Affairs
Center for Complex Chronic Care Management
Hines, Illinois

**Gina M. Wingood, ScD**
Rollins School of Public Health
Emory University
Atlanta, Georgia

**Kim Witte, PhD**
Department of Communication
Michigan State University
East Lansing, Michigan

**Rick S. Zimmerman, PhD**
Department of Communication
University of Kentucky
Lexington, Kentucky

# I

*Review Chapters*

# 1

## The Role of Partner Communication in Safer Sexual Behavior
### *A Theoretical and Empirical Review*

*Seth M. Noar*
University of Kentucky

*Timothy Edgar*
Emerson College

> Having a number of strategies at one's disposal is not only the sign of a skilled communicator but also may, in the case of the AIDS crisis, literally save one's life.
>
> Edgar and Fitzpatrick (1988)

> The immediate threat to the relationship might discourage talk about a potential health crisis, the impact of which will not be detectable for some time.
>
> Bowen and Michal-Johnson (1989)

> Sex ... is good for selling everything from shampoo, office machinery, hotel rooms, and beer to prime-time series and made-for-TV movies ... but a product that would prevent the tragedy of teenage pregnancy—the dreaded "c-word"—must never darken America's television screens.
>
> Strasburger and Wilson (2002)

Partner communication about safer sex, or the discussions and negotiations that sexual partners have with one another about their sexual histories, AIDS and sexually transmitted diseases (STDs), and condom use, is both a fascinating and a vitally important topic of study. Why is this topic so important? We would argue that to fail to understand these communication practices would be to fail to understand

3

sexual interactions at large, and if, how, whether, and why safer sex is integrated into such interactions. In addition, if we lack an understanding of these sexual interactions, we will likely fail in creating interventions that effectively promote safer sexual behavior.

Moreover, the quotations at the start of this chapter reveal an interesting dichotomy in the area of partner communication. On the one hand, the ability to communicate and negotiate with a sexual partner is a key set of skills that may often be necessary in bringing about safer sexual behaviors (e.g., Cline, 2003; Noar, Carlyle, & Cole, 2006). For instance, if in a sexual situation, how does one express the desire to use a condom without some type of communication, be it verbal or nonverbal? On the other hand, although the mass media is chock full of sexual content, there is a paucity of modeling of safer sexual skills of any kind (e.g., Strasburger & Wilson, 2002). And, there remain numerous social and interpersonal barriers to discussing condom use and safer sex, some of which are implicit in intimate relationships (see Cline, 2003; Misovich, Fisher, & Fisher, 1997; Noar, Zimmerman, & Atwood, 2004). Thus, although communication skills are vitally important for sexually active persons, there are few facilitators for and many barriers to such communication skills being both learned and utilized in sexual situations.

The purpose of the current chapter is to provide an overview of and suggest future directions for research on (a) theoretical perspectives used to understand the role of partner communication in safer sexual behavior, and (b) empirical data on the association of partner communication to safer sexual behavior. Our primary focus is with regard to communication about *safer sex* and *condom use*, although related topics are considered as well (e.g., communication about STDs). Over the more than two decades in which this topic has been studied, theoretical perspectives have grown and basic empirical data has continued to be generated. This chapter provides a review of what we are learning in this important area and points to gaps in the literature that deserve increased research attention.

## Theoretical Perspectives on Safer Sexual Communication

A number of theoretical perspectives have been used to understand the role of partner communication in safer sexual behavior. We divide these into three classes of perspectives, including (a) social cognitive,

(b) compliance gaining, and (c) sexual scripts. As suggested in Table 1.1 and discussed herein, these perspectives examine different aspects of partner communication. Thus, in many ways they are complementary rather than competing explanations of the role of partner communication in safer sexual encounters.

## Social Cognitive Perspectives

A number of social cognitive-oriented theories have been applied to health behavior in general and safer sexual behavior in particular. These theories include the health belief model (HBM) (Janz & Becker, 1984), theory of reasoned action (TRA) (Fishbein & Ajzen, 1975) and planned behavior (TPB) (Ajzen & Madden, 1986), social cognitive theory (SCT) (Bandura, 1986), information-motivation-behavioral skills model (IMB) (Fisher & Fisher, 1992), AIDS risk reduction model (ARRM) (Catania, Kegeles, & Coates, 1990), and the transtheoretical or "stages of change" model (TTM) (Prochaska, DiClemente, & Norcross, 1992). All of these theories have been widely applied to the study of safer sexual behavior, and though the empirical evidence for them varies, all enjoy some level of empirical support in the literature (see Fisher & Fisher, 2000; Noar, 2007).

The social cognitive perspective on safer sexual behavior tends to focus on the role of information, attitudes, and beliefs in an understanding of behaviors such as condom use. Though all of these theories have been applied to the safer-sex area and have implications for partner communication, some theories have focused more on communication practices than others. For instance, both the ARRM and IMB were specifically proposed to provide an understanding of sexual risk-taking behavior, and as such much of their attention is focused on behavioral skills such as partner communication. The ARRM (Catania et al., 1990) suggests that individuals progress through three stages on the way toward maintenance of safer sexual behavior: *labeling, commitment,* and *enactment.* In the first stage, individuals must *label* their behavior as putting them at risk for HIV or other STDs before they move to the next stage, *commitment,* during which time individuals weigh the benefits and costs of particular actions and begin to make a *commitment* to safer sex. One particularly important influence during this second stage is self-efficacy (Bandura, 1986), which is one's perceived ability to engage in a behavior across a variety of challenging

**TABLE 1.1    Theoretical Perspectives for Understanding the Role of Partner Communication in Sexual Encounters**

| Theoretical Perspective | Theories in This Area Include... | Questions Asked by This Perspective | Basic Answers Provided by Empirical Data | Implications for Interventions |
|---|---|---|---|---|
| Social Cognitive Perspectives | Health Belief Model Expanded Theories of Reasoned Action and Planned Behavior Transtheoretical or "stages of change" Model AIDS Risk Reduction Model Information-Motivation-Behavioral Skills Model | *Under what conditions* does safer sexual communication take place? | When individuals are motivated to use condoms and thus to discuss the topic. "Motivation" is defined in various (though often overlapping) ways by the many theories in this area, including having safer-sex information, viewing HIV/STDs as a threat, holding positive attitudes toward safer sex, viewing social norms in support of safer sex, having high self-efficacy to engage in safer sex, having strong intentions to use condoms, and being in an advanced stage of change for condom use. | Partner communication is an important skill necessary for the performance of condom use. However, individuals will likely use these kinds of skills (which they might learn from skills-training interventions) only if they are sufficiently motivated to engage in safe sex. If individuals are not motivated to have safe sex, appealing to their motivation should take place before working on behavioral skills. |

| Compliance-Gaining Perspective | A variety of compliance-gaining typologies | *How* do individuals attempt to persuade a partner to use a condom? | A variety of strategies are used to persuade partners to use condoms, both verbal and nonverbal (see Table 1.3). A variety of factors may influence one's choice of strategy, including gender, age, race, and perceived power in the situation. | There are a variety of ways to attempt to persuade a partner to have safer sex, and some strategies appear to be more effective than others. Individuals might try a variety of strategies with a sexual partner, especially using strategies that one is comfortable with and that are well suited to the context and situation. |
|---|---|---|---|---|
| Sexual Scripts Perspective | Sexual Scripts | *When* do individuals negotiate condom use, and what do sexual interactions look like? *Where* do individuals learn how to negotiate condom use? (e.g., movies, television) | The studies using this perspective suggest that in casual sexual situations, individuals do not bring up the topic of condom use until far into foreplay, when sexual intercourse is essentially imminent. Few studies have examined where individuals learn scripts to use when talking to sexual partners, perhaps because there are so few visible scripts for discussing safer sex in the mass media. | Many individuals wait until sex is literally about to happen to talk about condom use. Discussing condom use before things get to this point, as well as being prepared in terms of actually having a condom available, will likely increase the chances of safer sex taking place. In addition, given the lack of scripts in the mass media for safer sexual communication, interventions should teach and provide such scripts. |

situations. Finally, in the last stage, individuals *enact* their risk reduction plans, and partner sexual communication plays an important role in that process, according to the theory. Furthermore, according to the ARRM, individuals may move forward and backward through these stages as a natural part of the change process, which includes relapse and cycling through the stages. The ARRM perspective clearly suggests that individuals need to be sufficiently motivated (i.e., have labeled their behavior as risky and made a commitment to safer sex) before they will discuss safer sex with a partner.

Fisher and Fisher's (1992) IMB suggests a similar process through which partner communication takes place. This theory suggests that three broad sets of factors are important to achieving safer sexual behavior change: (a) information with regard to safer sex, (b) motivation to engage in safer sex, and (c) safer sexual behavioral skills. The behavioral skills do not become important until an individual has sufficient information to know which risk reduction measures to implement as well as having sufficient motivation to do so. "Motivation" is conceptualized in this theory as viewing HIV/STDs as a threat, holding positive attitudes toward safer sex, and perceiving normative pressure to engage in safer sexual behavior.

In addition, expanded versions of both the TRA (Sheeran, Abraham, & Orbell, 1999) and TPB (Bryan, Fisher, & Fisher, 2002) have been proposed in the safer-sex area, and each includes partner communication as a key factor. The expanded TPB is particularly well specified, and includes partner communication as one of a set of "preparatory behaviors" that comprise other behavioral skills such as obtaining and carrying condoms. The TPB suggests that if one has positive safer-sex attitudes, has positive social norms, and perceives that the behavior is under one's control, the individual will have strong intentions to engage in the behavior and will subsequently do so. Moreover, the expanded TPB suggests that "preparatory behaviors" mediate the relationship between intention and behavior, such that behavioral intentions are put into action through preparatory behaviors such as carrying and obtaining condoms, and discussing condom use (Bryan et al., 2002). This ultimately leads to engagement in the behavior (e.g., condom use).

Finally, an additional theory that has amended itself in the area of safer sex to include partner communication is the TTM (Grimley, Prochaska, & Prochaska, 1997). Similar to the ARRM, this theory holds that individuals progress through a number of stages of readiness on their way toward changing an unhealthy behavior to a healthy one. The stages include *precontemplation* (not intending to engage in safer sex), *contemplation* (intending to engage in safer sex in the near future), *preparation* (planning to engage in safer sex in the very near future and currently taking steps toward that goal), *action* (currently engaging in safer sex), and *maintenance* (currently engaging in safer sex and have been for a sustained period of time). The TTM suggests that sexual assertiveness with a partner is an important skill that is increasingly utilized by individuals as they progress through the stages of change, and is necessary for stage progression toward the maintenance of safer sex. Furthermore, data on the TTM suggest that individuals tend to be increasingly sexually assertive as they become increasingly motivated to practice safer sex, with motivation in this context meaning movement into advanced stages of change such as the preparation or action stage (Grimley et al., 1997; Noar, Morokoff, & Redding, 2002).

Comment on Social Cognitive Perspectives.    The social cognitive perspective helps us to understand the conditions under which partner communication is likely to take place (see Table 1.1). Namely, a common theme across these various theories is the following: Individuals will communicate with a partner about safer sex only if they are *sufficiently motivated* to actually engage in safer sexual behavior. Such "motivation" is conceptualized and measured in a variety of ways among these theories, although there is much overlap here and the theories tend to use a combination of information, attitudes, and beliefs to measure this concept. Moreover, this perspective tends to suggest a direct link between communication and safer sexual behavior, such that communication leads directly to safer sexual behaviors such as condom use. However, beyond data on that basic association and insight into the attitudes and beliefs that may lead to partner communication, the perspective provides limited insight into the nature of communication in sexual situations.

## Compliance-Gaining Perspective

The compliance-gaining perspective is derived from communication research as well as research in related disciplines such as social psychology. Such a perspective examines partner communication using the following question as a guide: "If you wanted to persuade a partner to use a condom, how would you do so?" A number of compliance-gaining typologies exist, some of which were developed decades ago (e.g., Falbo & Peplau, 1980; French & Raven, 1959; Howard, Blumstein, & Schwartz, 1986; Marwell & Schmitt, 1967). Each typology focuses on different ways in which individuals attempt to persuade others, including their romantic partners, to engage in a variety of activities. Furthermore, a variety of tactics with many underlying mechanisms including reward, manipulation, bargaining, coercion, suggestion, identification, and use of persuasive information is included in these typologies.

Marwell and Schmitt (1967) developed one of the most widely used typologies of compliance gaining. Their work resulted in five clusters of techniques that can be used to gain compliance, including: (a) rewarding activities, (b) punishing activities, (c) expertise, (d) activation of impersonal commitments, and (e) activation of personal commitments. Rewarding refers to promising or the providing of a variety of positive consequences if the individual complies with the request, whereas punishing refers to the promise or providing of negative consequences if the individual does *not* comply. Expertise refers to techniques that show one's expert knowledge in an area in order to gain compliance. Activation of *personal* commitments refers to a range of strategies of appealing to an individual's perceived commitment to help one in order to gain compliance (e.g., you should comply because you owe me a favor), whereas activation of *impersonal* commitments is similar except the requests are more impersonal in nature (e.g., a "good" person would comply with my request). Marwell and Schmitt developed this typology through empirical research, and it as well as others have subsequently been widely applied in compliance-gaining studies (Perloff, 2003).

In addition, these researchers observed that their compliance-gaining strategies were quite similar to French and Raven's (1959) bases of social power. What was further observed was the following: Individuals may choose a compliance-gaining technique based on the amount and type of power that they believe they possess. Thus, power dynamics quickly come into play and may help explain the choice of exactly *which* compliance-gaining techniques an individual chooses to utilize in a particular context.

Comment on Compliance-Gaining Perspectives.    Nearly two decades ago, Edgar and Fitzpatrick (1988) argued that existing typologies generated for general compliance gaining do not translate well to the area of safer sexual partner communication and negotiation. For instance, because this area is emotionally sensitive and because a request for compliance (to use condoms) may come after another request for compliance (to have sex), they argue that it is quite different than other areas of compliance-gaining research. In addition, other authors appear to agree with this assessment (e.g., Monahan, Miller, & Rothspan, 1997). Thus, the studies using this perspective, though often inspired by existing and widely used compliance-gaining typologies, often do not strictly adhere to such typologies.

What does this theoretical perspective offer in terms of an understanding of partner communication about safer sex (see Table 1.1)? Compliance-gaining theory and research suggests actual communication strategies that individuals can and do use to persuade sexual partners to use condoms. Such a perspective has helped to identify *how* individuals are negotiating safer sex, and has been suggestive of strategies that may be more effective as compared to other strategies. In addition, this perspective allows one to look at differences in strategy use across important variables, such as gender and perceived power, to see how these variables influence strategy choice and frequency of use. The results of compliance-gaining studies on partner communication about condom use will be reviewed when we consider the empirical evidence on how individuals negotiate condom use.

*Sexual Scripts*

The sexual-scripts perspective was proposed by Gagnon and Simon (1973; also see Gagnon, 1990; Simon & Gagnon, 1986), and has its roots in sociology. According to the theory, sexual scripts exist at three levels—cultural, interpersonal, and intrapsychic—and these three levels are not independent but, rather, interact with one another. Cultural scenarios operate in the abstract and are at the broadest level of the theory. They represent the broader cultural context in which the interpersonal scripts operate, and are necessary to understanding the meaning of the interpersonal interactions. Interpersonal scripts are the words, gestures, and actions that are executed in particular sequences by individuals in particular situations, and in the sexual situation might be referred to as a sexual interaction. In using these scripts, an individual is in many ways meeting the expectations of others within that situation. However, individuals do not always simply take cultural scripts and put them into action exactly as they are perceived to be. Rather, often there are multiple cultural scripts and one's interpersonal script includes some variation on these scripts, and perhaps some improvisation. This improvisation and integration is what is meant by the concept of intrapsychic scripts.

A concrete example of interpersonal scripts comes from literature on the negotiation of sex. Studies have examined the traditional "sexual script" for college students' sexual interactions—which includes the male making sexual advances and the female avoiding sex altogether or acting as a sexual limit setter. In fact, college-age men and women report both using a traditional sexual script that includes these elements, as well as being influenced by it (LaPlante, McCormick, & Brannigan, 1980). The LaPlante et al. study concluded that the interpersonal scripts of college students lagged behind the cultural terrain, given that the changing roles of women in the 1970s were not being reflected in the interpersonal scripts found to be at play in the study. Other studies have examined sexual scripts and described in greater detail what such a script looks like, including play-by-play descriptions of nonverbal gestures, movements, and discussions that take place in intimate sexual interactions (see McCormick, 1987).

Comment on Sexual Scripts.    What can this perspective bring to bear on interactions that include *safer* sexual behavior? Individuals often act according to interpersonal scripts that are derived from the cultural context around them. Thus, whether or not individuals negotiate safe sex, how they talk about it, and so forth, is shaped by the many social forces around us, according to the theory. This perspective takes a much broader point of view of safer sexual communication when compared to the social cognitive and compliance-gaining perspectives, which are more focused on the individual. It also suggests that we must look at the entire sexual interaction, and how talk about safer sex is (or is not) integrated into it, in order to achieve a full understanding of this communication. Moreover, it elucidates the *timing* of when sexual communication happens—

something not well addressed by the other perspectives. Two studies conducted on safer sexual communication and guided by this perspective are discussed later, and further illustrate the usefulness of such a perspective.

## Empirical Data on Partner Communication in the Context of Safer Sex

What do we know about partner communication and safer sexual behavior? Much data has been generated in this area, and here we focus on (a) the impact of partner communication on condom use, (b) *how* individuals negotiate condom use with sexual partners, and (c) how the sexual-scripts perspective has been used to examine partner communication in safer sexual interactions.

### Impact of Partner Communication on Safer Sex

A large number of studies now exist on the association of partner communication to safer sexual behavior (e.g., condom use), which suggest that partner communication has a strong impact on safer sexual behavior. Noar, Carlyle, and Cole (2006) recently conducted a comprehensive meta-analysis of the literature on this association, quantitatively synthesizing 55 studies on the topic. The studies obtained through a systematic literature review were quite diverse in nature, and included (a) a variety of populations recruited from a variety of venues, including schools, clinics, and community-based sites; (b) samples of men, women, and both combined; (c) racial and ethnic diversity (67% of studies were of non-White participants); (d) samples of gay/bisexual men and HIV-positive individuals, though the literature contained only a small number of such studies (5% to 7% of studies); (e) samples from a number of countries besides the United States (15% of studies); and (f) longitudinal (5% of studies) as well as cross-sectional studies, though most studies were cross-sectional. In addition, the articles were published in 27 different journals, showing the interdisciplinary nature of this topic of study.

The independent variable of interest in this meta-analysis was partner safer sexual communication, which was conceptualized and measured in a variety of ways. The dependent variable of interest was safer sex, which was measured in most studies by condom use and in a smaller number of studies by unprotected sex. All studies were coded on a number of conceptual, methodological, and other characteristics by two independent coders. Furthermore, analysis revealed that the coders had excellent consistency in coding, with 96% agreement among them (Cohen's kappa = .92).

Overall, results indicated that the mean sample-size weighted effect size of the partner communication-condom use relationship was $r = .22$ (95% confidence interval, .20 – .23). This association is of greater magnitude than a number of other theoretical condom use predictors examined in other meta-analyses (Sheeran et al., 1999), including safer-sex knowledge and perceived susceptibility of HIV/STDs (both $r = .06$), perceived severity of HIV/STDs ($r = .02$), various cues to action ($r = .02 – .10$), perceived barriers to condom use ($r = .13$), HIV/AIDS self-efficacy ($r = .12$), and perceived interpersonal consequences of using condoms ($r = -.10$). Furthermore, this value is similar to effect sizes for subjective normative beliefs about condom use ($r = .26$) and condom use self-efficacy ($r = .25$) and only slightly smaller than condom attitudes ($r = .32$) and previous condom use ($r = .36$; Sheeran et al., 1999).

Moreover, a number of conceptual moderators of the overall association were examined, including communication topic, conceptualization, and other factors. Table 1.2 reveals that partner communication about condom use or sexual history/HIV/STDs was more strongly associated with condom use than was communication about general safer sex (general safer sex was a "catch all" term used to describe measures that blended items from the other two categories [condom use and sexual history/HIV/STDs] together). Furthermore, partner communication *behavior* was found to be most strongly associated with condom use, followed by *behavioral intention* and finally by *self-efficacy*. Thus, stronger associations were observed with condom use when the partner communication measure was specific to condom use and when it measured behavior as opposed to intention or self-efficacy. In fact, when examining only measures on the topic of *condom use* that were conceptualized as *behavior* ($k = 12$ studies), the association with condom use was $r = .34$.

As can also been seen from Table 1.2, no differences were found when comparing the effect sizes of studies examining a safer-sex information exchange versus a safer-sex persuasion attempt; although, the measures used in these studies may not have been concrete and

**TABLE 1.2    Moderating Influences of the Partner Communication-Condom Use Association Examined in the Noar et al. (2006) Meta-Analysis**

| Variable | $N$ | $k$ | $r$ | 95% CI |
|---|---|---|---|---|
| **Communication Topic** | | | | |
| Condom use | 7,112 | 26 | .25[a] | [.23, .27] |
| Safer sex | 6,292 | 16 | .18[b] | [.16, .21] |
| Sexual history, HIV/STDs | 4,215 | 10 | .23[a] | [.21, .26] |
| Total | 17,619 | 52 | — | — |
| **Measurement Operationalization** | | | | |
| Past behavior | 9,328 | 27 | .29[a] | [.27, .31] |
| Self-efficacy | 8,001 | 21 | .13[b] | [.11, .15] |
| Intention | 1,019 | 6 | .18[c] | [.12, .24] |
| Total | 18,348 | 54 | — | — |
| **Communication Focus (past behavior studies only)** | | | | |
| Informational exchange | 6,215 | 17 | .29[a] | [.26, .31] |
| Persuasion attempt | 2,064 | 7 | .28[a] | [.24, .32] |
| Total | 8,279 | 24 | — | — |
| **Gender** | | | | |
| Male | 2,053 | 9 | .20[a] | [.16, .25] |
| Female | 4,412 | 16 | .19[a] | [.16, .22] |
| Total | 6,465 | 25 | — | — |

*Note:* $N$ = sample size, $k$ = number of studies, $r$ = sample size-weighted mean correlation, CI = confidence interval.

[a,b,c] Effect sizes with different subscripts were significantly different from one another at $p < .05$ or better.

specific enough to tease apart this difference. In addition, no gender differences were found, suggesting that if we accept the causal interpretation that partner communication leads to condom use, this outcome is no different for men or women. However, this does *not* speak to the question of *how often* men and women communicate about safer sex. In fact, some studies suggest that women are more likely to bring up the topic and discuss safer sex than are men (e.g., Debro, Campbell, & Peplau, 1994; Noar, Morokoff, & Harlow, 2002).

Finally, methodological moderators of this association were examined. These analyses revealed that longitudinal studies ($r = .20$), which measured partner communication at one time point and correlated it with condom use at a second time point, had very similar effect sizes to cross-sectional studies ($r = .22$), suggesting a robust effect. In addition, whereas the number of scale items in the communication scales had no impact on the association with condom use, coefficient alpha did have an impact. In fact, those studies with higher coefficient alphas for the partner communication scales had stronger relationships with condom use.

What does this meta-analysis tell us about the literature on partner communication about safer sex? Across a variety of populations recruited from a variety of settings, partner communication appears to be a moderately strong correlate of safer sexual behavior. In addition, how such communication is measured has clear implications for how it may relate to condom use. Investigators should think clearly about what aspect(s) of partner communication they are interested in before selecting and/or creating measures in this area, as differing conceptualizations and topics have implications for the association with safer sex. In addition, methodological aspects of these measures influence study outcomes. In fact, a number of the studies used one-item partner communication measures, which have unknown reliability. Among those studies that utilized multiple-item scales, those with higher coefficient alphas had stronger associations with condom use, reinforcing the fact that strong and robust measurement of variables is important. Finally, we note that other meta-analyses of condom use correlates, including those of both heterosexuals (Allen, Emmers-Sommer, & Crowell, 2002; Sheeran et al., 1999) and gay/bisexual men (Flowers, Sheeran, Beail, & Smith, 1997), have come to similar conclusions regarding the moderately strong association between partner communication and condom use (Noar et al., 2006).

## How Do Individuals Negotiate Condom Use?

Although the preceding review suggests a clear link between partner communication and condom use, it does not inform us as to the ways in which individuals negotiate condom use. For answers to the question of *how* individuals negotiate condom use, we turn to studies that have examined such strategies. These kinds of studies are both qualitative and quantitative in nature, and have used a variety of organizing frameworks to guide the study of these strategies, with many being rooted in the compliance-gaining literature (see Edgar, 1992).

One of the simplest divisions of strategies is *verbal* as opposed to *nonverbal* strategies. Verbal strategies, as the name implies, are those in which verbal discussion takes place, whereas nonverbal influence strategies are those in which no verbal discussion occurs. Though nearly all studies of condom influence strategies examine some aspect of *verbal* strategies, a small but growing number of studies have also examined nonverbal strategies (e.g., Bird & Harvey, 2001; Bird, Harvey, Beckman, & Johnson, 2001; Choi, Wojcicki, & Valencia-Garcia, 2004; Debro, Campbell, & Peplau, 1994; Edgar, Freimuth, Hammond, McDonald, & Fink, 1992; Lam, Mak, Lindsay, & Russell, 2004; Noar, Morokoff, & Harlow, 2002; Noar, Morokoff, & Harlow, 2004; Reel & Thompson, 2004). These studies find support for the proposition that individuals use (or say they would use) *nonverbal* strategies for condom influence, including taking out a condom and presuming to use it, presenting a condom to a sexual partner, or placing a condom in clear view of their partner such as on a dresser or pillow. In addition, given that condoms are a "male controlled" method in that men are the ones who actually wear condoms (except in the case of the female condom, which is not widely used), it is not surprising that some studies of heterosexuals suggest men to be more likely to use nonverbal strategies than women (Debro et al., 1994; Edgar et al., 1992; Noar, Morokoff, & Harlow, 2002).

These findings on nonverbal influence make a strong and important point about partner communication: Sexual partners do not have to have a long conversation about safe sex, or even *any conversation at all,* in order for partner influence to take place. In fact, a study of men who have sex with men in bathhouses found a "norm of silence" in which safer sex and condom use were *not* verbally discussed (Elwood, Greene, & Carter, 2003). How can one use condoms with a new partner, in this case an anonymous partner of unknown HIV/STD risk, when *verbal* interactions about condom use are forbidden by social norms? Many of the men did use condoms in these situations, and apparently used nonverbal influence strategies to achieve this goal of condom use (Elwood et al., 2003).

In addition, another simple division often made in this literature is between *direct* and *indirect* strategies. Direct strategies can be characterized as those that are clear in terms of their purpose, such as directly asking a person to use a condom, whereas indirect strategies are more subtle, and may consist of dropping hints, using deception, or using humor or flattery (e.g., Lam et al., 2004). Though some studies are very clear about a division of direct versus indirect strategies, other studies are not as clear as to this division.

What can the literature tell us about direct versus indirect strategies? Nearly all studies in this area find support for the idea that individuals both have used and say they would use a variety of direct and indirect strategies to negotiate condom use. However, a problem here is that there simply have not been enough studies examining direct versus indirect strategies, and in many studies direct/indirect is confounded with verbal/nonverbal. In fact, the choice of which strategy types might be used is an issue related to communication styles, and is likely complex and influenced by a variety of variables including age, gender, race, sexual orientation, personality, type of relationship (e.g., intimate, casual), length of relationship, and perceived power, as well as characteristics of the situation including whether alcohol or drugs have been used. Studies have only examined the tip of the iceberg in terms of understanding differences in use of direct/indirect strategies (and for that matter, verbal/nonverbal strategies) for condom use influence, and results thus far are not entirely conclusive. For instance, some studies of heterosexuals suggest that women are more likely to use indirect strategies than men (e.g., Lam et al., 2004), and also more likely to use indirect as opposed to direct strategies in general (Williams, Gardos, Ortiz-Torres, Tross, & Ehrhardt, 2001). However, other studies find women to very often use direct strategies (Edgar et al., 1992; Noar, Morokoff, & Harlow, 2002). Overall, there has simply not been enough large-scale studies that have examined the prevalence of both direct/indirect as well as verbal/nonverbal strategies and potential differences by many of the variables proposed here.

A number of additional studies in this literature have examined specific compliance-gaining strategies for condom influence, many derived from compliance-gaining typologies, whereas others derived from exploratory work with a target audience. These studies have revealed a number of different strategies that are used to persuade partners to use condoms, and many of the common strategies appearing in the literature are summarized in Table 1.3. As can be seen, a variety of strategies to persuade a partner to use a condom exist and have been captured in this literature.

**TABLE 1.3    Condom Negotiation Strategies Identified in the Literature**

| Strategy | V/N | Evidence in the Literature of Intended or Actual Use |
| --- | --- | --- |
| Verbal or nonverbal *direct requests* to use condoms | V/N | Bird & Harvey (2001), Bird et al. (2001), Choi et al. (2004), Edgar & Fitzpatrick (1988), Edgar et al. (1992), Harvey & Bird (2003), Lam et al. (2004), Noar, Morokoff, & Harlow (2002); Noar, Morokoff et al. (2004), Reel & Thompson (1994, 2004) |
| *Withholding sex* from a sexual partner unless a condom is used | V | Bird & Harvey (2001), Bird et al. (2001), Choi et al. (2004); Debro et al. (1994), Edgar & Fitzpatrick (1988), Edgar et al. (1992), Harvey & Bird (2003), Kline, Kline, & Oken (1992), Lam et al. (2004), Margillo & Imahori (1998), Noar, Morokoff, & Harlow (2002), Noar, Morokoff et al. (2004); Williams et al. (2001), Wingood, Hunter-Gamble, & DiClemente (1993), Wong et al. (1994) |
| *Presenting risk information about HIV, STDs, or pregnancy* to gain partner compliance | V | Bird & Harvey (2001), Bird et al. (2001), Debro et al. (1994), Edgar & Fitzpatrick (1988), Harvey & Bird (2003), Kline et al. (1992), Lam et al. (2004), Margillo & Imahori (1998), Noar, Morokoff, & Harlow (2002); Noar, Morokoff et al. (2004), O'Leary et al. (2003), Reel & Thompson (1994), Williams et al. (2001), Wingood et al. (1993), Wong et al. (1994) |
| *Deceiving a partner* in order to gain compliance | V | Bird & Harvey (2001), Debro et al. (1994), Edgar et al. (1992), Lam et al. (2004), Noar, Morokoff, & Harlow (2002), Noar, Morokoff et al. (2004); Wong et al. (1994) |
| *Using a focus on the relationship* and caring to persuade the partner | V | Bird & Harvey (2001), Kline et al. (1992), Margillo & Imahori (1998), Noar, Morokoff, & Harlow (2002), Noar, Morokoff et al. (2004), Reel & Thompson (1994) |
| *Seducing the partner* or eroticizing sex in order to gain compliance | V/N | Bird & Harvey (2001), Bird et al. (2001), Debro et al. (1994), Edgar & Fitzpatrick (1988), Edgar et al. (1992), Kline et al. (1992), Margillo & Imahori (1998), Noar, Morokoff, & Harlow (2002), Noar, Morokoff et al. (2004); Williams et al. (2001) |
| *Begging or crying* in order to persuade partner | V | Debro et al. (1994), Lam et al. (2004), Margillo & Imahori (1998) |
| *Using flattery, humor, or other means to reward partner* in order to gain compliance | V | Bird & Harvey (2001), Choi et al. (2004), Debro et al. (1994), Edgar & Fitzpatrick (1988), Edgar et al. (1992), Lam et al. (2004), Margillo & Imahori (1998), Reel & Thompson (2004), Wong et al. (1994) |

**TABLE 1.3 Condom Negotiation Strategies Identified in the Literature (continued)**

| Strategy | V/N | Evidence in the Literature of Intended or Actual Use |
|---|---|---|
| *Dropping hints* that a condom should be used in order to gain compliance | V | Bird & Harvey (2001), Harvey & Bird (2003), Lam et al. (2004) |

*Note:* V= Primarily a verbal strategy, V = primarily a nonverbal strategy, V/N = strategy can be carried out in either a verbal or nonverbal manner.

Furthermore, individuals often have a preference for a certain strategy that they might try first, such as a direct request, and report also having "back-up" strategies ready should the first attempt fail (e.g., Williams et al., 2001). In fact, some studies suggest that having an arsenal of strategies may be very important in condom use negotiation, as a first attempt at persuasion is likely to fail and needs to be followed up with additional persuasive tactics (Edgar, 1992; Edgar & Fitzpatrick, 1988). Thus, it is clear that condom negotiation is much more complex than simply using one strategy and having it be effective, and the complexity of this area is sometimes difficult to capture in survey research studies.

In addition, although it is difficult to say for sure which strategy or strategies in the current literature are truly *most effective,* a number of the quantitative studies have empirically examined associations between negotiation strategies and self-reported condom use behavior (Edgar et al., 1992; Noar, Morokoff et al., 2004; Noar, Morokoff, & Harlow, 2002; O'Leary et al., 2003) or have provided data on individual ratings of the perceived effectiveness of the strategies (e.g., Bird et al., 2001; Debro et al., 1994; Lam et al., 2004; Reel & Thompson, 1994, 2004). These data *suggest* that strategies such as verbal and nonverbal direct requests; presenting risk information about HIV, other STDs, or pregnancy; withholding sex unless condoms are used; focusing on caring and commitment for the relationship; and deceiving a partner regarding the reason to use condoms may be among the most effective negotiation strategies. Furthermore, this may vary by population. For instance, studies of male inmates' responses to their primary partner's requests to use a condom suggest that the most effective strategies (and those least likely to result in violence) would be those that would *not* hint at any sort of infidelity, such as using deception (e.g., saying a condom must be used because of a yeast infection or allergy to "acidic" sperm; Neighbors & O'Leary, 2003; Neighbors, O'Leary, & Labouvie, 1999). A study of commercial sex workers suggested that an effective strategy might also be deception, namely complaining about currently having STD symptoms (Wong et al., 1994). To date, few studies have made strong conclusions about strategies that should be avoided when negotiating condom use, but this, too, remains important.

Overall, the data from these studies make it very clear: There are a great variety of ways to negotiate condom use with a partner, with approaches that are verbal, nonverbal, direct, and indirect, and approaches that vary on a number of other dimensions. Interventions should not simply offer a *one-size-fits-all* approach to negotiation, such as suggesting that direct-verbal approaches are the only manner in which condom use can be negotiated (e.g., Lam et al., 2004). Rather, there are a number of ways that this can be achieved, and interventions should be reflective of this diversity (for a review of communication skills training in HIV prevention interventions, see chap. 2, this volume).

## Understanding Sexual Interactions Using a Sexual-Scripts Approach

Very few studies have examined how partner communication about safer sex might be a part of existing sexual scripts, and here we discuss two studies that did exactly that (Edgar & Fitzpatrick, 1993; Miller, Bettencourt, Debro, & Hoffman, 1993). Edgar and Fitzpatrick examined sexual scripts for *casual sexual encounters* among college students and constructed play-by-play interactions that might take place in both typical public (e.g., a bar) and private (e.g., an apartment) settings. The scripts developed by both men and women were quite similar in nature, and in the public setting included: the individuals noticing one another, eye contact, approaching and greeting one another, him buying her a drink, conversation between them, dancing, him complimenting her, nonintimate followed by intimate touching, and the suggestion to go somewhere private followed by the couple leaving together. There was much agreement regarding these actions taking place as well as the order of such interactions. The private script is where this interaction continued, and included:

one person inviting the guest in to their apartment, the host offering the guest a drink, questions and compliments about the apartment and roommates, eye contact, him moving closer to her and initiating nonintimate touching, her showing some reluctance, him kissing her, intimate touching taking place, and him asking her either directly or indirectly to have sex. She agrees, they lie down together, he undresses her, and she helps him undress. Then, if communication about birth control and condom use take place at all, it occurs at this time (Edgar & Fitzpatrick, 1993).

These scripts, particularly the private script, reveal much about sexual interactions, including the expectation that men are the initiators of intimate activities and sex and that women show some token resistance in this casual "one night stand" script. Most interesting, and contrary to Edgar and Fitzpatrick's (1993) hypothesis, partner communication about safer sex did *not* take place until the individuals both had taken their clothes off. It is difficult to overstate the implications of this result for prevention interventions. If the majority of such communication and negotiation takes place when individuals are in such a sexually excited state, this is a very different context than if individuals have a discussion much earlier in the interaction with their clothes on. For instance, nearly all of the social cognitive theories discussed in this review suggest quite a rational process of decision making with regard to using condoms, weighing the benefits and barriers to condom use in making a decision about using them. However, if such discussions and negotiations are taking place in a highly sexually charged context, such a rational decision-making model may not be an accurate theoretical description of the process that leads to safe sex. Moreover, if individuals are under the influence of alcohol and/or other drugs during such interactions, this changes the context further. In fact, correlations among such attitudinal and decision-making variables and condom use may result in part from "after the fact" reasoning about why condoms were or were not used, such as is suggested by cognitive dissonance theory. The implications here are so great because these social cognitive models serve as the basis for many if not most of the HIV prevention interventions in the literature (e.g., Peterson & DiClemente, 2000).

Although only two studies that we were able to locate have examined these issues from a sexual-scripts perspective, it is heartening that the study conducted by Miller et al. (1993) found nearly identical results to Edgar and Fitzpatrick (1993). These researchers examined the one-night-stand casual-sex script for young adults, and concluded that "the 'window' within which to introduce and use condoms... may be very small and involve high levels of sexual arousal..." (Miller et al., 1993, p. 98). Unfortunately, it appears that few studies have taken note of the Edgar and Fitzpatrick and Miller et al. findings, as studies have *not* tended to follow up on these results in order to gain a broader understanding of the context of partner communication within sexual interactions. This may be in part because of such a strong focus on individual-level social psychological models in HIV prevention research (e.g., see Noar, 2007), perhaps at the expense of other diverse theoretical perspectives such as sexual scripts.

What can we learn from this sexual-scripts perspective? Certainly, it suggests that we need to take the entire sexual interaction into account when attempting to understand partner communication around sex. Although prevention researchers and practitioners may prefer that individuals discuss condom use well before sex is imminent, this may not be what tends to happen in practice. Thus, one implication for interventions would be to encourage individuals to have condoms with them or very close by in sexual situations because, if this is not the case, condom use may be very unlikely to take place. In addition, in some cases individuals may be able to negotiate condom use earlier in the sequence of this script, but this might be more explicitly addressed within interventions. Finally, both of these studies examined scripts for casual sex, with neither examining sexual scripts within longer term, intimate relationships. The literature to date does suggest that individuals negotiate condom use early on in relationships and then either use or do not use condoms based on that early safer sex "agreement," although more data on how this process operates would be useful (see Kippax, 2002; Noar, Zimmerman et al., 2004).

## Conclusion and Implications

This chapter has reviewed theoretical perspectives and empirical data in the area of partner communication about safer sex. There are a number of subareas within this domain that are ripe for further research. For instance, as already discussed, a greater understanding of sexual interactions using perspectives such as sexual scripts would benefit this area of research, and help us to better understand the timing of safer sexual communication within a sexual interaction. In addition, a recent study that examined persuasion attempts to *dissuade* individuals from using condoms reminds us that an attempt to persuade one to use a condom may be responded to with a similar attempt to dissuade the use of condoms (Oncale & King, 2001). The lesson here is that negotiation is complex and we should strive to better understand both sides of the social-influence process—persuader and persuadee—as well as the interplay among the two. Along these same lines, negotiation is a two-person process and yet nearly all studies in this area are based on the perspective of an individual. A recent couples study suggests that partners do not always see eye-to-eye in terms of their perceptions of sexual decision making and their actual knowledge of sexual histories (Harvey, Bird, Henderson, Beckman, & Huszti, 2004). Thus, including both members of a couple in future studies may be very useful. In fact, laboratory studies in which safer sexual conversations are simulated could be very interesting in learning more about the dynamics of this fascinating and important social influence process.

Furthermore, although much of the HIV prevention literature has rapidly moved to the intervention stage (see chap. 2, this volume), gaps still remain in basic knowledge such as these important areas of sexual interactions and partner communication. Intervention efforts can only be as effective as the theories and findings upon which they are built. Thus, continued investment and inquiry into areas such as partner communication about safer sex will likely pay dividends down the road in terms of intervention effectiveness and ultimately in terms of impact on at-risk populations.

## References

Ajzen, I., & Madden, T. J. (1986). Prediction of goal-directed behavior: Attitudes, intentions, and perceived behavioral control. *Journal of Experimental Social Psychology, 22,* 453–474.

Allen, M., Emmers-Sommer, T. M., & Crowell, T. L. (2002). Couples negotiating safer sex behaviors: A meta-analysis of the impact of conversation and gender. In M. Allen, R. W. Preiss, B. M. Gayle, & N. A. Burrell (Eds.), *Interpersonal communication research: Advances through meta-analysis* (pp. 263–279). Mahwah, NJ: Lawrence Erlbaum Associates.

Bandura, A. (1986). *Social foundations of thought and action: A social cognitive theory.* Englewood Cliffs, NJ: Prentice-Hall.

Bird, S. T., & Harvey, S. M. (2001). "No glove, no love": Cultural beliefs of African-American women regarding influencing strategies for condom use. *International Quarterly of Community Health Education, 20*(3), 237–251.

Bird, S. T., Harvey, S. M., Beckman, L. J., & Johnson, C. H. (2001). Getting your partner to use condoms: Interviews with men and women at risk of HIV/STDs. *Journal of Sex Research, 38*(3), 233–240.

Bowen, S. P., & Michal-Johnson, P. (1989). The crisis of communicating in relationships: Confronting the threat of AIDS. *AIDS & Public Policy Journal, 4*(1), 10–19.

Bryan, A., Fisher, J. D., & Fisher, W. A. (2002). Tests of the mediational role of preparatory safer sexual behavior in the context of the theory of planned behavior. *Health Psychology, 21*(1), 71–80.

Catania, J. A., Kegeles, S. M., & Coates, T. J. (1990). Towards an understanding of risk behavior: An AIDS risk reduction model (ARRM). *Health Education Quarterly, 17*(1), 53–72.

Choi, K. H., Wojcicki, J., & Valencia-Garcia, D. (2004). Introducing and negotiating the use of female condoms in sexual relationships: Qualitative interviews with women attending a family planning clinic. *AIDS and Behavior, 8*(3), 251–261.

Cline, R. J. W. (2003). Everyday interpersonal communication and health. In T. L. Thompson, A. M. Dorsey, K. I. Miller, & R. Parrott (Eds.), *Handbook of health communication* (pp. 285–313). Mahwah, NJ: Lawrence Erlbaum Associates.

Debro, S. C., Campbell, S. M., & Peplau, L. A. (1994). Influencing a partner to use a condom: A college student perspective. *Psychology of Women Quarterly, 18*, 165–182.

Edgar, T. (1992). A compliance-based approach to the study of condom use. In T. Edgar, M. A. Fitzpatrick, & V. S. Freimuth (Eds.), *AIDS: A communication perspective* (pp. 47–67). Hillsdale, NJ: Lawrence Erlbaum Associates.

Edgar, T., & Fitzpatrick, M. A. (1988). Compliance-gaining in relational interaction: When your life depends on it. *The Southern Speech Communication Journal, 53*, 385–405.

Edgar, T., & Fitzpatrick, M. A. (1993). Expectations for sexual interaction: A cognitive test of the sequencing of sexual communication behaviors. *Health Communication, 5*(4), 239–261.

Edgar, T., Freimuth, V S., Hammond, S. L., McDonald, D. A., & Fink, E. L. (1992). Strategic sexual communication: Condom use resistance and response. *Health Communication, 4*(2), 83–104.

Elwood, W. N., Greene, K., & Carter, K. K. (2003). Gentlemen don't speak: Communication norms and condom use in bathhouses. *Journal of Applied Communication Research, 31*(4), 277–297.

Falbo, T., & Peplau, L. A. (1980). Power strategies in intimate relationships. *Journal of Personality and Social Psychology, 38*(4), 618–628.

Fishbein, M., & Ajzen, I. (1975). *Belief, attitude, intention and behavior: An introduction to theory and research.* Reading, MA: Addison-Wesley.

Fisher, J. D., & Fisher, W. A. (1992). Changing AIDS-risk behavior. *Psychological Bulletin, 111*(3), 455–474.

Fisher, J. D., & Fisher, W. A. (2000). Theoretical approaches to individual-level change in HIV risk behavior. In J. L. Peterson & R. J. DiClemente (Eds.), *Handbook of HIV prevention* (pp. 3–55). New York: Kluwer Academic /Plenum.

Flowers, P., Sheeran, P., Beail, N., & Smith, J. A. (1997). The role of psychosocial factors in HIV risk-reduction among gay and bisexual men: A quantitative review. *Psychology and Health, 12,* 197–230.

French, J. R. P., & Raven, B. (1959). The bases of social power. In D. Cartright (Ed.), *Studies in social power* (pp. 150–167). Ann Arbor: University of Michigan Press.

Gagnon, J. H. (1990). The explicit and implicit use of the scripting perspective in sex research. *Annual Review of Sex Research, 1,* 1–43.

Gagnon, J. H., & Simon, W. (1973). *Sexual conduct: The social sources of human sexuality.* Chicago: Transaction.

Grimley, D. M., Prochaska, G. E., & Prochaska, J. O. (1997). Condom use adoption and continuation: A transtheoretical approach. *Health Education Research, 12*(1), 61–75.

Harvey, S. M., & Bird, S. T. (2003). Power in relationships and influencing strategies for condom use: Exploring cultural beliefs among African American men. *International Quarterly of Community Health Education, 21*(2), 147–162.

Harvey, S. M., Bird, S. T., Henderson, J. T., Beckman, L. J., & Huszti, H. C. (2004). He said, she said: Concordance between sexual partners. *Sexually Transmitted Diseases, 31*(3), 185–191.

Howard, J. A., Blumstein, P., & Schwartz, P. (1986). Sex, power, and influence tactics in intimate relationships. *Journal of Personality and Social Psychology, 51*(1), 102–109.

Janz, N. K., & Becker, M. H. (1984). The health belief model: A decade later. *Health Education Quarterly, 11*(1), 1–47.

Kippax, S. (2002). Negotiated safety agreements among gay men. In A. O'Leary (Ed.), *Beyond condoms: Alternative approaches to HIV prevention* (pp. 1–15). New York: Kluwer Academic/Plenum.

Kline, A., Kline, E., & Oken, E. (1992). Minority women and sexual choice in the age of AIDS. *Social Science and Medicine, 34*(4), 447–457.

Lam, A. G., Mak, A., Lindsay, P. D., & Russell, S. T. (2004). What really works? An exploratory study of condom negotiation strategies. *AIDS Education and Prevention, 16*(2), 160–171.

LaPlante, M. N., McCormick, N., & Brannigan, G. G. (1980). Living the sexual script: College students' views of influence in sexual encounters. *The Journal of Sex Research, 16*(4), 338–355.

Margillo, G. A., & Imahori, T. T. (1998). Understanding safer sex negotiation in a group of low-income African American women. In N. L. Roth & L. K. Fuller (Eds.), *Women and AIDS: Negotiating safer practices, care, and representation* (pp. 43–69). New York: Harrington Park Press.

Marwell, G., & Schmitt, D. R. (1967). Dimensions of compliance gaining behavior: An empirical analysis. *Sociometry, 30*, 350–364.

McCormick, N. B. (1987). Sexual scripts: Social and therapeutic implications. *Sexual and Marital Therapy, 2*(1), 3–27.

Miller, L. C., Bettencourt, B. A., DeBro, S. C., & Hoffman, V. (1993). Negotiating safer sex: Interpersonal dynamics. In J. B. Pryor & G. D. Reeder (Eds.), *The social psychology of HIV infection* (pp. 85–123). Hillsdale, NJ: Lawrence Erlbaum Associates.

Misovich, S. J., Fisher, J. D., & Fisher, W. A. (1997). Close relationships and elevated HIV risk behavior: Evidence and possible underlying psychological processes. *Review of General Psychology, 1*(1), 72–107.

Monahan, J. L., Miller, L. C., & Rothspan, S. (1997). Power and intimacy: On the dynamics of risky sex. *Health Communication, 9*(4), 303–321.

Neighbors, C. J., & O'Leary, A. (2003). Response of male inmates to primary partner requests for condom use: Effects of message content and domestic violence history. *AIDS Education and Prevention, 15*(1), 93–108.

Neighbors, C. J., O'Leary, A., & Labouvie, E. (1999). Domestically violent and non-violent male inmates' evaluations and responses to their partner's requests for condom use: Testing a social-information processing model. *Health Psychology, 18*, 427–431.

Noar, S. M. (2007). An interventionist's guide to AIDS behavioral theories. *AIDS Care, 19*, 392–402.

Noar, S. M., Carlyle, K., & Cole, C. (2006). Why communication is crucial: Meta-analysis of the relationship between safer sexual communication and condom use. *Journal of Health Communication, 11*(4), 365–390.

Noar, S. M., Morokoff, P. J., & Harlow, L. L. (2002). Condom negotiation in heterosexually active men and women: Development and validation of a condom influence strategy questionnaire. *Psychology and Health, 17*, 711–735.

Noar, S. M., Morokoff, P. J., & Harlow, L. L. (2004). Condom influence strategies in a community sample of ethnically diverse men and women. *Journal of Applied Social Psychology 34*(8), 1730–1751 .

Noar, S. M., Morokoff, P. J., & Redding, C. A. (2002). Sexual assertiveness in heterosexually active men: A test of three samples. *AIDS Education and Prevention, 14*(4), 330–342.

Noar, S. M., Zimmerman, R. S., & Atwood, K. A. (2004). Safer sex and sexually transmitted infections from a relationship perspective. In J. H. Harvey, A. Wenzel, & S. Sprecher (Eds.), *Handbook of sexuality in close relationships* (pp. 519–544). Mahwah, NJ: Lawrence Erlbaum.

O'Leary, A., Moore, J. S., Khumalo-Sakutukwa, G., Loeb, L., Cobb, D., Hruschka, D. et al. (2003). Association of negotiation strategies with consistent use of male condoms by women receiving an HIV prevention intervention in Zimbabwe. *AIDS, 17*(11), 1705–1707.

Oncale, R. M., & King, B. M. (2001). Comparison of men's and women's attempts to dissuade sexual partners from the couple using condoms. *Archives of Sexual Behavior, 30*(4), 379–391.

Perloff, R. M. (2003). *The dynamics of persuasion: Communication and attitudes in the 21st century* (2nd ed.). Mahwah, NJ: Lawrence Erlbaum Associates.

Peterson, J. L., & DiClemente, R. J. (Eds.). (2000). *Handbook of HIV prevention.* New York: Kluwer Academic/Plenum.

Prochaska, J. O., DiClemente, C. C., & Norcross, J. C. (1992). In search of how people change: Applications to addictive behaviors. *American Psychologist, 47*(9), 1102–1114.

Reel, B. W., & Thompson, T. L. (1994). A test of the effectiveness of strategies for talking about AIDS and condom use. *Journal of Applied Communication Research, 22,* 127–140.

Reel, B., & Thompson, T. L. (2004). Is it a matter of politeness?: Face and the effectiveness of messages about condom use. *Southern Communication Journal, 69*(2), 99–120.

Sheeran, P., Abraham, C., & Orbell, S. (1999). Psychosocial correlates of heterosexual condom use: A meta-analysis. *Psychological Bulletin, 125*(1), 90–132.

Simon, W., & Gagnon, J. H. (1986). Sexual scripts: Permanence and change. *Archives of Sexual Behavior, 15*(2), 97–120.

Strasburger, V. C., & Wilson, B. J. (2002). *Children, adolescents, & the media.* Thousand Oaks, CA: Sage.

Williams, S. P., Gardos, P. S., Ortiz-Torres, B., Tross, S., & Ehrhardt, A. A. (2001). Urban women's negotiation strategies for safer sex with their male partners. *Women & Health, 33*(3/4), 133–148.

Wingood, G. M., Hunter-Gamble, D., & DiClemente, R. J. (1993). A pilot study of sexual communication and negotiation among young African American women: Implications for HIV prevention. *Journal of Black Psychology, 19*(2), 190–203.

Wong, M. L., Archibald, C., Chan Roy, K. W., Goh, A., Tan, T. C., & Goh, C. L. (1994). Condom use negotiation among sex workers in Singapore: Findings from qualitative research. *Health Education Research, 9*(1), 57–67.

# 2

# Communication Skills Training in HIV Prevention Interventions

*Timothy Edgar*
Emerson College

*Seth M. Noar*
University of Kentucky

*Bryan Murphy*
Emerson College

In the previous chapter, Noar and Edgar reviewed a large body of literature that demonstrates that effective communication between partners is a key ingredient to the enactment of safer-sex practices. The entire corpus of research, however, has limited value in the fight against the further spread of HIV unless individuals at risk learn the "good news" about the efficacy of communication in sexual encounters and have the opportunity to improve and use their skills. That is, it is essential that researchers and health communication practitioners take the next step and develop interventions that provide instruction on how to best communicate with a partner. In the edited volume that served as the precursor to this book (Edgar, Fitzpatrick, & Freimuth, 1992), this chapter's first author wrote a review of the extant literature on sexual-communication skills in which he included a section on interventions that featured a training component aimed at improving the ability of participants to communicate with a partner about condom use (Edgar, 1992). At that point in the early 1990s, only three such studies existed (Kelly, St. Lawrence, Betts, Brasfield, & Hood, 1990; Kelly, St. Lawrence, Hood, & Brasfield, 1989; Solomon & DeJong, 1989). The results showed promise in that they met with early success, but at that point, the knowledge base was only in its infancy.

Since that time, the number of published HIV prevention intervention studies has multiplied substantially. And, fortunately, the populations that have been included in the interventions range far beyond the ubiquitous college sophomore. College students have not been excluded from interventions (see, e.g., Fisher, Fisher, Misovich, Kimble, & Mallory, 1996; Jaworski & Carey, 2001; Tulloch, McCaul, Miltenberger, & Smyth, 2004), but they are in the minority. Because this research stream has been well funded, intervention teams have been afforded the luxury of testing instructional designs within populations as diverse as Asian Americans (Choi et al., 1996); African Americans attending a sexually transmitted disease (STD) clinic (Kalichman, Williams, & Nachimson, 1999); adolescents in substance abuse treatment (St. Lawrence et al., 1994); adults in substance abuse treatment (Elwood & Vega, 2005); gay and bisexual men (Kegles, Hays, & Coates, 1996; Kelly et al., 1997; Peterson et al., 1996); African-American women (DiClemente et al., 2004; DiClemente & Wingood, 1995; Kalichman, Rompa, & Coley, 1996); high school students (Walter & Vaughn, 1993); junior high students (Coyle, Kirby, Marín, Gómez, & Gregorich, 2004); teenagers in juvenile detention (Gillmore et al., 1997; St. Lawrence, Crosby, Belcher, Yazdani, & Brasfield, 1999); psychiatric patients (Carey et al., 2004; Otto-Salaj, Kelly, Stevenson, Hoffman, & Kalichman, 2001); male prostitutes (Miller, Klotz, & Eckholdt, 1998); Mexican American women (Shain et al., 1999); and youth infected with an STD (Orr, Langefeld, Katz, & Cain, 1996; Rotheram-Borus et al., 2001; Shrier et al., 2001).

Overall, the results from intervention studies are very positive in that compelling evidence exists that the communication skills necessary for successfully interacting with a sexual partner are teachable and that the acquisition of these skills contributes to desired attitudinal and behavioral outcomes. This chapter reviews that literature in detail to help understand the variety of approaches that have been employed. First, we review the different categories of skills that intervention teams have included in their training, the ways in which those categories have been operationalized, and methodological techniques used to determine if participants truly acquired taught skills. Second, we examine the variety of ways in which intervention teams have approached instructional design. Third, we try to glean from the literature how much skills training is necessary for success. And, fourth, we offer suggestions for future directions. The studies discussed in this chapter were collected after a major literature review in this area that included combing the lists of numerous reviews and meta-analyses of the HIV prevention literature as well as conducting database searches of the literature. Although we cannot guarantee that we located every article in the literature that includes communication skills training, we feel confident that we identified the majority of the published reports that allow us to draw conclusions about the state of the literature.

## Types of Skills Taught

Throughout the intervention literature, teams have taught a variety of skills including assertion, negotiation, eroticization, refusal skills, and nonverbal skills. In this section, we review the key studies that have identified the exact skills research teams have intended to teach their participants. Although published reports typically identify skills by name, and there is consistency across the literature in the labels used, too often they leave the reader with questions about how particular skills were operationalized. That is, a published report might, for instance, state that participants received instruction on how to negotiate condom use successfully with a partner, but the reader does not necessarily learn how to recognize a negotiation skill or understand the key components of the message type that differentiate it from another skill form. As a result, the typical report provides insufficient information to allow others to duplicate the success of an effective training initiative without directly contacting the authors for more details. Although the literature does not provide as much detail as it could, there still are significant insights to be gleaned. In the paragraphs that follow, we examine the major skill categories one at a time.

### Assertiveness Skills

One of the two skills most commonly included in HIV-related interventions is assertion (see, e.g., Aarons et al., 2000; Carey et al., 2004; DiClemente & Wingood, 1995; Jaworski & Carey, 2001; Kalichman et al., 1996; Kelly et al., 1990; Kelly, St. Lawrence, Hood, &

Brasfield, 1989; Kipke, Boyer, & Hein, 1993; Metzler, Biglan, Noell, Ary, & Ochs, 2000; Morrison-Beedy, Carey, Kowalski, & Tu, 2005; Otto-Salaj et al., 2001; Peterson et al., 1996; Rosser et al., 2002; St. Lawrence et al., 1994, 1995; Workman, Robinson, Cotler, & Harper, 1996). The frequent inclusion of assertiveness skills suggests that sexually active individuals often find themselves in situations where either they actually meet resistance when attempting to convince a partner to agree to safe sex or, at the very least, they have reason to believe that resistance is likely. As a result, some teams have taught assertiveness skills by modeling them within specific situations such as encounters where a potential partner has been drinking (DiClemente & Wingood, 1995).

A complementary approach to teaching assertiveness skills has been to contrast assertion with other forms of expression. For example, DiClemente and Wingood (1995) taught the African-American women in their intervention how to differentiate assertion in sexual situations from passive and aggressive communication styles, and St. Lawrence et al. (1994) included exactly the same comparison in their approach with adolescents in a treatment facility for drug abuse. Jaworski and Carey (2001), on the other hand, explained to undergraduate women how to see the difference between anger and assertion when communicating with their partners. In all three studies, however, the authors offered limited information about how they illustrated the differences between assertion and other ways of communicating a message.

One of the most elaborate operational definitions of assertiveness found in the literature was developed by Kelly et al. (1990) for an intervention with gay men. Their definition, which identifies multiple components of the assertion process, said that assertiveness is effectively resisting coercion or pressure from a partner to engage in unprotected intercourse by acknowledging the partner's wish but firmly refusing it, providing a reason or rationale, noting the need to be safe, and proposing an alternative (e.g., using a condom, engaging in an alternative practice, or refraining from sex). Using this approach to assertiveness as their guide, they also instructed the men in the study to establish safe-sex concurrence with a partner prior to the possibility of sex. Members of the same intervention team and other research teams have used a very similar definition to guide their assertiveness training with other populations (Roffman et al., 1998; St. Lawrence et al., 1994, 1995).

In an interesting addition to the typical approach to assertiveness training, St. Lawrence et al. (1995) recognized that asserting one's self in a sexual encounter is not necessarily an easy fit for all personality types and might require some adjustment to work effectively. St. Lawrence and her colleagues first provided instruction on assertiveness skills to African-American adolescents and then engaged them in discussion about their individual comfort level with actually using the new skill if they encountered a situation similar to the role-play scenario employed in training. After the discussion on comfort, facilitators encouraged individuals to practice the skills during the upcoming week, and then they had the opportunity the following week to return to a group session to discuss their experience with being assertive. In another study, which used a more gradual approach to learning about assertion, Carey et al. (2004) first provided participants a chance to practice assertiveness skills through role plays not related to sexual matters. In two subsequent training sessions, participants translated the more general assertiveness skills learned in the initial session to scenarios involving sexual behavior.

## Negotiation Skills

The very use of the term negotiation to describe communication between sex partners implies that individuals work toward a mutually agreed upon outcome. In the book that preceded this one (Edgar et al., 1992), Mara Adelman (1992) contributed a provocative chapter in which she challenged communication researchers to avoid the use of negotiation as a metaphor for conceptualizing research about communication surrounding safer-sex practices. According to Adelman:

> This focus [on negotiation] suggests a highly scripted, rule-governed, premeditative, goal-driven account of the sexual encounter. The metaphor is understandably appealing to social scientists because it emphasizes control and management of the interaction. This emphasis is closely aligned with the highly prized outcomes of a positivist paradigm for research—to control and predict human behavior. However, the metaphor seems glaringly out of synch when one tries to imagine actual people lying down and negotiating their sex lives. Quite frankly, it lacks "emotive potential," an ability to evoke or satisfy the particular emotions. (p. 70)

Adelman's depiction of the extant research no doubt was accurate. Negotiation became the concept that framed the bulk of the interpersonal communication literature on HIV issues in the late 1980s and early 1990s as researchers began a quest to isolate, measure, and describe the interaction surrounding condom use. However, a review of the intervention studies from the last decade and a half suggests that either most of the intervention teams did not read Adelman's essay or her arguments fell on deaf ears. Along with assertiveness skills, the communication intervention literature related to HIV has focused more on negotiation skills (and negotiation is the term used) than any other strategy. A substantial number of studies have reported the inclusion of condom negotiation as a key component of their educational approach to reducing risk through more effective communication between partners (see, e.g., Choi et al., 1996; Cohen, MacKinnon, Dent, Mason, & Sullivan, 1992; Elwood & Vega, 2005; Fisher et al., 1996; Gillmore et al., 1997; Hovell et al., 1998; Imrie et al., 2001; Jemmott, Jemmott, & Fong, 1998; Levy et al., 1995; Lou, Wang, Shen, & Gao, 2004; Maher, Peterman, Osewe, Odusanya, & Scerba, 2002; Malow, West, Corrigan, Pena, & Cunningham, 1994; Morrison-Beedy et al., 2005; O'Donnell, Doval, Duran, & O'Donnell, 1995; Otto-Salaj et al., 2001; Patterson, Shaw, & Semple, 2003; Peragallo et al., 2005; Peterson et al., 1996; Rosser, 1990; Rotheram-Borus, Gwadz, Fernandez, & Srinivasan, 1998; Rotheram-Borus et al., 2001; Rotheram-Borus et al., 2004; St. Lawrence et al., 1999; St. Lawrence, Crosby, Brasfield, & O'Bannon, 2002; Sampaio, Brites, Stall, Hudes, & Hearst, 2002; Shain et al., 1999; Shrier et al., 2001; Stall, Paul, Barrett, Crosby, & Bein, 1999; Stanton et al., 1996; Toro-Alfonso, Varas-Díaz, & Andújar-Bello, 2002; Tudiver et al., 1992; Walter & Vaughn, 1993).

Much like the studies that include assertiveness skills in their training, there is an inevitable frustration that scholars such as the authors of this chapter encounter when reviewing the body of literature that addresses negotiation skills. Intervention teams report that they taught negotiation, but the details about precisely what their participants learned often remains vague in their descriptions of these skills. There are, however, a few published articles that shed some light. For example, through the use of a computer program (see more detail in the subsection Instruction Through Interactive Technologies), Thomas, Cahill, and Santilli (1997) asked their participants to respond to seven different situations that the intervention team characterized as negotiation tasks. For the first two, they voiced how they would turn down sex and how they would ask a partner to use a condom. In the final set of tasks, respondents replied through a microphone to each of the following lines from a hypothetical partner: (a) "Let's just do it natural ... I don't want to spoil the feeling"; (b) "I haven't been with anyone but you ... you don't need to worry"; (c) "Come on ... I'm clean"; (d) "Just this once ... we'll use one the next time"; and (e) "We are using the pill ... we don't need a condom" (p. 76). Thomas et al. did not report if they gave the participants precise instruction prior to the exercise on ideal negotiation strategies.

A study that provided greater detail on how a team instructed participants to negotiate effectively was an elaborate intervention designed by Gillmore et al. (1997). They divided sexually active teenagers recruited through an STD clinic into three different groups so that each group received instruction about negotiation skills through one of three channels—a comic book, a 27-minute video, or an 8-hour group skill-training format led by facilitators. For each type of instructional format, other teens (fictional characters in the case of the comic book) modeled an approach to negotiating condom use that involved four stages. The first stage they labeled as "Think it up," which means that individuals should plan in advance what to say, where and when to say it, and what the bottom line will be if one's partner refuses to use a condom. The second stage, which they called "Bring it up," instructed the teenagers to take the initiative to express their desire to use a condom. For the third stage, which was  known as "Keep it up," the models demonstrated that one should repeat the request and give reasons if a partner resists. Finally, Gillmore et al. referred to the final stage as "Reward it," which means that regardless of the outcome the person who initiated the negotiation should give him or herself credit for having the courage to bring up the topic and, if one's partner agrees to use a condom, to communicate appreciation.

By far, the greatest detail we identified that is readily available about the operationalization of negotiation skills comes from an intervention conducted by Rotheram-Borus et al. (2004) with young people in Los Angeles living with HIV. In the text of their publication, Rotheram-Borus and her colleagues provided few insights about the negotiation skills they taught their participants, but they did include a link in the body of the article to a Web site where readers can access the lengthy training manual they used for a session on "Should I try to get my partner to accept our using a condom?" In their description of the intervention in the text of the article, the authors used the term *negotiation skills* to identify what they taught their participants, and the objectives outlined at the beginning of the manual intended only for the eyes of the facilitators also used the word *negotiation*. But at no point did the manual instruct the facilitators to describe the new skill set being taught as a negotiation process. Instead, facilitators told the young people in the intervention that they would learn to "influence" or "convince" a partner to use a condom.

During the training, the participants first learned an eight-step process of negotiation designed specifically for use with new partners. The steps included:

1. Decide when and where to ask (e.g., select a safe place).
2. Know your strategy (e.g., have a specific reason why a condom should be used such as "your partner says he loves you and will do anything for you").
3. State your needs (e.g., "I want to feel good about myself by knowing that I have protected my partner").
4. State how you feel (e.g., "I will feel happy when...").
5. State what you want from the other person (e.g., say exactly what you want your partner to do).
6. State the other person's point of view (e.g., "Let him hear what he's telling you; he'll know you are listening").
7. Repeat what you need to say as often as needed (the participants were told that "sometimes it's OK to sound like a broken record").
8. Stay firm (e.g., "You have the right to protect yourself").

Later during the session, the facilitators switched from guidance on negotiation with a new partner to skill development for negotiating with a steady partner. They presented the negotiation process in three parts: how to prepare, things to say and do, and things not to say and do. For the "get ready" phase, facilitators taught participants to think of when you got your partner to do something you wanted in the past; decide your bottom line such as asking yourself if keeping your partner is more important than protecting your partner and yourself; think of ways to build your partner's feeling good about himself; and pick a good time and place to talk about it. For the communication actions they wanted participants to adopt, facilitators told them to start with something positive; tell your partner how you feel and what you want; repeat back to your partner what he says he wants from you; tell your partner when he says something you like; and stop the moment the discussion gets negative. And for behaviors to avoid during negotiation, participants learned to never put a partner down; never keep trying to talk to a partner if he makes nasty comments about you; and never let your rights be violated. Throughout the negotiation training, the participants had the opportunity to practice new skills through role plays.

Eroticizing Condom Use.   In the preceding section on negotiation skills, we cited the essay by Adelman (1992) in which she criticized the ubiquitous use of the negotiation metaphor in the research on sexual communication and condom use. In the same chapter, she recommended that health communicators can achieve success in changing the behavior of individuals who either forego the use of condoms completely or use them inconsistently by reframing condom use as a form of play instead of as a negotiation. As an alternative to viewing communication about condoms formally, Adelman lobbied for a new way of thinking that made condom use a more playful act that enhances the erotic nature of the encounter through improvisation and spontaneity. More specifically, she argued:

> Unlike its more strategic counterpart, negotiation, the metaphor and study of safer sex as play may shed light on the emergent, novel, and contextual features of the sexual episode. Furthermore, this emphasis on the improvisational is crucial to understanding the new demands on erotic reality posed by the harsh threat of AIDS. (p. 73)

Despite the persuasive case that Adelman made 15 years ago, there are few examples in the intervention literature of teams incorporating the eroticization of condoms into an overall arsenal of strategies for communicating with a partner. The few who have chosen this direction for their instruction have tended to suggest eroticism of condoms as a tool of personal invention rather than presenting it as a precise skill that can be taught in the same manner as negotiation or assertiveness. For example, a training session that Kegeles et al. (1996) labeled as *Eroticizing Safe Sex* included a group exercise in which they asked young gay men "to think more creatively about safer sex" (p. 1131). The team, however, did not specify in their report what ideas the participants generated nor did they say how they instructed the men to translate their creative thoughts into meaningful behavior change. In a similar vein, Choi et al. (1996) developed an activity for gay men of Asian or Pacific Islander heritage in which the men wrote down on slips of paper a list of erotic but safe ways of touching. Like Kegeles and her colleagues, Choi et al. did not report the strategies that the men identified. Several other studies (Carey et al., 1997; Morrison-Beedy et al., 2005; Shain et al., 1999; Toro-Alfonso et al., 2002) also listed eroticization as a component of their overall educational strategy to improve communication, but all teams reported even fewer details than did Choi et al. and Kegeles et al.

Refusal Skills.    Numerous studies have included refusal skills or what are sometimes known as "no" statements (Coyle et al., 1996, 2004; Fisher, Fisher, Bryan, & Misovich, 2002; Hovell et al., 1998; Kalichman et al., 1996; Kelly et al., 1997; Kirby et al., 2004; Levy et al., 1995; Roberto, Zimmerman, Carlyle, & Abner, 2007; St. Lawrence et al., 2002; Sampaio et al., 2002; Weeks et al., 1995). Rarely do investigators provide any further detail about how they explain a refusal skill to a participant. This is likely because the skill is no more complicated than urging people to exercise their veto power over sexual intercourse if a partner is not willing to practice safe sex. For example, through interactive technologies, Roberto et al. asked high school students in rural Appalachia to participate in a Refusal Skills Activity in which they had the opportunity to "practice" online their best original refusal skill line. The intervention team apparently gave the students the freedom to be creative but did provide instruction on refusal skills beforehand. Coyle et al. (1996) provided some clues about instruction when they said that they taught the 9th- and 10th-grade students who were their participants that refusal statements must be clear and communicated in the proper context, but Coyle et al. did not specify what the students learned about how to identify when the context is appropriate.

## Nonverbal Skills

Although the self-report literature on sexual communication related to condom use tells us that nonverbal behavior is an integral component of the interaction that takes place between partners (see chap. 1, this volume), the published reports on HIV-related interventions provide little information about how trainers include instruction (if in fact they do at all) on the role of nonverbal communication in negotiating condom use. The most frequently cited estimate is that 93% of all information exchanged between humans is nonverbal in nature (Mehrabian, 1971), and other research (and common sense) informs us that eye contact, facial expression, and touching behavior play a major part in any sexual encounter regardless of whether or not couples use condoms (see Edgar & Fitzpatrick, 1992, e.g., on how the research subjects describe nonverbal communication in sexual scripts). Of the few studies that say they incorporated specific instruction about nonverbal communication in their interventions (Fisher et al., 1996; Kegeles et al., 1996; Kirby, Korpi, Adivi, & Weissman, 1997), we identified only one that actually describes what facilitators taught individuals. As part of the training on nonverbal behavior, Fisher et al. told the heterosexual undergraduate students in their study that one message option is to forego discussion about safe sex and simply put on a condom (they do not say if they gave this advice only to men or if they also told women to put a condom on their male partners without asking), and they also presented them with the possibility of nonverbally communicating a wish to practice safer sex by leaving condoms in full view for a partner to see prior to intercourse.

## Other Skills

In addition to the ones already mentioned, a few other terms have been used with much less regularity by researchers to describe the types of skills they taught the participants in their studies. For example, some have characterized the nature of the communication-training component by relying on very general descriptors such as the phrase "sexual communication" (Lou et al., 2004; Otto-Salaj et al., 2001; Rosser et al., 2002) or by using the most nondescript term of all— *communication skills* (Baker et al., 2003; Stanton et al., 1998; Workman et al., 1996; Zimmerman, Ramirez-Valles, Sarez, de la Rosa, & Castro, 1997). Still others such as Coyle et al. (2004) referred to the communication portion of their intervention as "skills to maintain limits"; both Jemmott, Jemmott, Fong, and McCaffree (1999) and Miller et al. (1998) described teaching persuasive communication skills; Weeks et al. (1997) identified the communication portion of their training as "resistance skills"; and a few studies included "listening skills" in their training (Roffman et al., 1997, 1998).

As with so many of the other studies in this body of literature, these published reports tend to provide few, if any, details to help the reader more precisely understand the nature of the advice they gave to the participants. An exception is the study by Tulloch et al. (2004) in which they used the simple term *communication skills* to describe the interaction-based portion of their intervention, but they did give some clues as to what the undergraduate students in their training sessions learned. Specifically, Tulloch et al. taught their subjects communication skills through instruction on how to raise the topic of condom use, how to discuss the benefits of using or costs of not using condoms, how to request one's sexual partner to use a condom, and how to respond effectively if a partner says that he or she does not want to use a condom. Still, the reader craves more information because we do not know, for instance, what Tulloch et al. identified as the most effective strategies for countering refusal.

One other descriptor of note in the literature that we mention here because of its conspicuous absence is compliance gaining. A large corpus of literature exists in the domain of persuasion research in which scholars have developed typologies of messages that people use on a daily basis to convince others to respond in a desired manner. In the early days of the research that linked communication skills to safer-sex practices, scholars, especially those from the communication discipline, often grounded their methodological approach conceptually within the compliance-gaining literature, which differentiates message types based on the persuasive force of individual messages (see, e.g., Edgar & Fitzpatrick, 1988; Edgar, Freimuth, Hammond, McDonald, & Fink, 1992). Few research teams, however, have developed communication-based interventions that draw specifically, at least on the surface, from the realm of compliance-gaining research. Only a small number of studies even use the word *compliance* (e.g., Bayne-Smith, 1994; Orr et al., 1996) in their reports. One explanation for this may be that the majority of scholars who have published the results of HIV-related interventions with a communication component typically are individuals trained in related disciplines such as public health and social and health psychology, but scholars from the field of communication (or even other social scientists who devote their research to understanding the dynamics of the persuasion process) have had minimal participation on these interventions teams.

*Measuring Change in Communication Skills*

Regardless of the exact type of communication skills that researchers attempt to teach participants in an HIV-related intervention, the inclusion of skills training has little merit unless individuals can actually apply the skills after they receive instruction. Unfortunately, a substantial number of the studies in the intervention literature have failed to provide any measure of change in communication behavior. For these studies, they either incorporated no outcome measures of any kind, or their outcome assessment focused strictly on safer sex practices (e.g., condom use, number of new partners) and/or health outcomes (e.g., number of reported new cases of HIV or STD infection). Studies with no measure for detecting changes in communication behavior typically assume that if risky behaviors decrease and incidence of new infections is minimal within an intervention group that received communication training, then one can infer that communication skills improved and contributed in a meaningful way to larger outcomes. The assumption might be a valid one, but the argument for the positive role of communication behavior in safer-sex practices is more powerful if there is direct evidence that those who received communication training were better communicators after instruction than they were before.

For those studies that have provided a measure of change in communication behavior, the methodological approaches have varied with a mix of both self-report and observational techniques. Within the domain of self-report, some have relied on measures that the research team typically administers to participants prior to the intervention and at single or multiple follow-up assessments to gauge actual behavior change. Choi et al. (1996), for example, asked their participants to report on the extent to which they had talked about safer-sex practices with partners in the 3 months following the intervention, and Peragallo et al. (2005) used a 10-item scale at both 3 and 6 months after training to determine how often participants discussed health protective topics with first-time partners. Other researchers, meanwhile, have collected self-report data that focused on intentions and confidence in one's ability to implement newly acquired skills in the future. For example, Otto-Salaj et al. (2001) asked participants to respond to an item on a questionnaire immediately after training that asked them to indicate the likelihood that they would "insist on condom use even if my partner is resistant," and Thomas et al. (1997) asked their trainees how ready they felt they were to handle situations such as asking a new partner to use a condom during a first sexual encounter; asking a long-time partner to start using condoms; and convincing a partner to use a condom, even if the partner did not want to use one at first.

In contrast to the self-report method of skills assessment, numerous teams have asked trainees to respond to different hypothetical scenarios in which communication about safer-sex practices would be an appropriate option and then rated the responses along various dimensions (e.g., Hovell et al., 1998, 2001; Jaworski & Carey, 2001; Kelly et al., 1990; Kipke et al., 1993; Metzler et al., 2000; St. Lawrence et al., 1994, 1995; Tulloch et al., 2004). In most studies of this type, the intervention team then has compared the ratings of those who participated in communication skills training to those in a control group not exposed to the training to determine if the instruction resulted in a higher skill level for participants. In some studies, coders rated written responses (e.g., Jaworski & Carey, 2001), but in most interventions of this type, members of the research team rated live role plays, listened to audio recordings, or watched videotapes of role plays in which a participant interacts with either another trainee or a facilitator. For example, Tulloch et al. (2004) used raters to observe participants engaged in role plays with a research assistant of the opposite sex. At the conclusion of the role plays, the coders classified the interaction in one of four ways: inappropriate/ineffective; states something about using a condom, but does not provide an argument about condom use; gives an argument for using a condom, but does not specifically respond to the partner's refusal statement; or responds effectively by addressing the partner's refusal statement and gives an argument for using a condom. As an example of a somewhat different rating scheme, coders for St. Lawrence et al. (1994) listened to audio recordings of role plays and then provided an effectiveness rating for each of the following five communication behaviors: acknowledgment of the other person's point of view; specific refusal of an unsafe invitation or action; providing a reason or rationale for the refusal; specifically stating the need for safety; and proposing a lower risk alternative to the proposed action.

## Instructional Techniques

Regardless of the type of communication skill the intervention team is trying to teach, researchers must make a decision about the most appropriate instructional strategy for maximizing the odds that participants will depart the training with skills they realistically can translate to real-life situations. The general literature on teaching communication skills provides guidance on an ideal approach. In a comprehensive review of the communication skills training literature, Segrin and Givertz (2003) concluded that the most effective training programs "generally employ multiple procedures, often in a sequential fashion" (p. 139). Noting that much of the skills-training literature draws heavily from Bandura's social learning theory (Bandura, 1977), Segrin and Givertz identified six phases for an ideal communication skills training curriculum to be followed in order:

- Assessment: Trainers should first determine if a population is capable of being taught communication skills and, if so, which skills to focus on.
- Direct Instruction and Coaching: The skills training should begin with an explanation of the specific communication behavior being taught, how to use it effectively, and the rationale for acquiring the targeted skill.
- Modeling: The purpose of modeling in communication skills training is to provide the trainee a template for his or her own behavior by observing an "other" successfully enact the desired skill. "People who have difficulty saying and doing certain things when in the presence of others are sometimes more comfortable doing so after seeing someone else do it first" (Segrin & Givertz, 2003, p. 140). The literature suggests, however, that the model presented to trainees should not necessarily be flawless. As Segrin and Givertz noted, "Watching others struggle through these challenges may create more realistic and less perfectionistic expectations, in addition to demonstrating the value of perseverance in the face of difficulties" (p. 142).
- Role Playing: The purpose of role playing is for trainees to produce the targeted behavior in a controlled setting in which they are observed and receive corrective feedback and positive reinforcement.
- Homework Assignments: In this phase, the trainee puts into actual practice the targeted skill outside the controlled setting where the instruction, modeling, and role playing occurred.
- Follow-Up: Because communication skills are complex behaviors to learn and maintain, continued monitoring of a trainee's successes and failures and subsequent corrective feedback and reinforcement are highly recommended.

A review of the HIV-related intervention literature reveals that the principles described by Segrin and Gervitz (2003), especially coaching, modeling, and role playing, have been followed, at least in part, within a variety of instructional formats for delivering sexual–communication skills training. Very few studies have incorporated homework assignments and follow-up or booster training.[1] In the current section, we examine the inclusion (and exclusion) of coaching, modeling, and role playing in their various forms within the context of four approaches to instruction: (a) traditional teacher–student interactions, (b) noninteractive video, (c) interactive technologies, and (d) opinion leaders.

### Instruction Through Traditional Classroom Techniques

The most common approach to teaching communication skills to intervention participants has been to rely on a traditional instructor–student environment in which a trained facilitator provides direct instruction and coaching of the appropriate skills. In some studies, the instructional component ends with the instruction/coaching (e.g., Solomon & DeJong, 1989), but in more elaborate designs, researchers have added other key elements of the ideal skills training paradigm such as modeling and role playing. For example, Morrison-Beedy et al. (2005) conducted a multisession intervention with adolescent girls in which facilitators taught sexual assertiveness skills to groups of six to eight participants. They emphasized improvement of self-efficacy, negotiation of condom use with a partner, and eroticization of condom use. Although the published report does not say whether facilitators explicitly modeled the behaviors for the girls, the participants did have the opportunity to role-play their new skills. Following the role plays, the instructors provided corrective feedback to help the girls further improve their ability to communicate effectively with partners. At a 3-month follow-up, Morrison-Beedy and her colleagues found that the girls in the intervention group were significantly more likely to have talked with a partner about safer sex than were those in a control group.

Other studies clearly have incorporated both modeling and post-coaching role plays into their designs, but there have been variations in approach to the role-playing portion of the training. For example, DiClemente and Wingood (1995) had educators model sexual-assertiveness skills for African-American women, and then the participants practiced in *dyads* with one of the educators who played the role of a potential sexual partner. Those who received the more comprehensive skills training reported more consistent condom use at a follow-up data collection point. In contrast, St. Lawrence et al. (1994) placed substance-dependent youth in *triads* for role plays after initial coaching and modeling of behaviors. Using written scenarios as a guide, one of the youth role-played the part of a coercive partner while another participant attempted to respond assertively with skills just acquired in training. The third member of the triad was a facilitator who coached and offered suggestions to the other two. For those who participated in the triads, the researchers found that there was a reduction in the percentage that was coerced into unwanted sexual activity at a 2-month follow-up.

## Instruction Through Watching Video

Although the majority of interventions aimed at teaching participants safer-sex negotiation skills have relied on a more traditional trainer–trainee approach, others have used technologies in various forms to sharpen communication competence. Several studies have facilitated learning by presenting information through video. For example, although Kalichman, Williams, and Nachimson (1999) did not create new video material for their intervention, they did present African-American women recruited from an STD clinic with scenes from five popular films lasting 2 to 3 minutes that depicted interactions between fictional African-American characters that the researchers identified as preludes to sexual encounters. The clips, which were shown after communication skills coaching by facilitators, did not actually model behavior but did serve as a stimulus for role plays. The intervention team stopped the clips at points and asked participants to role-play responses to what they observed onscreen, and they then received feedback from both group members and facilitators. Kalichman et al. found at a 1-month follow-up that, compared to a control group, those who participated in the intervention were more likely to report talking to a partner about condoms. Kalichman and his colleagues described a similar procedure with studies they conducted with African-American men (Kalichman, Cherry, & Browne-Sperling, 1999) and HIV-positive men and women (Kalichman et al.,

2001), and in both studies, follow-up assessments showed significant differences in risk reduction behaviors when compared to control groups. For an intervention targeted to Latino and Anglo teenagers, Hovell et al. (1998) created their own videos in which adolescents modeled communication skills onscreen. After watching the videos, a facilitator provided students with a rationale for each skill and then gave students the opportunity to role-play the new skill shown in the video. Results showed that teens who received communication training improved their skills more than youth in other conditions.

## Instruction Through Interactive Technologies

Some studies have incorporated more sophisticated interactive technologies into their interventions, especially when developing training for younger populations. For example, Thomas et al. (1997) created a computer program called "Life Challenge" for adolescents that allowed users to consider multiple strategies when learning negotiation skills. Through a voice capture and playback mechanism, participants had the chance to "talk" to (or role-play with) imaginary partners and hear their recorded statements played back to them. After listening to their own responses, the adolescents judged their attempt at persuasion by clicking on either a "try again" or a "sounds OK" button. Thomas et al. also included a game show segment in the interactive video in which students identified the fictionalized contestant they felt communicated the most effective message to a sexual partner. Unfortunately, Thomas et al. did not assess any behavioral outcomes.

More recently, Downs et al. (2004) designed an interactive system for teenage women in which a male character on video models an attempt to convince his female partner to engage in unsafe sex. In response, the video's female characters modeled less-risky choices. The participant was able to interact with the video (a form of role play) through the presentation of choice points and behavioral alternatives. After watching the scenes, the system also permitted users to perform "cognitive rehearsals" where they imagined what they would say or do in a similar situation while the screen froze for 30 seconds. Participants in the study who used the interactive video reported at follow-up that they had completely avoided risky behaviors. (For other studies using interactive video, see chaps. 14 and 24, this volume.)

*Instruction Through Opinion Leaders*

In addition to the more direct intervention approaches, there also exists a small but compelling body of research based on a "go between" model, where the goal of the interventions was to train opinion leaders within the communities who then were tasked with disseminating information about HIV prevention, including sexual-communication skills, to others. This strategy relies less on techniques grounded in social learning theory and more on the diffusion of innovations model, which asserts that behavior is mediated by perceived peer norms (Rogers, 2003). By identifying and training the opinion leaders to alter their own norms and adopt new behaviors, they begin to shift the perception of what is normative with the expectation that subsequent members of the community will adopt the behaviors regardless of whether they had direct contact with the original opinion leaders. Modeling as a strategy for change still exists in this approach but occurs in a somewhat different form than in approaches using traditional classroom instruction or new technologies.

In one of the earliest interventions of this type, Kelly et al. (1991) trained bartenders in one of three U.S. cities to select a team of opinion leaders from the patrons of the gay clubs in which they worked (a subsequent study by Kelly and his colleagues in 1992 evaluated the intervention after it was conducted in two other cities). Following four weekly 90-minute training sessions, which included communication skills training on how to discuss safe sex practices in advance and how to assertively refuse unsafe sexual coercion, these opinion leaders were contracted to serve as risk reduction endorsers and have conversations with their peers in the club setting. To stimulate the conversations, the opinion leaders wore buttons depicting a red, yellow, and green traffic light logo (but with no text) that corresponded with posters placed throughout the club. The study authors hoped that these opinion leaders would not only convey communication and behavior strategies for sexual risk reduction, but also establish the norm within the community that safe-sex behavior changes are important and acceptable to adopt. The study revealed that both the opinion leaders and those who received the peer-facilitated intervention reduced their high-risk sexual behavior (Kelly et al., 1992).

Miller et al. (1998) attempted to replicate the work of Kelly and his colleagues by targeting a peer-facilitated intervention at male prostitutes and patrons of hustler bars. Because part of this study was to test the feasibility of implementing the intervention design of Kelly et al., Miller et al. followed a virtually identical protocol for selecting and training peer opinion leaders to communicate safe-sex strategies and norms. Trainers taught the opinion leaders how to generate specific methods for eroticizing condom use and how to convince a paying partner to use a condom, which they were then to convey in conversations at the bars. Not only did this study find that the intervention design of Kelly et al. was "relatively easy" to implement, Miller and colleagues also reported reductions in the involvement in and frequency of paid, unprotected sex among men who received the peer-facilitated interventions.

In a third study that followed a similar model, Kegeles et al. (1996) described an intervention that developed a network of social settings and events for the community of gay men in Eugene, Oregon. The Mpowerment Project was designed by a group of 12 to 15 young gay men with assistance from a community advisory board. The young men conducted informal outreach through day-to-day conversations between themselves and their friends where they talked about the need to adopt safe-sex practices. The men invited their peers to small group meetings where more formal outreach was conducted. Teaching communication skills was an element of these meetings where leaders modeled verbal and nonverbal safer-sex strategies (with scenarios for both casual partners and boyfriends included) and ways to eroticize safe sex. Kegeles et al. reported reductions in unprotected anal intercourse with men in general, with boyfriends, and with secondary partners in the 2 months prior to assessment for men who received the intervention.

## Amount of Training

In addition to making decisions about the specific types of skills to teach and the format through which training gets delivered, intervention designers must also determine how much communication training is needed in order to have the desired effect. The answer is not a simple one because the research data provide contradictory results. Some evidence suggests that one training session can lead to success. For instance, Orr et al. (1996) provided a single-session intervention for female adolescents infected with an STD in which a facilitator discussed the infection with the teenagers using a pamphlet as a guide, showed how to use a condom correctly, and then provided communication instruction in a structured rehearsal scenario in which a young woman attempts to persuade her sexual partner to use a condom. Orr et al. found that the adolescents in the intervention group reported a threefold greater use of condoms 6 months later than did their counterparts in the study's control group. Interventions in addition to the one by Orr et al. have also reported some success with behavioral change based on single-session instruction on sexual communication (see, e.g., Choi et al., 1996; Kalichman, Williams, & Nachimson, 1999; Kipke et al., 1993).

In contrast, other researchers have had limited effect with single-dose interventions. For example, a training strategy devised by Tulloch et al. (2004) resulted in a disappointing outcome when they sought to increase condom use among heterosexual college students by providing them with a single session of communication skills training. Specifically, Tulloch et al. taught negotiation skills to participants and then had them engage in two role plays with a research assistant of the opposite sex in which the students practiced their new skills. When the students had the opportunity to use the skills in a hypothetical situation, data from coded observations indicated that the skill level increased for most of the participants. However, the follow-up portion of the study, which occurred 2 months later, found little change in condom use among those who received the communication training. Tulloch et al. speculated that the training lacked the necessary intensity and was not thorough enough to produce the desired result. In yet another single-session communication-based intervention, Jaworski and Carey (2001) focused on modeling for female undergraduates through role plays highlighting the differences between angry and assertive approaches to communicating with a partner about requesting that the couple use a condom. Although their follow-up data showed that participants in the intervention group reduced their number of sexual partners, there was no improvement in attitudes toward condoms or actual condom use. Jaworski and Carey surmised that sustained practice is the key to translating newly acquired communication skills into meaningful behavior change for protection against STD infection. They believed the students in their study had insufficient opportunity to practice the skills both in the training session and in their everyday lives following the intervention. Their conclusion is consistent with the findings from the general literature on communication skills training that suggests that homework assignments and follow-up training increase the likelihood of sustained skill acquisition (Segrin & Givertz, 2003).

Although many interventions have provided only a single lesson on effective means of communicating with a partner about safer-sex practices, there have been interventions in which individuals received communication training through more intense interventions, but the results for these studies also provide some ambiguity about how much training is enough to provide the desired outcome. Workman et al. (1996), for example, designed an intervention for African-American and Hispanic adolescent women that included two sessions on sexual assertiveness skills that each lasted 30 minutes. When they compared skill levels after the training to baseline measures, Workman et al. found no significant differences in the ability of participants to use assertiveness skills. They concluded that a total of 60 minutes of training is not enough to effect meaningful change. Likewise, Hovell et al. (2001) found little evidence for sustained change based on two sessions of communication training. After adolescents participated in negotiation role plays, observations from coders revealed that the teenagers immediately improved their communication skills when they had the chance to demonstrate competence in a hypothetical scenario, but an assessment of their skills 6 months later showed that the adolescents had not retained the negotiation skill level achieved at the time of the original training.

In contrast, other research teams have developed approaches incorporating multiple doses of communication skills training that resulted in change, at least for a period of months, in safer-sex behaviors. A prime example is the study conducted by Otto-Salaj et al. (2001) in which they created an intervention for severely mentally ill outpatients at a psychiatric clinic in which they included instruction on sexual communication in three of the seven sessions they devoted to HIV-related issues. The team then provided the participants with booster training at both 1- and 2-month follow-up sessions after the initial intervention, which follows the recommendation of the skills-training literature on adding a follow-up component to instruction (Segrin & Givertz, 2003). In the booster sessions, participants had the opportunity to discuss with other trainees and facilitators how they had handled risk reduction situations since their last session. Otto-Salaj et al. found that those who participated in the intervention group significantly increased their frequency of condom-protected sex at 3-, 6-, and 9-month follow-up assessments; however, the behavior change effects diminished when they measured the same variables 12 months after the original intervention. A key question that arose from the results was whether or not long-term change can be sustained more easily within a population not challenged by serious psychiatric disorders.

Although Otto-Salaj et al. employed a more intensive approach to communication training with some success, they did not systematically compare their version of the intervention to a less intense method, but at least one research team has. Using a design with multiple experimental conditions intended specifically to help answer the "How much is enough?" question, Peterson et al. (1996) assigned African-American homosexual and bisexual men to one of three conditions: a wait-list control group, a one-session intervention, or a three-session intervention. In both intervention groups, participants learned about assertiveness skills for negotiating low-risk sexual behaviors and then had the opportunity to rehearse the skills in role plays. The research team exposed participants in the single-session group to the same types of communication activities developed for those in the three-session group, but the single-session participants received the information in a compacted format. Peterson and his colleagues found that individuals in the three-session group greatly reduced their frequency of unprotected anal intercourse at both 12- and 18-month follow-up assessments, whereas levels of risky behavior for the single-session group decreased only slightly at both the 12- and 18-month evaluations. Rotheram-Borus et al. (1998) also conducted an experiment in which they varied the timing of their overall training approach to HIV education (i.e., seven sessions of 1.5 hours each versus three sessions of 3.5 hours each). Although the total amount of time devoted to instruction on sexual communication was comparable in both conditions, there was greater behavior change for those who attended the shorter sessions offered over the longer period of time.

One of the challenges of making sense of the lessons learned from the intervention literature is that communication training is always just one of multiple components of an overall instructional approach to effecting behavior change. That is, the intent of the team that creates the intervention is to produce one or more attitudinal outcomes (e.g., more positive attitudes toward condoms, intention to use condoms, increased confidence in one's ability to initiate conversation about safer sex with a partner) and/or behavioral outcomes (e.g., reduction in number of risky sexual encounters, decrease in number of sexual partners, improved sexual negotiation skills). However, the instructional design model for interventions is a multifaceted one.

An example of an intervention that perfectly illustrates this point is one created by DiClemente and Wingood (1995). Using an experiment designed to reduce the risk of HIV infection among heterosexual African-American women, DiClemente and Wingood provided participants in their experimental group with five 2-hour sessions of training spread over a 5-week period. The third session emphasized sexual assertiveness and communication training where participants learned how to differentiate assertive, passive, and aggressive communication styles, and with facilitators on hand to provide corrective feedback, they practiced their new skills through role plays. In the fifth session, the same facilitators introduced cognitive rehearsals to the instructional mix by describing sexual scenarios to the women that involved a noncompliant sexual partner. To solve the hypothetical problems, the women applied the assertiveness strategies they learned in the third session. However, in the midst of the intense communication training, they also acquired other skills and knowledge in the first, second, and fourth sessions. For instance, the first class emphasized pride in their womanhood and their African-American heritage; the second session provided information about HIV-associated risk behaviors; and the fourth meeting emphasized proper condom use skills and positive norms toward consistent condom use. When DiClemente and Wingood assessed multiple outcome variables at a 3-month follow-up, comparison data to another group that only received standard HIV education information (i.e., information similar to what the women in the experimental group received in their second session) revealed that the women in the five-session group demonstrated increased condom use, greater sexual self-control, greater use of sexual communication, greater sexual assertiveness, and increased partners' adoption of norms supporting consistent condom use.[2]

The results from the DiClemente and Wingood (1995) study and others with similar designs (e.g., Metzler et al., 2000; Walter & Vaughn, 1993) provide persuasive evidence that communication training is a powerful component of a comprehensive educational strategy for helping individuals make behavioral choices that can prevent serious illness, but there remains a question of how much variance can be attributed to the communication-based instruction. For example, how impressive would the results have been for DiClemente and Wingood without the addition of the discussion of gender and ethnic pride and the information on condom use skills and positive norms? And, on the flip side, how much power to effect positive change would have been lost if the communication training had not been included? Several literature reviews and meta-analyses have concluded that the communication skills component is without doubt a key ingredient in the intervention mix (i.e., Herbst et al., 2005; Johnson, Carey, Marsh, Levin, & Scott-Sheldon, 2003; Johnson et al., 2002; Pedlow & Carey, 2004), but no analyses have estimated the degree to which communication training makes a difference.

## Implications for Future HIV Prevention Interventions Involving Skills Training

In this final section, we summarize by first offering suggestions on how best to report results for those who publish new articles on intervention studies so that other scholars with similar interests can derive the maximum benefit from the literature. We then close by providing recommendations for future studies.

### Recommendations for Future Reporting of Intervention Studies

Although the body of literature as a whole has much to teach us, this review was limited somewhat by the lack of detail provided in the primary articles on the overall design of interventions and on the operationalization of skill types. In many articles, there were significant omissions in the reporting on the communication skills–training components. Because of this, the current review has focused more on those articles that provided fuller reporting of skills-training components. We hope to see more information appear in published reports in the future. But we understand that there are inherent barriers to realizing that goal, and we do not mean to suggest that authors of published articles intentionally seek to be vague. The fault more likely lies within the inherent constraints of the editorial process where journal editors must insist that the final versions of manuscripts conform to a standard length. Thus, publishing an intervention team's entire training protocol in most cases is simply impractical. In the future, we hope to see more journals implement a system where readers can link to the journal's Web site to find more detailed materials for which there was insufficient space in the published form of the article. For example, in an intervention study with Latino women recently published in *Nursing Research,* within the article the editor included a URL that directs the reader to a comprehensive outline of the authors' training protocol complete with session objectives, discussion points, and assignments (Peragallo et al., 2005). Information of this sort has great benefit for others who wish to learn more about a program that has strong evidence of success.

The current chapter also reviewed a number of modes through which communication skills are taught in interventions, including traditional classroom techniques, use of video, interactive technologies, and opinion leaders. As we argued earlier in the chapter, the training techniques most commonly reflect principles described in social learning theory or the diffusion of innovations model. Some intervention designers explicitly connect their approach to training to established behavior change frameworks, but most do not. Many implicitly ground their approaches to training within accepted models by incorporating techniques such as modeling and role playing, but often it is not clear if intervention designers made choices based on intuition or if decisions are connected to a large conceptual framework for thinking about the acquisition and maintenance of communication competence. We urge future researchers to provide clear rationales in their manuscripts for their pedagogical choices.

Finally, there is now a large body of literature on basic issues in safer sexual communication and negotiation that can be drawn on to inform this component of intervention efforts (for reviews, see chap. 1, this volume; Noar, Carlyle, & Cole, 2006). For instance, are interventions fusing knowledge from this basic literature in their skills-training components, such as teaching individuals the variety of strategies that at-risk men and women report utilizing to negotiate safer sex (i.e., Noar, Morokoff, & Harlow, 2004)? Although some reports clearly rely on this literature to inform communication skills training, we suspect that interventions may be underutilizing this knowledge.

## Future Research Directions

There are a number of important directions for future research in the area of sexual communication skills training. For instance, each of the modes of intervention—traditional classroom, use of video, interactive technologies, and opinion leaders—are modes that are widely used in the HIV prevention intervention literature at large. When such interventions involve skills training, however, a number of questions arise. For instance, how can each of these modes be enhanced to make the most of its potential in the skills-training area? Which of these intervention modes is most effective for teaching sexual communication skills? And, how can these methods for teaching skills be integrated into the many intervention contexts that exist in the HIV prevention literature (i.e., individual-level, community based, media campaigns, policy initiatives, etc.)? Future research might address a number of these questions in order to give us a broader and more systematic understanding of communication skills training for safer sex. For instance, a simple but valuable study would be one that compares a number of these approaches side by side and examines their individual (and perhaps combined) abilities to successfully impart sexual communication skills to at-risk audiences. Gillmore et al. (1997) conducted a study of this sort in 1997 by comparing skills training delivered through a videotape, a comic book, and face-to-face instruction, but the delivery options have expanded dramatically within the last 10 years with an increased sophistication in technology. The efficacy of content delivery through the Internet will be especially key as a point of comparison in future studies (Bull, McFarlane, & King, 2001; Cassell, Jackson, & Cheuvront, 1998; Noar, Clark, Cole, & Lustria, 2006).

This review also has raised other key questions for further research, such as how much intervention "dose" is needed to successfully teach sexual communication and negotiation skills. This, of course, is a question for the intervention literature at large. In the context of a conversation about communication skills, though, it raises the issue of not only how long an intervention must be but also how much time might be devoted to communication skills training. Interventions can last only so long and teaching skills must be balanced with other issues such as motivating individuals to engage in safer sex in the first place. If individuals are not motivated to engage in safer sex, then any skills that they learn will likely *not* be put to use. How a balance of content is achieved in any intervention context is a complex issue, and one with which the literature must continue to struggle. For instance, the Otto-Salaj et al. (2001) study discussed earlier in this chapter included seven sessions, three of which focused on skills training, and gave individuals an opportunity to "try out" skills with their actual sexual partners through "homework assignments" and then come back to the intervention group and report on their experiences. The general literature on communication skills training tells us that this kind of rehearsal in a real-life situation along with sharing with the group to gain feedback is likely a powerful way in which to learn and maintain such skills. However, is the "payoff" from this kind of intervention worth the time and resources that must be devoted to incorporating the extra components? Can a more time-condensed intervention achieve similar outcomes if the training follows other core instructional principles that consume less time?

Finally, although overwhelming evidence exists that communication training is a key component to the success of an HIV-related intervention, we still do not know for sure *how much* of a contribution communication training adds to the overall mix of elements typically incorporated into an instructional design (e.g., basic information about HIV transmission, condom use skills, empowerment training, etc.). We propose that future studies include experimental designs that permit researchers to tease out the communication-training aspect of a more complex intervention. For instance, Kalichman et al. (1996, 2005) have used a component analysis paradigm to examine the independent and interactive effects of different intervention components. In one study based on the information-motivation-behavioral skills model, various HIV prevention counseling conditions were compared, including (a) information only, (b) information plus motivational enhancement, (c) information plus behavioral-skills training, and (d) information plus motivational enhancement *and* behavioral-skills training (Kalichman et al., 2005). Using such a design, one can tease apart the individual and interactive effects of these differing intervention components, and thus can "unpack" and isolate the effects of these differing components. A similar study applied to this area and using a theory like the theory of reasoned action might compare (a) no-treatment control or usual care, (b) safer-sex attitudes component only, (c) safer-sex norms component only, (d) communication skills training only, and (e) safe-sex attitudes, norms, and communication skills training. In this manner, researchers can understand whether communication skills training works by itself as compared to other intervention approaches as well as how it operates in the context of other intervention components.

## Notes

1. For a description of a study that included a homework assignment, see the summary of St. Lawrence et al. (1995) in the earlier subsection Assertiveness Skills. For a description of a study that included a follow-up or booster session, see the summary of Otto-Salaj et al. (2001) in the Amount of Training section later in this chapter.
2. For more detail on the work of DiClemente and his colleagues, see chapter 16 in this volume.

## References

Aarons, S. J., Jenkins, R. R., Raine, T. R., El-Khorazaty, M. N., Woodward, K. M., Williams, R. L., et al. (2000). Postponing sexual intercourse among urban junior high school students—a randomized controlled evaluation. *Journal of Adolescent Health, 27,* 236–247.

Adelman, M. B. (1992). Healthy passions: Safer sex as play. In T. Edgar, M. A. Fitzpatrick, & V.S. Freimuth (Eds.), *AIDS: A communication perspective* (pp. 69–89). Hillsdale, NJ: Lawrence Erlbaum Associates.

Baker, S. A., Beadnell, B., Stoner, S., Morrison, D. M, Gordon, J., Collier, C., et al. (2003). Skills training versus health education to prevent STDs/HIV in heterosexual women: A randomized controlled trial utilizing biological outcomes. *AIDS Education and Prevention, 15,* 1–14.

Bandura, A. (1977). *Social learning theory.* Englewood Cliffs, NJ: Prentice-Hall.

Bayne-Smith, M. A. (1994). Teen incentives program: Evaluation of a health promotion model for adolescent pregnancy prevention. *Journal of Health Education, 25,* 24–29.

Bull, S. S., McFarlane, M., & King, D. (2001). Barriers to STD/HIV prevention on the Internet. *Health Education Research, 16,* 661–670.

Carey, M. P., Carey, K. B., Maisto, S. A., Gordon, C. M., Schroder, K. E. E., & Vanable, P. A. (2004). Reducing HIV-risk behavior among adults receiving outpatient psychiatric treatment: Results from a randomized controlled trial. *Journal of Consulting and Clinical Psychology, 72,* 252–268.

Carey, M. P., Maisto, S. A., Kalichman, S. C., Forsyth, A. D., Wright, E. M., & Johnson, B. T. (1997). Enhancing motivation to reduce the risk of HIV infection for economically disadvantaged urban women. *Journal of Consulting and Clinical Psychology, 65,* 531–541.

Cassell, M. M., Jackson, C., & Cheuvront, B. (1998). Health communication on the Internet: An effective channel for health behavior change? *Journal of Health Communication, 3,* 71–79.

Choi, K., Lew, S., Vittinghoff, E., Catania, J. A., Barrett, D. C., & Coates, T. J. (1996). The efficacy of brief group counseling in HIV risk reduction among homosexual Asian and Pacific Islander men. *AIDS, 10,* 81–87.

Cohen, D. A., MacKinnon, D. P., Dent, C., Mason, H. R. C., & Sullivan, E. (1992). Group counseling at STD clinics to promote use of condoms. *Public Health Reports, 107,* 727–731.

Coyle, K. K., Kirby, D. B., Marín, B. V., Gómez, C. A., & Gregorich, S. E. (2004). Draw the line/respect the line: A randomized trial of middle school intervention to reduce sexual risk behaviors. *Research and Practice, 94,* 843–851.

Coyle, K., Kirby, D., Parcel, G., Basen-Engquist, K., Bansoach, S., Rugg, D., et al. (1996). Safer choices: A multicomponent school-based HIV/STD and pregnancy prevention program for adolescents. *Journal of School Health, 66,* 89–94.

DiClemente, R. J., & Wingood, G. M. (1995). A randomized controlled trial of an HIV sexual risk-reduction intervention for young African-American women. *Journal of the American Medical Association, 274,* 1271–1276.

DiClemente, R. J., Wingood, G. M., Harrington, K. F., Lang, D. L, Davies, S. L., et al. (2004). Efficacy of an HIV prevention intervention for African American adolescent girls: A randomized controlled trial. *Journal of the American Medical Association, 292,* 171–179.

Downs, J. S., Murray, P. J., Bruine de Bruin, W., Penrose, J., Palmgren, C., & Fischhoff, B. (2004). Interactive video behavioral intervention to reduce adolescent females' STD risk: A randomized controlled trial. *Social Science & Medicine, 59,* 1561–1572.

Edgar, T. (1992). A compliance-based approach to the study of condom use. In T. Edgar, M. A. Fitzpatrick, & V. S. Freimuth (Eds.), *AIDS: A communication perspective* (pp. 47–67). Hillsdale, NJ: Lawrence Erlbaum Associates.

Edgar, T., & Fitzpatrick, M. A. (1988). Compliance-gaining in relational interaction: When your life depends on it. *Southern Speech Communication Journal, 53,* 385–405.

Edgar, T., Fitzpatrick, M. A., & Freimuth, V. S. (1992). *AIDS: A communication perspective.* Hillsdale, NJ: Lawrence Erlbaum Associates.

Edgar, T., & Fitzpatrick, M. A. (1993). Expectations for sexual interaction: A cognitive test of the sequencing of sexual communication behaviors. *Health Communication, 5,* 239–261.

Edgar, T., Freimuth, V. S., Hammond, S. L., McDonald, D., & Fink, E. L. (1992). Strategic sexual communication: Condom use resistance and response. *Health Communication, 4,* 83–104.

Elwood, W. N., & Vega, M. (2005). Process evaluation results from a condom use intervention with substance abusers in treatment: From "Cinderella" to "Show me!" *Alcoholism Treatment Quarterly, 23,* 47–62.

Fisher, J. D., Fisher, W. A., Bryan, A. D., & Misovich, S. J. (2002). Information-motivation-behavioral skills model-based HIV risk behavior change intervention for inner-city high school youth. *Health Psychology, 21,* 177–186.

Fisher, J. D., Fisher, W. A., Misovich, S. J., Kimble, D. L., & Malloy, T. E. (1996). Changing AIDS risk behavior: Effects of an intervention emphasizing AIDS risk reduction information, motivation, and behavioral skills in a college student population. *Health Psychology, 15,* 114–123.

Gillmore, M. R., Morrison, D. M., Richey, C. A., Balassone, M. L., Gutierrez, L., & Farris, M. (1997). Effects of a skill-based intervention to encourage condom use among high risk heterosexually active adolescents. *AIDS Education and Prevention, 9,* 22–43.

Herbst, J. H., Sherba, R. T., Crepaz, N., DeLuca, J. B., Zohrabyan, L., Stall, R. D., et al. (2005). A meta-analytic review of HIV behavioral interventions for reducing sexual risk behavior of men who have sex with men. *Journal of Acquired Immune Deficiency Syndromes, 39,* 228–241.

Hovell, M. F., Blumberg, E. J., Liles, S., Powell, L., Morrison, T. C., Duran, G., et al. (2001). Training AIDS and anger prevention social skills in at-risk adolescents. *Journal of Counseling & Development, 79,* 347–355.

Hovell, M., Blumberg, E., Sipan, C., Hofstetter, C. R., Burkham, S., Atkins, C., et al. (1998). Skills training for pregnancy and AIDS prevention in Anglo and Latino youth. *Journal of Adolescent Health, 23,* 139–149.

Imrie, J., Stephenson, J. M., Cowan, F. M., Wanigaratne, S., Billingon, A. J. P., Copas, A. J., et al. (2001). A cognitive behavioral intervention to reduce sexually transmitted infections among gay men: Randomised trial. *British Medical Journal, 322,* 1451–1456.

Jaworski, B. C., & Carey, M. P. (2001). Effects of a brief, theory-based STD-prevention program for female college students. *Society for Adolescent Medicine, 2,* 417–425.

Jemmott, J. B., III, Jemmott, L. S., & Fong, G. T. (1998). Abstinence and safer sex HIV risk-reduction interventions for African American adolescents: A randomized controlled trial. *Journal of the American Medical Association, 279,* 1529–1536.

Jemmott, J. B., Jemmott, L.S., Fong, G. T., & McCaffree, K. (1999). Reducing HIV risk-associated sexual behavior among African American adolescents: Testing the generality of intervention effects. *American Journal of Community Psychology, 27,* 161–187.

Johnson, B. T., Carey, M. P., Marsh, K. L., Levin, K. D., & Scott-Sheldon, L. A. J. (2003). Interventions to reduce sexual risk for the human immunodeficiency virus in adolescents, 1985–2000: A research synthesis. *Archives of Pediatric and Adolescent Medicine, 157,* 381–388.

Johnson, W. D., Hedges, L. V., Ramirez, G., Semaan, S., Norman, L. R., Sogolow, E., et al. (2002). HIV prevention research for men who have sex with men: A systematic review and meta-analysis. *Journal of Acquired Immune Deficiency Syndromes, 30,* S118–S129.

Kalichman, S. C., Cain, D., Weinhardt, L., Benotsch, E., Presser, K., Zweben, A., et al. (2005). Experimental components analysis of brief theory-based HIV/AIDS risk-reduction counseling for sexually transmitted infection patients. *Health Psychology, 24*(2), 198–208.

Kalichman, S. C., Cherry, C., & Browne-Sperling, F. (1999a). Effectiveness of a video-based motivational skills-building HIV risk-reduction intervention for inner-city African American men. *Journal of Consulting and Clinical Psychology, 67,* 959–966.

Kalichman, S. C., Rompa, D., Cage, M., DiFonzo, K., Simpson, D., Austin, J., et al. (2001). Effectiveness of an intervention to reduce HIV transmission risks in HIV-positive people. *American Journal of Preventive Medicine, 21,* 84–92.

Kalichman, S. C., Rompa, D., & Coley, B. (1996). Experimental component analysis of a behavioral HIV-AIDS prevention intervention for inner-city women. *Journal of Consulting and Clinical Psychology, 64,* 687–693.

Kalichman, S. C., Williams, E., & Nachimson, D. (1999). Brief behavioral skills building intervention for female controlled methods of STD-HIV prevention: Outcomes of a randomized clinical field trial. *International Journal of STD and AIDS, 10,* 174–181.

Kegeles, S. M., Hays, R. B., & Coates, T. J. (1996). The Mpowerment project: A community-level HIV prevention intervention for young gay men. *American Journal of Public Health, 86,* 1129–1136.

Kelly, J. A., Murphy, D. A., Sikkema, K. J., McAuliffe, T. L., Roffman, R. A., Solomon, L. J., et al. (1997). Randomized, controlled, community-level HIV-prevention intervention for sexual-risk behavior among homosexual men in U.S. cities. *The Lancet, 350,* 1500–1505.

Kelly, J. A., St. Lawrence, J. S., Betts, R., Brasfield, T. L., & Hood, H. V. (1990). A skills-training group intervention model to assist persons in reducing risk behaviors for HIV infection. *AIDS Education and Prevention, 2,* 24–35.

Kelly, J. A., St. Lawrence, J. S., Betts, R., Hood, H. V., & Brasfield, T. L. (1989). Behavioral intention to reduce AIDS risk activities. *Journal of Consulting and Clinical Psychology, 57,* 60–67.

Kelly, J. A., St. Lawrence, J. S., Diaz, Y. E., Stevenson, L. Y., Hauth, A. C., Brasfield, T. L., et al. (1991). HIV risk behavior reduction following intervention with key opinion leaders of population: An experimental analysis. *American Journal of Public Health, 81,* 168–171.

Kelly, J. A., St. Lawrence, J. S., Hood, H. V., & Brasfield, T. L. (1989). Behavioral intervention to reduce AIDS risk activities. *Journal of Consulting and Clinical Psychology, 57,* 60–67.

Kelly, J. A., St. Lawrence, J. S., Stevenson, Y., Hauth, A. C., Kalichman, S. C., Diaz, Y. E., et al. (1992). Community AIDS/HIV risk reduction: The effects of endorsements by popular people in three cities. *American Journal of Public Health, 82,* 1483–1489.

Kipke, M. D., Boyer, C., & Hein, K. (1993). An evaluation of an AIDS risk reduction education and skills training (arrest) program. *Journal of Adolescent Health, 14,* 533–539.

Kirby, D. B., Baumler, E., Coyle, K. K., Basen-Engquist, K., Parcel, G. S., Harrist, R., et al. (2004). The "Safer Choices" intervention: Its impact on the sexual behavior of different subgroups of high school students. *Journal of Adolescent Health, 35,* 442–452.

Kirby, D., Korpi, M., Adivi, C., & Weissman, J. (1997). An impact evaluation of project SNAPP: An AIDS and pregnancy prevention middle school program. *AIDS Education and Prevention, 9,* 44–61.

Levy, S. R., Perhats, C., Weeks, K., Handler, A. S., Zhu, C., & Flay, B. R. (1995). Impact of a school-based AIDS prevention program on risk and protective behavior for newly sexually active students. *Journal of School Health, 65,* 145–151.

Lou, C., Wang, B., Shen, Y., & Gao, E. (2004). Effects of a community-based sex education and reproductive health service program on contraceptive use of unmarried youths in Shanghai. *Journal of Adolescent Health, 34,* 433–440.

Maher, J. E., Peterman, T. A., Osewe, P. L., Odusanya, S., & Scerba, J. R. (2003). Evaluation of a community-based organization's intervention to reduce the incidence of sexually transmitted diseases: A randomized, controlled trial. *Southern Medical Journal, 96,* 248–253.

Malow, R. M., West, J. A., Corrigan, S. A., Pena, J. M., & Cunningham, S. C. (1994). Outcome of psychoeducation for HIV risk reduction. *AIDS Education and Prevention, 6,* 113–125.

Mehrabian, A. (1971). *Silent messages.* Belmont, CA: Wadsworth.

Metzler, C. W., Biglan, A., Noell, J., Ary, D. V., & Ochs, L. (2000). A randomized controlled trial of a behavioral intervention to reduce high-risk sexual behavior among adolescents in STD clinics. *Behavior Therapy, 31,* 27–54.

Miller, R. L., Klotz, D., & Eckholdt, H. M. (1998). HIV prevention with male prostitutes and patrons of hustler bars: Replication of an HIV prevention intervention. *American Journal of Community Psychology, 26,* 97–131.

Morrison-Beedy, D., Carey, M. P., Kowalski, J., & Tu, X. (2005). Group-based HIV risk reduction intervention for adolescent girls: Evidence of feasibility and efficacy. *Research in Nursing & Health, 28,* 3–15.

Noar, S. M., Carlyle, K., & Cole, C. (2006). Why communication is crucial: Meta-analysis of the relationship between safer sexual communication and condom use. *Journal of Health Communication, 11*(4), 365–390.

Noar, S. M., Clark, A., Cole, C., & Lustria, M. (2006). Review of interactive safer sex websites: Practice and potential. *Health Communication, 20,* 233–241.

Noar, S. M., Morokoff, P. J., & Harlow, L. L. (2004). Condom influence strategies in a community sample of ethnically diverse men and women. *Journal of Applied Social Psychology, 34,* 1730–1751.

O'Donnell, L. N., Doval, A., Duran, R., & O'Donnell, C. (1995). Video-based sexually transmitted disease patient education: Its impact on condom acquisition. *American Public Health Association, 85,* 817–822.

Orr, D. P., Langefeld, C. D., Katz, B. P., & Caine, V. A. (1996). Behavioral intervention to increase condom use among high-risk female adolescents. *The Journal of Pediatrics, 128,* 288–295.

Otto-Salaj, L. L., Kelly, J. A., Stevenson, L. Y., Hoffmann, R., & Kalichman, S. C. (2001). Outcomes of a randomized small-group HIV prevention intervention trial for people with serious mental illness. *Community Mental Health Journal, 37,* 123–144.

Patterson, T. L., Shaw, W. S., & Semple, S. J., (2003). Reducing the sexual risk behaviors of HIV+ individuals: Outcome of a randomized controlled trial. *Annals of Behavioral Medicine, 25,* 137–145.

Pedlow, C. T., & Carey, M. P. (2004). Developmentally appropriate sexual risk reduction interventions for adolescents: Rationale, review of interventions, and recommendations for research and practice. *Annals of Behavioral Medicine, 27,* 172–184.

Peragallo, N., DeForge, B., O'Campo, P., Lee, S. M., Kim, Y. J., Cianelli, R., et al. (2005). A randomized clinical trial of an HIV-risk-reduction intervention among low-income Latina women. *Nursing Research, 54,* 108–118.

Peterson, J. L., Coates, T. J., Catania, J., Hauck, W. W., Acree, M., Daigle, D., et al. (1996). Evaluation of an HIV risk reduction intervention among African-American homosexual and bisexual men. *AIDS, 10,* 319–325.

Roberto, A. J., Zimmerman, R. S., Carlyle, K. E., & Abner, E. L. (2007). The effects of a computer-based pregnancy, STD, and HIV prevention program on rural adolescents. *Journal of Health Communication, 12,* 53–76.

Roffman, R. A., Downey, L., Beadnell, B., Gordon, J. R., Craver, J. N., & Stephens, R. S. (1997). Cognitive-behavioral group counseling to prevent HIV transmission in gay and bisexual men: Factors contributing to successful risk reduction. *Research on Social Work Practice, 7,* 165–186.

Roffman, R. A., Stephens, R. S., Curtin, L., Gordon, J. R., Craver, J. N., Stern, M., et al. (1998). Relapse prevention as an interventive model for HIV risk reduction in gay and bisexual men. *AIDS Education and Prevention, 10,* 1–18.

Rogers, E. M. (2003). *Diffusion of innovation* (5th ed.). New York: The Free Press.

Rosser, B. R. S. (1990). Evaluation of the efficacy of AIDS education interventions for homosexually active men. *Health Education Research, 5,* 299–308.

Rosser, B. R. S., Bockting, W. O., Rugg, D. L, Robinson, B. E., Ross, M. W., Bauer, G. R., et al. (2002). A randomized controlled intervention trial of a sexual health approach to long-term HIV risk reduction for men who have sex with men: Effects of the intervention on unsafe sexual behavior. *AIDS Education and Prevention, 14,* 59–71.

Rotheram-Borus, M. J., Gwadz, M., Fernandez, M. I., & Srinivasan, S. (1998). Timing of HIV interventions on reductions in sexual risk among adolescents. *American Journal of Community Psychology, 26,* 73–96.

Rotheram-Borus, M. J., Lee, M. B., Murphy, D. A., Futterman, D., Duan, N., Birnbaum, J. M., et al. (2001). Efficacy of a preventive intervention for youths living with HIV. *American Public Health Association, 91,* 400–405.

Rotheram-Borus, M. J., Swendeman, D., Comulada, W. S., Weiss, R. E., Lee, M., & Lightfoot, M. (2004). Prevention for substance-using HIV-positive young people. *Acquired Immune Deficiency Syndromes, 37*(Suppl. 2), S68–S77.

St. Lawrence, J. S., Brasfield, T. L., Jefferson, K. W., Alleyne, E., O'Bannon, R. E., & Shirley, A. (1995). Cognitive-behavioral intervention to reduce African American adolescents' risk for HIV infection. *Journal of Consulting and Clinical Psychology, 63,* 221–237.

St. Lawrence, J. S., Crosby, R. A., Belcher, L., Yazdini, N., & Brasfield, T. L. (1999). Sexual risk reduction and anger management interventions for incarcerated male adolescents: A randomized controlled trial of two interventions. *Journal of Sex Education and Therapy, 24,* 9–17.

St. Lawrence, J. S., Crosby, R. A., Brasfield, T. L., & O'Bannon, R. E., III. (2002). Reducing STD and HIV risk behavior of substance-dependent adolescents: A randomized trial. *Journal of Consulting and Clinical Psychology, 70,* 1010–1021.

St. Lawrence, J. S., Jefferson, K. W., Banks, P. G., Cline, T. R., Alleyne, E., & Brasfield, T. L. (1994). Cognitive-behavioral group intervention to assist substance-development adolescents in lowering HIV infection risk. *AIDS Education and Prevention, 6,* 424–435.

Sampaio, M., Brites, C., Stall, R., Hudes, E. S., & Hearst, N. (2002). Reducing AIDS risk among men who have sex with men in Salvador, Brazil. *AIDS and Behavior, 6,* 173–181.

Segrin, C., & Givertz, M. (2003). Methods of social skills training and development. In J. O. Greene & B. R. Burleson (Eds.), *Handbook of communication and social interaction skills* (pp. 135–176.). Mahwah, NJ: Lawrence Erlbaum Associates.

Shain, R. N., Piper, J. M., Newton, E. R., Perdue, S. T., Ramos, R., Champion, J. D., et al. (1999). A randomized, controlled trial of a behavioral intervention to prevent sexually transmitted disease among minority women. *New England Journal of Medicine, 340,* 93–100.

Shrier, L. A., Ancheta, R., Goodman, E., Chiou, V. M., Lyden, M. R., & Emans, S. J. (2001). Randomized controlled trial of a safer sex intervention for high-risk adolescent girls. *Archives of Pediatric Adolescent Medicine, 155,* 73–79.

Solomon, M. Z., & DeJong, W. (1989). Preventing AIDS and other STDs through condom promotion: A patient education intervention. *American Journal of Public Health, 79,* 453–458.

Stall, R. D., Paul, J. P., Barrett, D. C., Crosby, G. M., & Bein, E. (1999) An outcome evaluation to measure changes in sexual risk-taking among gay men undergoing substance use disorder treatment. *Journal of Studies on Alcohol, 60,* 837–845.

Stanton, B. F., Li, X., Kahihuata, J., Fitzgerald, A. M., Neumbo, S., Kanduuombe, G., et al. (1998). Increased protected sex and abstinence among Namibian youth following a HIV risk-reduction intervention: A randomized, longitudinal study. *AIDS, 12,* 2473–2480.

Stanton, B. F., Li, X., Ricardo, I., Galbraith, J., Feigelman, S., & Kaljee, L. (1996). A randomized, controlled effectiveness trial of an AIDS prevention program for low-income African-American youths. *Archives of Pediatric Adolescent Medicine, 150,* 363–372.

Thomas, R., Cahill, J., & Santilli, L. ( 1997). Using an interactive computer game to increase skill and self-efficacy regarding safer sex negotiation: Field test results. *Health Education & Behavior, 24,* 71–86.

Toro-Alfonso, J., Varas-Díaz, N., & Andújar-Bello, I. (2002). Evaluation of an HIV/AIDS prevention intervention targeting Latino gay men and men who have sex with men in Puerto Rico. *AIDS Education and Prevention, 14,* 445–546.

Tudiver, F., Myers, T., Kurtz, R. G., Orr, K., Rowe, C., & Jackson, E. (1992). The Talking Sex Project: Results of a randomized controlled trial of small-group AIDS education for 612 gay and bisexual men. *Evaluation & the Health Professions, 15,* 26–42.

Tulloch, H. E., McCaul, K. D., Miltenberger, R. G., & Smyth, J. M. (2004). Partner communication skills and condom use among college couples. *Journal of American College Health, 52,* 263–267.

Walter, H. J., & Vaughan, R.D. (1993). AIDS risk reduction among a multiethnic sample of urban high school students. *Journal of the American Medical Association, 270*, 725–730.

Weeks, K., Levy, S. R., Gordon, A. K., Handler, A., Perhats, C., & Flay, B. R. (1997). Does parental involvement make a difference? The impact of parental interactive activities on students in a school-based AIDS prevention program. *AIDS Education and Prevention, 9*, 90–106.

Weeks, K., Levy, S. R., Zhu, C., Perhats, C., Handler, A., & Flay, B. R. (1995). Impact of a school-based AIDS prevention program on young adolescents' self-efficacy skills. *Health Education Research Theory and Practice, 10*, 329–344.

Workman, G. M., Robinson, W. L., Cotler, S., & Harper, G. W. (1996). A school-based approach to HIV prevention for inner-city African-American and Hispanic adolescent females. *Journal of Prevention & Intervention in the Community, 14*, 41–60.

Zimmerman, M. A., Ramirez-Valles, J., Suarez, E., de la Rosa, G., & Castro, M. A. (1997). An HIV/AIDS prevention project for Mexican homosexual men: An empowerment approach. *Health Education and Behavior, 2*, 177–190.

# 3

# The Social and Personal Dynamics of HIV Stigma

*Lance S. Rintamaki*
State University of New York at Buffalo

*Frances M. Weaver*
Department of Veteran Affairs

Advances in antiretroviral treatments have dramatically increased the life span of those infected with HIV to such a degree that HIV, which was once seen as a terminal illness, is now treated by health professionals as a chronic, but manageable, condition (e.g., Burgoyne, Rourke, Behrens, & Salit, 2004; Hogg et al., 1998). As a result, added emphasis is now being placed on managing quality-of-life factors beyond the physiological concerns of those infected with the virus. One issue of considerable importance to quality of life for people living with HIV is the social stigma that accompanies infection. Studies show that large portions of the U.S. public misunderstand HIV and its routes of transmission, express fear and disgust toward those infected with the virus, and support public policies that would deprive people living with HIV of their civil rights (e.g., Herek & Capitanio, 1999; Herek, Capitanio, & Widmann, 2002). Many people living with HIV are greatly concerned about the impact such stigma may have in their lives, report being stigmatized and, as a result, experience stress, anxiety, and a general disruption in their positive social interactions with others (D'Augelli, 1989; Derlega, Lovejoy, & Winstead, 1998). Subsequently, stigma has been labeled as the most important social and psychological issue of the HIV experience (Chung & McGraw, 1992; Crandall & Coleman, 1992; Moneyham et al., 1996).

Researchers in many fields have taken up the task of studying HIV stigma (e.g., Bennett, 1990; Chung & Magraw, 1992; Crandall & Coleman, 1992; King, 1989; McCain & Grambling, 1992; Siegel & Krauss, 1991; Weitz, 1989, 1993). They have defined HIV stigma (e.g., Herek & Glunt, 1988), identified its sources (e.g., Alonzo & Reynolds, 1995), and provided evidence of how it affects the social, psychological, and physical experiences of those living with HIV (e.g., Blendon & Donelan, 1988; Burris, 1999). Despite the value of this foundational work, far more research is required to better understand the broad range of HIV stigma's psychosocial dynamics. In particular, research that explores the intersection of communication and psychosocial outcomes would greatly elucidate how HIV stigma functions in the lives of people infected with the virus. As such, the purpose of this chapter is to synthesize the extant literature on HIV stigma to provide a review of the sources, forms, and prevalence of HIV stigma within the United States, as well as the documented effects stigma has on people living with HIV, culminating in the presentation of unfulfilled areas of social interaction research still needed to address the challenging and pervasive epidemic of HIV stigma.


## Definitions of HIV Stigma

Herek and Glunt (1988) coined one of the first and most widely cited definitions of HIV stigma, describing it as "stigma directed at persons perceived to be infected with HIV, regardless of whether they are actually infected or whether they manifest symptoms of AIDS or AIDS-related complex" (p. 886). This early definition guided much of the subsequent research on HIV stigma and includes three important elements: (a) Anyone perceived to be HIV positive (and not just those who are infected) may become a target of stigmatizing behavior from others; (b) infection with HIV provokes stigmatization from others, regardless of the stage of infection or if the immune system has been compromised to the point of AIDS classification; and (c) an in-group versus out-group paradigm exists in which people with HIV are relegated to a disenfranchised social out-group (Devine, Plant, & Harrison, 1999).

Although these three elements are important to understanding the phenomenon of HIV stigma, Herek and Glunt's (1998) early definition did not describe how HIV stigma is enacted or performed.

This definition also neglected how society stigmatizes not only those who are infected with HIV, but also the social groups disproportionately affected by the virus. Herek and his colleagues (Herek, 1990; Herek & Capatanio, 1999), along with researchers such as Alonzo and Reynolds (1995) and Pryor, Reeder, and Landau (1999), identified these limitations and moved toward a more inclusive description of the phenomenon. Subsequently, the operational definition of HIV stigma has evolved to account for these omissions, which now includes "prejudice, discounting, discrediting, and discrimination directed at people perceived to have AIDS or HIV, and the individuals, groups, and communities with which they are associated" (Herek, 1999, p. 1107).

## Sources of HIV Stigma

All illness is stigmatized to varying degrees and those who are ill (or perceived to be ill) may confront bias and diminished acceptance from those around them (Vash, 1981). Illness itself has been defined as a form of deviancy and, from a structural-functionalist perspective, those who become ill are seen to disrupt social order (Parsons, 1951). Therefore, it is not surprising that a disease as threatening and complex as HIV would provoke considerable stigmatization, placing a significant social burden on those already facing the debilitating physical effects of HIV infection (Frierson, Lippmann, & Johnson, 1987). Building on the dimensions of stigma delineated by Goffman (1963), Katz (1981), and Jones et al. (1984), Alonzo and Reynolds (1995) developed a framework for understanding the primary sources of HIV stigma, which include (a) association with deviant groups, (b) responsibility for infection, (c) religion and morality, (d) (mis)perceptions regarding contagion, and (e) association with death. Each source by itself would cause an illness to be stigmatized, but when taken together their gestalt explains the depth and intensity with which HIV stigma pervades the general social climate.

### Association with Deviant Groups

Since the outbreak of HIV in the United States in the early 1980s, the virus has been associated with disenfranchised social groups, including gay men, intravenous drug users and, to some extent, African and Latino Americans (Herek & Capitanio, 1997, 1999; Herek & Glunt, 1988; Price & Hsu, 1992; Pryor, Reeder, Vinacco, & Kott, 1989). Sexual activity (particularly between same-sex male partners) and intravenous drug use are viewed as deviant behaviors by much of the general public and also are the most frequent routes of HIV transmission in the United States. In particular, a strong relationship exists between the stigmatization of gay people and the stigmatization of HIV. Work by Pryor and colleagues (Pryor et al., 1989; Pryor, Reeder, & McManus, 1991) has demonstrated how people's reactions to those living with HIV are influenced by their attitudes toward gay people. Those with high levels of homophobia are less willing to interact with those who have HIV, regardless of how a person with HIV actually acquired the virus (see also Le Poire, 1994; Le Poire, Ota, & Hajek, 1997).

Derogation of people living with HIV and the perception that the disease is unique to "deviant groups" may serve as a psychological coping strategy for dealing with the threat of HIV. Pittam and Gallois (1997, 2000) have suggested that placing the blame on social groups to which one does not belong may free people from the anxiety that they also may be at risk of infection. Although this may serve to mitigate anxiety over the threat of HIV, it can ultimately prove self-defeating and decrease the likelihood of using protective strategies when engaged in behaviors that place someone at risk for HIV infection.

### Responsibility for Infection

Individuals are more likely to be greeted with contempt and anger, rather than empathy or concern, when they contract an illness through their own actions, particularly if these involve non-normative behaviors (Weiner, 1993). Because the primary transmission routes for HIV involve behaviors believed to be performed of one's own free will, infected individuals are often blamed for contracting the virus (e.g., Cobb & DeChambert, 2002; Dodds, 2002; Frierson et al., 1987; Herek & Capitanio, 1999; Pittam & Gallois, 1997). Consistent with this, people who acquire HIV through routes that are outside their control (e.g., through blood transfusions or postnatally from HIV-positive mothers) are shown to evoke less stigma from the general public (e.g., Dowell, Lo Presto, & Sherman, 1991; Herek, 1990; Lewis & Range, 1992). People who acquire the virus through such routes may even be labeled as "innocent victims" of the disease (e.g., Rehm & Franck, 2000; Weiner, 1993; Wiener, Battles, & Heilman, 2000).

Herek et al. (2002) examined the extent to which the general public in the 1990s placed blame on those who contracted HIV, during which blame peaked in the last half of that decade. In 1997, one half of the respondents believed people with HIV were responsible for having contracted the virus, whereas one in four believed that those with HIV "got what they deserved." Unfortunately, these numbers waned only slightly by the end of the 20th century.

## Religion and Morality

HIV stigma also derives from the moral denouncement of behaviors that serve as major transmission routes for the virus. This denouncement stems from a normative morality that is partly accounted for by the doctrine and influence of religious institutions. Various churches have been found to perpetuate HIV stigma and condemn those living with the virus (Kennamer, Honnold, Bradford, & Hendricks, 2000; Swain, 1999). In areas where religious institutions have a pervasive influence, such as rural communities, greater stigmatization of HIV is reported (Heckman, Somlai, Kalichman, Franzoi, & Kelly, 1998). Presumably due to religious influences, some people even view HIV as a divine punishment for sin (Weitz, 1993).

## Contagion

Although any illness may be stigmatized, communicable diseases such as HIV evoke the strongest reactions from the general public (Pryor et al., 1989; Scheper-Hughes & Lock, 1991). Several studies have demonstrated that stigmatizing attitudes are tied closely to misperceptions about how HIV is transmitted (e.g., Herek & Capitanio, 1997, 1999; Price & Hsu, 1992). Perceptions of danger and fears of contagion have surrounded HIV since the beginning of the epidemic (Herek, 1990) and are evident in Americans' continuing overestimation of the risks posed by casual contact with those who are HIV-positive (Herek & Capitanio, 1999; Herek et al., 2002). This fear of contagion, also referred to as the instrumental function of HIV stigma (Pryor et al., 1989), is central to many of the negative social interactions experienced by people living with HIV (e.g., Bennett, 1998; Botnick, 2000; Gerbert, Maguire, Bleecker, Coates, & McPhee, 1991).

Despite considerable efforts to educate the public, misunderstandings about HIV and how the virus is transmitted are prevalent. Herek and colleagues (Capitanio & Herek, 1999; Herek, 1999; Herek & Capitanio, 1993, 1994, 1997, 1999; Herek & Glunt, 1988; Herek et al., 1998, 2002) reported that, across the 1990s, the general public often correctly identified prominent HIV transmission routes (specifically, through sexual activity and exposure to blood products); however, illogical and wholly incorrect beliefs were also common, such as the perception that the virus could be transmitted by coming in contact with objects previously touched by people living with HIV (see also Rozin, Markwith, & Nemeroff, 1992). These misperceptions peaked late in the decade, despite public educators' significant efforts to address these issues. Concerns over such things as sharing a glass or being sneezed on by someone with HIV were common, with as many as half of the respondents believing these to be dangerous events (see also Herek & Capitanio, 1997). Fear over possible infection from the use of public toilets also increased over the decade, ending with as many as two out of every five people believing this to be a possible route of HIV transmission. Even socially benevolent actions such as donating blood were viewed with suspicion, with roughly one in three Americans believing the act of blood donation puts people at risk for contracting HIV. These misperceptions wrongly depict the communicability of HIV and unfairly paint those with the disease as a virulent threat to the general public.

### Association with Death

Despite the advances in combination drug therapies that have considerably extended the lives of those infected, HIV is still seen by many in the general public as a terminal disease. Being diagnosed with a life-threatening or terminal illness is regarded by many as the equivalent to dying, which may serve as an unwelcome reminder to people of their own mortality (e.g., Peters-Golden, 1982). Those who fear death and experience a sense of hopelessness in the face of fatal diseases have been shown to shun and avoid the terminally ill (e.g., Lerner & Miller, 1978; Peters-Golden, 1982). In addition, HIV infection has degenerative effects on the body, leading to outward signs of advanced immune system dysfunction, such as sarcomas and wasting syndromes (e.g., Tang, Jacobson, Spiegelman, Knox, & Wanke, 2005). Such outward symptoms often become readily apparent to observers, who may perceive them as repulsive and upsetting, further contributing to HIV's association with a frightening and repugnant form of death.

## Expressions and Effects of HIV Stigma

To better understand the stigmatized illness experience, it is important to consider both how stigma is expressed and the impact stigmatizing encounters have on stigmatized people (Taylor, 1995). The expression of stigma can be conceptualized as occurring at both macro- and microsocial levels. At the macrosocial level, the expression of HIV stigma takes the form of social policy or laws that impose on the rights of people living with HIV. At the microsocial level, the expression of HIV stigma occurs during interpersonal exchange and includes acts of rejection, isolation, and overt harassment. The relationship between these two levels may be cyclical, such that sweeping social policies influence how people treat and interact with those who have HIV, whereas the presence of pervasive discrimination at the interpersonal level may lead to the introduction and support of social polices that impair the lives of people infected with the virus. Consequently, the expression of HIV stigma at each level is discussed, followed by a review of how stigma may affect the physical, mental, and social well-being of people living with HIV.

At the macrosocial level in the United States, HIV stigma has led members of the general public to advocate for laws that would deprive people with HIV of their civil rights (e.g., Blendon & Donelan, 1988; Burris, 1999; Gostin & Webber, 1997, 1998). A variety of studies have demonstrated that throughout the 1990s a majority of the general public provided some level of support for punitive and invasive policies directed against people living with HIV (e.g., Capitanio & Herek, 1999; Herek, 1999; Herek & Capitanio, 1993, 1994, 1997, 1999; Herek & Glunt, 1988; Herek et al., 1998, 2002).

Although some legislation has been passed to protect the civil liberties of those infected with HIV (e.g., Burris, 1999; Gostin & Webber, 1998), in 1999 as many as one in five adults supported legislation that would enable the public identification or even the quarantine of people living with the virus (Herek et al., 2002). Furthermore, protective legislation is sometimes bypassed or even subverted, including by agents of the federal government. For instance, in 1996 legislation was passed that discharged enlisted military personnel found to be HIV-positive, but allowed personnel with comparable medical conditions to continue their service (Shenon, 1996).

At the microsocial level, people often express HIV stigma through their interpersonal behavior. People living with the virus report encountering a variety of problematic events when communicating with others, including social ostracism, personal rejection, or discrimination directed at them because of their HIV status (e.g., Bennett, 1990; Gostin, 1990; Herek & Capitanio, 1993, 1994, 1997; Herek & Glunt, 1991; Price & Hsu, 1992). These include such behaviors as people refusing to touch or shake hands with them, staring at them, and even openly ridiculing or mocking them for having HIV (e.g., Bennett, 1990; Moneyham et al., 1996). Like many potentially terminal diseases, the plague metaphors surrounding HIV and the fear they incite can lead to the dissolution of former social ties as people distance themselves from those who are infected with HIV (Cherry & Smith, 1993; Sontag, 1988), including friends and family (Bor, Miller, & Goldman, 1993; Demi, Bakeman, Moneyham, & Sowell, 1997; McDonell, Abell, & Miller, 1991). In addition, people living with HIV also report encountering subtle nonverbal behaviors from others, such as people using minimal eye contact or talking from afar to a person living with HIV, behaviors that alone may be explained away, but taken together lead people to feel stigmatized (Chapman, 2002). Stigmatizing behaviors can come from both strangers and family alike, as well as from employers and coworkers, on whom people with HIV are dependent for their livelihood (Fesko, 1998; Ortloff, 1996). In its extreme form, hostile expression of stigma has even driven people from their homes and led to acts of physical violence against them (Gielen, O'Campo, Faden, & Eke, 1997; Gostin, 1990; Hunter & Rubenstien, 1992; Zierler et al., 2000). Recent research demonstrates how such violence is an issue for both heterosexual and homosexual men (Zierler et al., 2000), but may be of particular significance for women, who too often report being beaten by their partners upon the disclosure of their HIV-positive status (e.g., Craft & Serovich, 2005; Gielen et al., 1997; Liebschutz, Geier, Horton, Chuang, & Samet, 2005).

## HIV Stigma and Health Care Provision

One of the most troubling outcomes of HIV stigma involves its effects among the medical providers on whom people living with HIV must depend. Although health care personnel have played a vital role in managing the HIV pandemic, some have also been found to openly report aversion and prejudice toward patients with HIV (McCann, 1997, 1999; Norton, Schwartzbaum, & Wheat, 1990) and even refuse to provide treatment for HIV-positive patients (Crawford, Humfleet, Ribordy, Ho, & Vickers, 1991; Kass, Faden, Fox, & Dudley, 1992; Levin, Krantz, Driscol, & Fleishman, 1995; Quam, 1990). Such prejudicial attitudes have been identified among a range of health care personnel, including practicing physicians, nurses, psychologists, and medical students (Breault & Polifroni, 1992; Dworkin, Albrecht, & Cooksey, 1991; Knox, Dow, & Cotton, 1989). Although such negative attitudes are shown to decrease as health care providers gain experience, they are sometimes prevalent even among those who spend considerable time with HIV-positive patients (Ficarrotto, Grade, & Zegans, 1991; Orlander, Samet, Kazis, Freedberg, & Libman, 1994).

These stigmatizing attitudes among health care personnel may be due, in part, to moral judgments regarding homosexuality or injection drug use (Breault & Polifroni, 1992; Cole & Slocumb, 1993; Peate, 1995). For instance, homophobia repeatedly has been shown to affect the attitudes of, and care provided by, various medical professionals (Crawford et al., 1991; Kopacz, Grossman, & Klamen, 1999). Consequently, stigma derived from (or compounded by) homophobia places patients with HIV at greater risk of being misunderstood and poorly received by the medical professionals on whom they depend (Peate, 1995; Rose, 1994).

Though most HIV stigma research in health care contexts tends to focus on the antecedents of stigma (e.g., attitudes toward people living with HIV) rather than how it is communicated (e.g., Parker & Aggleton, 2003), some research has identified the ways in which stigma shapes medical professionals' interactions with HIV-positive patients. Research by Chapman (2002), as well as Rintamaki and colleagues (Rintamaki, Scott, Kosenko, Jensen, & Jordon, 2005), has examined patients' reported perceptions of and experiences with HIV stigma in health care contexts. This work demonstrates that HIV-positive patients are mindful of health care personnel's behaviors and sensitive to anything that may indicate bias or stigmatization. Participants in these studies reported encountering what they perceived to be a variety of stigmatizing behaviors expressed by a wide range of health care personnel. Problematic behaviors included such things as awkward or nervous nonverbal behaviors, use of excessive safety precautions, avoidance, refusal to provide care, and anger at having to provide care for HIV-positive patients. In addition, participants also described events in which health care personnel openly mocked or blamed patients for their HIV status, unfairly labeled them or maligned them to other health care personnel, and even physically abused HIV-positive patients. These behaviors were observed in ambulances, doctor's offices, dental care facilities, in-patient hospital rooms, and the common areas of hospitals, such as hallways and reception desks.

In the general patient population, sensing subtle signals of dislike from care providers has been found to affect patients' perceptions of the quality of care they receive (e.g., Topacoglu et al., 2004), as well as their trust in and likelihood of returning to suspect care providers (e.g., Fiscella et al., 2004; Rowland, Coe, Burchard, & Pricolo, 2005). Participants in these studies reported experiencing far more than health care personnel's subtle signals of negative affect, however, with examples of overt hostility being as extreme as physical pummeling of patients by health care personnel. Although violence directed toward people living with HIV has been reported in earlier HIV research, it has been discussed primarily in the context of romantic relationships (e.g., Craft & Serovich, 2005; Liebschutz et al., 2005). These findings reveal a frightening dilemma, in which seeking health care may, in fact, put HIV-positive patients' health and safety at risk.

## Negative Health Effects

Stigma has been linked to negative health outcomes among people living with HIV. The social isolation that many stigmatized people experience may inhibit their ability to adjust and consequently diminish their overall well-being (Baumeister & Leary, 1995). HIV stigma can induce shame, stress, and depression (e.g., Lawless, Kippax, & Crawford, 1996; Moneyham et al., 1996), which, in turn, can have detrimental effects on mental and physical health, such as a greater likelihood of death (e.g., Clark & Bessinger, 1997; Kilbourne et al., 2002), including through suicide (e.g., Demi et al., 1997; Heckman et al., 2002).

Stress.   Most people have powerful needs to belong and affiliate with others, which unless fulfilled through positive, ongoing relationships, diminish a person's overall well-being (Baumeister & Leary, 1995). After diagnosis, however, people living with HIV often experience a loss of their former social networks. Rejection from one's social ties can lead to considerable negative affect and has been identified as one of the major stressors of the HIV experience (Bennett, 1990; Chung & Magraw, 1992; Crandall & Coleman, 1992; Demas, Schoenbaum, Wills, Doll, & Klein, 1995; McCain & Grambling, 1992; Moneyham et al., 1996; Siegel & Krauss, 1991; Sowell et al., 1997; Weitz, 1989). Alienation from former in-groups can be acutely felt by people living with HIV, as the desire to affiliate is accentuated for people dealing with negative experiences (Miller & Zimbardo, 1966; Schacter, 1959). From this, people living with HIV often report feeling rejected, alienated, isolated, and excluded (Bennett, 1990; Cherry & Smith, 1993; Sontag, 1988; Wolcott, Namir, Fawzy, Gottlieb, & Mitsuyasu, 1986). A frequent consequence of this alienation has been described as a staggering sense of loneliness (Cherry & Smith, 1993), which is not only distressing, but can lead to negative health effects, such as alcoholism or suicide among people living with HIV (e.g., Rundell, Kyle, Brown, & Thomason, 1992). Social isolation also can lead to poorer psychological health, inability to perform social functions (such as going to work), and even an increased risk of death (Bennett, 1990; Leslie, Stein, & Rotheram-Borus, 2002; Lichtenstein, Laska, & Clair, 2002).

Shame and Self-Esteem.   People with HIV may experience guilt, shame, and self-rejection as a result of losing friends and family or through internalizing the larger society's disparaging views of them (e.g., Bennett, 1990; Lawless et al., 1996; Lewis, 1998; Link & Phelan, 2001). This self-stigmatization is synonymous with shame and includes a person's acceptance of others' derogation of oneself or one's social group (Lewis, 1998). Although lowered self-esteem clearly has implications for overall quality of life, it also may undermine self-protection and HIV prevention efforts. For example, people with low self-esteem may inconsistently practice safer sex, court numerous sexual partners, and abuse alcohol and illegal drugs (Stokes & Peterson, 1998).

Depression.    Depression is another common psychological disorder with which people who have HIV must contend (Katz, 1996). Research suggests that the frequency of depression among people living with HIV varies, with estimates ranging from 40% to 60% (Belkin, Fleishman, Stein, Piette, & Mor, 1992; Lyketsos, Hanson, Fishman, McHugh, & Treisman, 1994). Although several factors may account for such depression, social stigma is one of the most prominent (Michels & Marzuk, 1993). Crandall and Coleman (1992) reported that depression is correlated with perceived stigma, such that people who deal with greater amounts of negative social interaction are also at greater psychological risk. The withdrawal of people's support networks, which often results from HIV stigma, compounds the problem of depression (Littlefield, Rodin, Murray, & Craven, 1990).

Depression brought on by HIV stigma can also lead to other serious problems. Depression has been found to increase patients' sense of hopelessness, demoralization, and impulsiveness (e.g., Angelino & Treisman, 2001; Suominen, Isometsa, Henriksson, Ostamo, & Lonnqvist, 1997). People with HIV who experience depression are more likely to engage in substance abuse (e.g., Crum, Brown, Liang, & Eaton, 2001; Greenfield, Rehm, & Rogers, 2002; Lehmann, Hubbard, & Martin, 2001) and risky behaviors (Joe, Knezek, Watson, & Simpson, 1991; Kelly et al., 1993; Nemoto, Foster, & Brown, 1991; Nyamathi, Bennett, & Leake, 1995), which may account, in part, for why depressed patients are also less likely to adhere to their treatment regimens (e.g., Singh et al., 1996). Failure to effectively manage their illness, in turn, may explain why depressed patients often experience more rapid disease progression and death than their affectively healthy peers (Burack et al., 1993; Ickovics et al., 2001).

Suicide.    Rates of suicidal thoughts, attempts at suicide, and successful suicide are exceedingly high among people living with HIV (e.g., Belkin et al., 1992; Cote, Biggar, & Dannenberg, 1992; Mancoske, Wadsworth, Dugas, & Hansey, 1995) and are higher than rates reported among the general public or even among people with comparably serious illnesses (e.g., Marzuk et al., 1997; Rundell et al., 1992). Some evidence suggests that the shock of diagnosis alone may be enough to compel some people to take their own lives (O'Dowd, Biderman, & McKegney, 1993; Rundell et al., 1992); however, other research demonstrates how social stigma and social isolation may well be the most important variables in the decision to commit suicide among people with HIV (e.g., Goldin, 1994; Marzuk et al., 1988). A lack of meaning in one's life can result from social isolation and diminished support (Wadland & Gleeson, 1991) and correlates with higher rates of suicide (Kinkel, Bailey, & Josef, 1989; Kinnier, Metha, Keim, & Okey, 1994). In short, through the elimination of social ties, stigma reduces the sources of meaning on which people with HIV depend to make sense of their lives, subsequently influencing suicidal behavior (Starace & Sherr, 1998).

## Managing HIV Stigma

Compared to the amount of research on the prevalence of stigmatizing attitudes or the forms of HIV stigma expressed during interaction, relatively little research has explored the ways in which people living with HIV manage the social stigma surrounding the virus. In general, however, stigmatized people know that others may judge them in light of their condition (Frable, Blackstone, & Scherbaum, 1990; Goffman, 1963). Concern over subsequent negative evaluations may affect how the bearers of visible stigmas feel about themselves and how they interact socially (e.g., Steele & Aronson, 1995). What's more, people prefer to feel good about themselves and work to avoid negative affect and self-evaluations (Abrams & Hogg, 1988). Consequently, they are likely to respond to the potential for stigma and stigmatizing encounters in ways that would protect their self-esteem (Scambler & Hopkins, 1990). Indeed, people belonging to stigmatized social groups are not powerless or complacent about their situation, but rather "they are strategists, expert managers, and negotiators who play active (although not always successful) roles" in managing social interaction (Herman, 1993, p. 324). It is reasonable, then, to assume that people living with HIV intentionally interact with others in ways that mitigate the impact of both the potential and performance of stigma. What little can be distilled from the HIV literature on stigma coping strategies pertains to (a) strategic concealment and disclosure of one's HIV status and (b) collective activism.

## Concealment and Disclosure

The difficulties and uncertainties of revealing personal information by a stigmatized individual are part of a complex process of concealment and disclosure (Dindia, 1998). If the stigmatizing attribute is visible to others, then concealment is no longer an option; however, if the stigmatizing condition is not readily apparent to others, then the individual may "pass" undetected within society (Dindia, 1998). Many people living with HIV, particularly if they are asymptomatic, attempt to pass as HIV-negative (Alonzo & Reynolds, 1995; Chesney & Smith, 1999); however, to access treatment, receive social support, or explain specific behaviors (e.g., going on disability or taking medications), they may need to disclose their HIV status to others. Deciding how and to whom one will disclose their HIV status includes serious dilemmas and can be both a challenging and prolonged process (e.g., Armistead, Tannenbaum, Forehand, Morse, & Morse, 2001; Greene & Serovich, 1996). Derlega and colleagues revealed people's awareness that they may face ignorance, social rejection, and even physical harm upon disclosure of their HIV status (e.g., Derlega et al., 1998; Derlega, Winstead, & Folk-Barron, 2000; Gielen et al., 1997; Squire, 1999; Zeirler et al., 2000). Subsequently, people who suspect others might stigmatize them can be reluctant to disclose their HIV-positive status, even to members of their own family (Derlega et al., 1998, 2000; Leary & Schreindorfer, 1998). People have even been shown to conceal their HIV status at the cost of foregoing medical treatment and other social services (Pizzi, 1992; Rintamaki, Hogan, & Weaver, 2005; Rintamaki, Davis, Skripkauskas, Bennet, & Wolf, 2006).

In addition to the immediate consequences of disclosing one's status, people living with HIV know that once their HIV status is revealed, control over that information is lost (Petronio, 2000; Simoni et al., 1995). In essence, every new person who learns of one's HIV status could potentially tell an unlimited number of other people, not all of whom may be accepting and supportive of the person with HIV. Thus, despite the relief or catharsis that disclosure can sometimes bring people with HIV (Derlega et al., 1998; Holt et al., 1998), concern over other people potentially misusing or spreading this information prevents many people from disclosing their HIV status (e.g., Derlega et al., 1998; Moneyham et al., 1996).

Although concealment may circumvent stigmatizing responses in some cases, people also may choose to actively disclose their status in an attempt to reduce stigma through the education of others (e.g., Paxton, 2002; Squire, 1999). In the previously cited study by Derlega and colleagues (Derlega et al., 1998), for instance, people with HIV reported engaging with others for the purpose of educating them about the disease and arguing against the stigmatization of HIV. Such disclosures also may prove self-affirming and serve to counteract stigma through asserting one's legitimacy as a member of the larger social system (Dindia, 1998; Holt et al., 1998; Kaufman, 1996).

## Collective Activism

Joining a collective for the purpose of political activism might also serve as a means to address HIV stigma. One of the most well-known HIV activist organizations is the AIDS Coalition to Unleash Power (ACT UP), which was formed to address the slow response of the federal government and pharmaceutical companies in addressing the HIV crisis (Gamson, 1989). ACT UP and similar organizations work to affect social policy, educate the public, advocate for drug and immunology research for HIV, and challenge social stigma (Epstein, 1995, 1996; Herman, 1993). Such collectives provide a less threatening environment in which people with HIV can interact with peers and learn strategies for coping with the physical and social consequences of HIV (Brashers, Neidig, & Goldsmith, 2004). This is achieved, in part, through training members in skills required for advocacy work, including protest and civil disobedience (Brashers, Haas, Neidig, & Rintamaki, 2002). Additionally, social interaction with peers in these organizations may bolster participants' sense of identity as one of many people living with HIV (Roth & Nelson, 1997). As a result of participation in these organizations, people may develop new coping styles for dealing with HIV stressors, such as social stigma. Brashers et al. (2002) found that people in AIDS activist organizations were more likely than those not in these organizations to use active, problem-focused coping strategies to address HIV stressors. These findings suggest that people join activist organizations in order to immerse themselves in affirming, peer-affiliated environments and to affect social change. At the interpersonal level, this suggests that members of such organizations will address HIV stigma directly, in active, possibly even contentious, ways (also see Brashers, Haas, Klingle, & Neidig, 2000).

## Future Directions

Considerable research has explored the sources and prevalence of HIV stigma. This work has shed light on the significance of the phenomenon and the effects it can have on those living with HIV. Yet, far more work remains in order to fully understand the many dynamics of HIV stigma and how to help those living with the virus when coping with the many stressors stigma entails. These include issues for which communication scholars and those who study social interaction are uniquely qualified to address. Specifically, such research involves a more nuanced exploration of how people interact with those who have HIV, coupled with how people living with HIV interact with others.

Regardless if stigmatizing behaviors are subtle or explicit, they are likely to be particularly salient for people with HIV (Bennett, 1990; Crandall & Coleman, 1992; King, 1989; Limandri, 1989). Research on people belonging to stigmatized groups (e.g., Frable et al., 1990), including people living with HIV (e.g., Chapman, 2002), suggests that belonging to a stigmatized group leads people to develop a keen awareness of any behaviors in others that may signal bias or discrimination. This heightened sensitivity has implications for how people interpret others' behaviors, particularly those that are quirky or ambiguous. Work by Crocker, Major, and colleagues (Crocker & Major, 1989; Crocker, Voelkl, Testa, & Major, 1991; Major & Crocker, 1993) suggests that people belonging to stigmatized groups struggle to decipher the meaning and motives behind other people's behavior, often wondering if other people's actions are in some way tied to social stigma.

Previous research has often focused on the more sensational expressions of HIV stigma, such as overt discrimination, physical violence, or people being fired from their jobs. Although important, these events are not necessarily the most frequent stigmatizing experiences encountered by people living with HIV. On a day-to-day basis, more subtle and ambiguous events (such as people using little eye contact or standing at a distance when speaking with someone who has HIV) may be common occurrences, yet have equally serious consequences for such things as relational and emotional well-being. Consider, for instance, if a patient meets with a nurse for the first time and this nurse uses clipped tones or seems a bit brusque, the patient may be prone to wonder if this behavior is caused by the nurse feeling uncomfortable or angry at having to work with an HIV-positive client. In the process, the patient may overlook or fail to consider other explanations for this behavior, such as these actions being the nurse's individual communication style or the nurse having a headache at the time of the encounter. Even if the patient does consider alternative explanations, lingering doubt may lead him or her to focus on stigma as the likely motivator behind the nurse's actions. We know very little about how these attribution processes play out for people living with HIV. Research has yet to determine if sensitivity or attribution processes change over time or in certain contexts, such as when interacting with new acquaintances. Also, research has yet to identify particular cues or comments that may trigger this attribution process or raise alarms that social stigma may be present. Additional research is needed to assess these more subtle phenomena, including their forms, frequencies, and the effects they may have on people living with HIV.

Similarly, more work can be done to examine the forms and effects of HIV stigma when performed in specific contexts or by specific groups of people. For instance, the recent work to identify problematic behaviors among health care providers demonstrates that people living with HIV are highly sensitive to potentially stigmatizing signals, particularly when interacting with those on whom they must depend or who have power over them (Chapman, 2002; Rintamaki, Scott, et al., 2005). Although the forms of these troublesome behaviors are currently being cataloged, research has not yet examined their frequencies or the types and magnitudes of effect these actions may have on people living with HIV. Conceivably, experiencing stigmatizing behavior from one's own care providers may lead people to minimize or even forego future health care. Similar research is needed with other groups of people who hold social power over those living with HIV, such as law enforcement personnel (Flavin, 1998). Given, for example, the fact that intravenous drug users with HIV often cross paths with the police, coupled with evidence that police may be prone to mistreat those infected with the virus (Rashbaum,

2000), assessment of the attitudes and actions of police toward people living with HIV is paramount.

In conjunction with identification of behaviors that signal someone is a threat, research is also needed to determine how people can effectively demonstrate their status as an ally to people living with HIV. Put differently, research has yet to determine what actions disarm a heightened sensitivity to stigma and send positive signals that someone is, in fact, comfortable with or supportive of people who have HIV. Identifying behaviors that signal someone is a safe and supportive HIV ally is of both great academic interest and practical value, as this knowledge may assist in preparing those who will work with or are supportive of people living with HIV on how to communicate openness and more quickly establish trusting relationships.

Questions have also gone unanswered on how best to provide support for someone dealing with the stigma surrounding HIV. For instance, what supportive actions best help people struggling with internalized HIV stigma? What supportive actions best help people who have just experienced overt discrimination or been mocked because of their HIV status? What attempts at support are perceived as unhelpful or even counterproductive in the eyes of people living with HIV? Research on these topics will benefit both people living with HIV and those who support them to better cope with the social stigma surrounding the virus.

Regardless if people living with HIV internalize or reject the social stigma surrounding the virus, their awareness of society's attitudes toward them may affect their communicative behaviors in a variety of ways. Concealing their HIV status to avoid persecution, in particular, is at the heart of much of the current research on HIV stigma and behavior outcomes; however, much of this work is incomplete or has yet to get off the ground. For instance, concern for HIV stigma can inhibit people from disclosing their positive status to those with whom they engage in potentially risky behaviors (Chesney & Smith, 1999; Derlega et al., 1998; Ford, Wirawan, Sumantera, Sawitri, & Stahre, 2004; Gaudioso, 2005; Gielen et al., 1997; Simoni et al., 1995). Although of critical importance, this work has mostly considered stigma's effects on status disclosure to prospective sexual partners, largely overlooking assessment of the effects stigma has on status disclosure to current and past sexual or IV drug–using partners. Similarly, evidence suggests that fear of being discovered as HIV-positive leads people to forego their HIV medications to avoid discovery of their HIV status (Golin, Isasi, Bontempi, & Eng, 2002; Rintamaki, Hogan, et al., 2005; Rintamaki et al., 2006), yet we have little insight on how pervasive such concerns are or how often they lead to non-adherence. Future research is required to expand on these important discoveries and tap into as yet unexplored connections between status concealment and health behavior outcomes.

Determining how internalized stigma affects the behavior of those living with HIV also requires additional attention. When such internalization occurs, little is known about the degree to which this affects such things as social networking, support seeking, or important health behaviors, such as health care utilization or treatment adherence. When coping with internalized stigma, are there specific strategies people living with HIV might utilize that are more or less helpful for managing these feelings? How, too, might the Internet play a role in helping cope with the social stigma surrounding HIV? Future research on these topics could shed light on how best to help people newly diagnosed with HIV cope with the negative feelings that result from internalizing HIV stigma.

A growing body of research on stereotype threat has interesting implications for the ways in which people living with HIV conduct themselves in the presence of others. A stereotype threat consists of knowledge that an undesirable stereotype exists about the social group to which one belongs, coupled with concern over doing anything that may confirm this negative stereotype in the eyes of others (e.g., Steele & Aronson, 1995). Ongoing research by the authors demonstrates how stereotypes exist regarding the types of people who have HIV and the means through which HIV was acquired (e.g., if you're a man and HIV-positive, you're probably gay, or if you're a woman, you're probably a prostitute). Knowing that such stereotypes exist, how do people living with HIV react? Do they feel compelled to challenge such stereotypes or are they unconcerned with larger society's perceptions of them? Preliminary findings from the authors' own research suggest that stereotypes about men with HIV being gay troubles many men who identify as heterosexual, leading them to go so far as to start physical altercations or to conspicuously have sex with many different women in attempts to prove their sexual identities to others.

Another underdeveloped area of HIV stigma research centers on how people living with the virus respond when they encounter stigmatizing behaviors in others. Do they avoid conflict or challenge their persecutors? Do they mobilize with HIV-positive peers to address injustice or do they isolate themselves to become less likely targets? Regardless of their actions, what dilemmas or issues do they consider when deciding how to respond to stigma and what goals are they pursuing when different response strategies are employed? What, from HIV-positive people's experiences, may be more or less effective strategies for accomplishing these different goals? These questions remain almost completely unanswered in the extant literature, yet understanding response strategies for managing HIV stigma may be exceptionally useful for equipping the newly diagnosed with skills to navigate tricky social situations they may someday encounter.

## Conclusion

Social stigma remains one of the most subversive and challenging aspects of the HIV experience. In this chapter, literature was reviewed on the sources, forms, and prevalence of HIV stigma within the United States, as well as the effects HIV stigma may have on general social interaction and those living with the virus. Though research has established the scope and effects of HIV stigma, far more is needed to better understand this phenomenon and assist people newly diagnosed with HIV to manage the difficult social burdens HIV stigma entails.

## References

Abrams, D., & Hogg, M. A. (1988). Comments on the motivational status of self-esteem in social identity and intergroup discrimination. *European Journal of Social Psychology, 18,* 317–334.

Alonzo, A. A., & Reynolds, N. R. (1995). Stigma, HIV and AIDS: An exploration and elaboration of a stigma trajectory. *Social Science & Medicine, 41,* 303–315.

Angelino, A. F., & Treisman, G. J. (2001). Management of psychiatric disorders in patients infected with human immunodeficiency virus. *Clinical Infectious Diseases, 33,* 847–856.

Armistead, L., Tannenbaum, L., Forehand, R., Morse, E., & Morse, P. (2001). Disclosing HIV status: Are mothers telling their children? *Journal of Pediatric Psychology, 26,* 11–20.

Baumeister, R. F., & Leary, M. R. (1995). The need to belong: Desire for interpersonal attachments as a fundamental human motivation. *Psychological Bulletin, 117,* 497–529.

Belkin, G. S., Fleishman, J. A., Stein, M. D., Piette, J., & Mor, D. (1992). Physical symptoms and depressive symptoms among individuals with HIV infection. *Psychosomatics, 33,* 416–427.

Bennett, J. (1998). Fear of contagion: A response to stress? *Advances in Nursing Science, 21,* 76–87.

Bennett, M. J. (1990). Stigmatization: Experiences of persons with acquired immune deficiency syndrome. *Issues in Mental Health Nursing, 11,* 141–154.

Blendon, R. J., & Donelan, K. (1988). Discrimination against people with AIDS: The public's perspective. *New England Journal of Medicine, 319,* 1022–1026.

Bor, R., Miller, R., & Goldman, E. (1993). HIV/AIDS and the family: A review of research in the first decade. *Journal of Family Therapy, 15,* 187–204.

Botnick, M. R. (2000). Part 2: Fear of contagion, fear of intimacy. *Journal of Homosexuality, 38,* 77–101.

Brashers, D. E., Haas, S. M., Klingle, R. S., & Neidig, J. L. (2000). Collective AIDS activism and individuals' perceived self-advocacy in physician–patient communication. *Human Communication Research, 2,* 372–402.

Brashers, D. E., Haas, S. M., Neidig, J. L., & Rintamaki, L. S. (2002). Social activism, self-advocacy, and coping with HIV illness. *Journal of Social & Personal Relationships, 19,* 113–134.

Brashers, D. E., Neidig, J. L., & Goldsmith, D. J. (2004). Social support and the management of uncertainty for persons living with HIV or AIDS. *Health Communication, 16,* 305–331.

Breault, A. J., & Polifroni, E. C. (1992). Caring for people with AIDS: Nurses' attitudes and feelings. *Journal of Advanced Nursing, 17,* 21–27.

Burack, J. H., Barrett, D. C., Stall, R. D., Chesney, M. A., Ekstrand, M. L., & Coates, T. J. (1993). Depressive symptoms and CD4 lymphocyte decline among HIV-infected men. *Journal of the American Medical Association, 270,* 256–257.

Burgoyne, R. W., Rourke, S. B., Behrens, D. M., & Salit, I. E. (2004). Long-term quality-of-life outcomes among adults living with HIV in the HAART era: The interplay of changes in clinical factors and symptom profile. *AIDS & Behavior, 8,* 151–163.

Burris, S. (1999). Studying the legal management of HIV-related stigma. *American Behavioral Scientist, 42,* 122–124.

Capitanio, J. P., & Herek, G. M. (1999). AIDS-related stigma and attitudes toward injecting drug users among Black and White Americans. *American Behavioral Scientist, 42*, 1148–1161.

Chapman, E. (2002). Patient impact of negative representations of HIV. *AIDS Patient Care & STDs, 16*, 173–177.

Cherry, K., & Smith, D. H. (1993). Sometimes I cry: The experience of loneliness for men with AIDS. *Health Communication, 5*, 181–208.

Chesney, M. A., & Smith, A. W. (1999). Critical delays in HIV testing and care: The potential role of stigma. *American Behavioral Scientist, 42*, 116–117.

Chung, J. Y., & Magraw, M. M. (1992). A group approach to psychosocial issues faced by HIV-positive women. *Hospital & Community Psychiatry, 43*, 891–894.

Clark, R. A., & Bessinger, R. (1997). Clinical manifestations and predictors of survival in older women infected with HIV. *Journal of Acquired Immune Deficiency Syndromes & Human Retrovirology, 15*, 341–345.

Cobb, M., & De Chabert, J. T. (2002). HIV/AIDS and care provider attributions: Who's to blame? *AIDS Care, 14*, 545–548.

Cole, F. L., & Slocumb, E. M. (1993). Nurses' attitudes toward patients with AIDS. *Journal of Advanced Nursing, 18*, 1112–1117.

Cote, T. R., Biggar, R. J., & Dannenberg, A. L. (1992). Risk of suicide among persons with AIDS: A national assessment. *Journal of the American Medical Association, 268*, 2066–2068.

Craft, S. M., & Serovich, J. M. (2005). Family-of-origin factors and partner violence in the intimate relationships of gay men who are HIV positive. *Journal of Interpersonal Violence, 20*, 777–791.

Crandall, C. S., & Coleman, R. (1992). AIDS-related stigmatization and the disruption of social relationships. *Journal of Social & Personal Relationships, 9*, 163–177.

Crawford, I., Humfleet, G., Ribordy, S. C., Ho, F. C., & Vickers, A. (1991). Stigmatization of AIDS patients by mental health professionals. *Professional Psychology Research & Practice, 22*, 357–361.

Crocker, J., & Major, B. (1989). Social stigma and self-esteem: The self-protective properties of stigma. *Psychological Review, 96*, 608–630.

Crocker, J., Voelkl, K., Testa, M., & Major, B. (1991). Social stigma: The affective consequences of attributional ambiguity. *Journal of Personality & Social Psychology, 60*, 218–228.

Crum, R. M., Brown, C., Liang, K.-Y., & Eaton, W. W. (2001). The association of depression and problem drinking: Analyses from the Baltimore ECA follow-up study. *Addictive Behaviors, 26*, 765–773.

D'Augelli, A. R. (1989). AIDS fears and homophobia among rural nursing personnel. *AIDS Education & Prevention, 1*, 277–284.

Demas, P., Schoenbaum, E. E., Wills, T. A., Doll, L. S., & Klein, R. S. (1995). Stress, coping, and attitudes toward HIV treatment in injecting drug users: a qualitative study. *AIDS Education & Prevention, 7*, 429–442.

Demi, A., Bakeman, R., Moneyham, L., & Sowell, R. (1997). Effects of resources and stressors on burden and depression of family members who provide care to an HIV-infected woman. *Journal of Family Psychology, 11*, 35–48.

Derlega, V. J., Lovejoy, D., & Winstead, B. A. (1998). Personal accounts on disclosing and concealing HIV-positive test results: Weighing the benefits and risks. In V. J. Derlega & A. P. Barbee (Eds.), *HIV and social interaction* (pp. 147–164). Thousand Oaks, CA: Sage.

Derlega, V. J., Winstead, B. A., & Folk-Barron, L. (2000). Reasons for and against disclosing HIV-seropositive test results to an intimate partner: A functional perspective. In S. Petronio (Ed.), *Balancing the secrets of private disclosures* (pp. 53–69). Mahwah, NJ: Lawrence Erlbaum Associates.

Devine, P. G., Plant, E. A., & Harrison, K. (1999). The problem of "us" versus "them" and AIDS stigma. *American Behavioral Scientist, 42,* 1212–1228.

Dindia, K. (1998). "Going into and coming out of the closet": The dialectics of stigma disclosure. In B. M. Montgomery & L. A. Baxter (Eds.), *Dialectical approaches to studying personal relationships* (pp. 83–108). Mahwah, NJ: Lawrence Erlbaum Associates.

Dodds, C. (2002). Messages of responsibility: HIV/AIDS prevention materials in England. *Health: An Interdisciplinary Journal for the Social Study of Health, Illness & Medicine, 6*, 139–171.

Dowell, K. A., Lo Presto, C. T., & Sherman, M. F. (1991). When are AIDS patients to blame for their disease? Effects of patients' sexual orientation and mode of transmission. *Psychological Reports, 69,* 211–219.

Dworkin, J., Albrecht, G., & Cooksey, J. (1991). Concern about AIDS among hospital physicians, nurses and social workers. *Social Science & Medicine, 33*, 239–248.

Epstein, S. (1995). The construction of lay expertise: AIDS activism and the forging of credibility in the reform of clinical trials. *Science, Technology & Human Values, 20*, 408–437.

Epstein, S. (1996). *Impure science: AIDS, activism, and the politics of knowledge.* Berkeley: University of California Press.

Fesko, S. L. (1998). Accommodation and discrimination: Workplace experiences of individuals who are HIV+ and individuals with cancer (Doctoral dissertation, Boston College, 1998). *Dissertation Abstracts International, 59*(6B), 2715.

Ficarrotto, T. J., Grade, M., & Zegans, L. S. (1991). Occupational and personal risk estimates for HIV contagion among incoming graduate nursing students. *Journal of the Association of Nurses in AIDS Care, 2*, 5–11.

Fiscella, K., Meldrum, S., Franks, P., Shields, C. G., Duberstein, P., McDaniel, S. H. et al. (2004). Patient trust: is it related to patient-centered behavior of primary care physicians? *Medical Care, 42*, 1049–1055.

Flavin, J. (1998). Police and HIV/AIDS: The risk, the reality, the response. *American Journal of Criminal Justice, 23*(1), 33–58.

Ford, K., Wirawan, D. N., Sumantera, G. M., Sawitri, A. A. S., & Stahre, M. (2004). Voluntary HIV testing, disclosure, and stigma among injection drug users in Bali, Indonesia. *AIDS Education and Prevention, 16*, 487–498.

Frable, D. E., Blackstone, T., & Scherbaum, C. (1990). Marginal and mindful: Deviants in social interactions. *Journal of Personality & Social Psychology, 59*, 140–149.

Frierson, R. L., Lippmann, S. B., & Johnson, J. (1987). AIDS: Psychological stresses on the family. *Psychosomatics, 28*, 65–68.

Gamson, J. (1989). Silence, death, and the invisible enemy: AIDS activism and social movement "newness." *Social Problems, 36*, 351–367.

Gaudioso, A. (2005). An investigation of misrepresented HIV status between sexual contacts (Doctoral dissertation, Barry University, 2005). *Dissertation Abstracts International, 66*(1A), 100.

Gerbert, B., Maguire, B. T., Bleecker, T., Coates, T. J., & McPhee, S. J. (1991). Primary care physicians and AIDS. Attitudinal and structural barriers to care. *Journal of the American Medical Association, 266*, 2837–2842.

Gielen, A. C., O'Campo, P., Faden, R. R., & Eke, A. (1997). Women's disclosure of HIV status: Experiences of mistreatment and violence in an urban setting. *Women & Health, 25*, 19–31.

Goffman, E. (1963). *Stigma: Notes on the management of spoiled identity.* Englewood Cliffs, NJ: Prentice-Hall.

Goldin, C. S. (1994). Stigmatization and AIDS: Critical issues in public health. *Social Science & Medicine, 39*, 1359-1366.

Golin, C., Isasi, F., Bontempi, J. B., & Eng, E. (2002). Secret pills: HIV-positive patients' experiences taking antiretroviral therapy in North Carolina. *AIDS Education and Prevention, 14*, 318–329.

Gostin, L. O. (1990). The AIDS Litigation Project. A national review of court and human rights commission decisions, Part I: The social impact of AIDS. *Journal of the American Medical Association, 263*, 1961–1970.

Gostin, L. O., & Webber, D. W. (1997). The AIDS Litigation Project: HIV/AIDS in the courts in the 1990s, Part 1. *AIDS & Public Policy Journal, 12*, 105–121.

Gostin, L. O., & Webber, D. W. (1998). The AIDS Litigation Project: HIV/ AIDS in the courts in the 1990s, Part 2. *AIDS & Public Policy Journal, 13,* 3–19.

Greene, K., & Serovich, J. (1996). Appropriateness of disclosure of HIV testing information: The perspective of PLWAs. *Journal of Applied Communication Research, 24,* 50–65.

Greenfield, T. K., Rehm, J., & Rogers, J. D. (2002). Effects of depression and social integration on the relationship between alcohol consumption and all-cause mortality. *Addiction, 97,* 29–38.

Heckman, T. G., Miller, J., Kochman, A., Kalichman, S. C., Carlson, B., & Silverthorn, M. (2002). Thoughts of suicide among HIV-infected rural persons enrolled in a telephone-delivered mental health intervention. *Annals of Behavioral Medicine, 24,* 141–148.

Heckman, T. G., Somlai, A. M., Kalichman, S. C., Franzoi, S. L., & Kelly, J. A. (1998). Psychosocial differences between urban and rural people living with HIV/AIDS. *Journal of Rural Health, 14,* 138–145.

Herek, G. M. (1990). Illness, stigma, and AIDS. In P. T. J. Costa & G. R. VandenBos (Eds.), *Psychological aspects of serious illness: Chronic conditions, fatal diseases, and clinical care* (pp. 103–150). Washington, DC: American Psychological Association.

Herek, G. M. (1999). AIDS and stigma. *American Behavioral Scientist, 42,* 1106–1116.

Herek, G. M., & Capitanio, J. P. (1993). Public reactions to AIDS in the United States: A second decade of stigma. *American Journal of Public Health, 83,* 574–577.

Herek, G. M., & Capitanio, J. P. (1994). Conspiracies, contagion, and compassion: trust and public reactions to AIDS. *AIDS Education & Prevention, 6,* 365–375.

Herek, G. M., & Capitanio, J. P. (1997). AIDS stigma and contact with persons with AIDS: Effects of direct and vicarious contact. *Journal of Applied Social Psychology, 27,* 1–36.

Herek, G. M., & Capitanio, J. P. (1999). AIDS stigma and sexual prejudice. *American Behavioral Scientist, 42,* 1130–1147.

Herek, G. M., Capitanio, J. P., & Widaman, K. F. (2002). HIV-related stigma and knowledge in the United States: Prevalence and trends, 1991–1999. *American Journal of Public Health, 92,* 371–377.

Herek, G. M., & Glunt, E. K. (1988). An epidemic of stigma: Public reactions to AIDS. *American Psychologist, 43,* 886–891.

Herek, G. M., & Glunt, E. K. (1991). AIDS-related attitudes in the United States: A preliminary conceptualization. *Journal of Sex Research, 28,* 99–123.

Herek, G. M., Mitnick, L., Burris, S., Chesney, M., Devine, P., Fullilove, M. T., et al. (1998). Workshop report: AIDS and stigma: A conceptual theory and research agenda. *AIDS & Public Policy Journal, 13,* 36–47.

Herman, N. J. (1993). Return to sender: Reintegrative stigma-management strategies of ex-psychiatric patients. *Journal of Contemporary Ethnography, 22,* 295–330.

Hogg, R. S., Heath, K. V., Yip, B., Craib, K. J., O'Shaughnessy, M. V., Schechter, M. T., et al. (1998). Improved survival among HIV-infected individuals following initiation of antiretroviral therapy. *Journal of the American Medical Association, 279,* 450–454.

Holt, R., Court, P., Vedhara, K., Nott, K. H., Holmes, J., & Snow, M. H. (1998). The role of disclosure in coping with HIV infection. *AIDS Care, 10,* 49–60.

Hunter, N. D., & Rubenstein, W. B. (1992). AIDS and civil rights: The new agenda. *AIDS & Public Policy Journal, 7,* 204–208.

Ickovics, J. R., Hamburger, M. E., Vlahov, D., Schoenbaum, E. E., Schuman, P., Boland, R. J., Moore, J., et al. (2001). Mortality, CD4 cell count decline, and depressive symptoms among HIV-seropositive women: Longitudinal analysis from the HIV Epidemiology Research Study. *Journal of the American Medical Association, 285,* 1466–1474.

Joe, G. W., Knezek, L., Watson, D., & Simpson, D. D. (1991). Depression and decision-making among intravenous drug users. *Psychological Reports, 68,* 339–347.

Jones, E. E., Farina, A., Hastorf, A. H., Markus, H., Miller, D. T., & Scott, R. A. (1984). *Social stigma: The psychology of marked relationships.* New York: Freeman.

Kass, N. E., Faden, R. R., Fox, R., & Dudley, J. (1992). Homosexual and bisexual men's perceptions of discrimination in health services. *American Journal of Public Health, 82,* 1277–1279.

Katz, A. (1996). Gaining a new perspective on life as a consequence of uncertainty in HIV infection. *Journal of the Association of Nurses in AIDS Care, 7,* 51–60.

Katz, I. (1981). *Stigma: A social psychological analysis.* Hillsdale, NJ: Lawrence Erlbaum Associates.

Kaufman, G. (1996). *The psychology of shame: Theory and treatment of shame-based syndromes* (2nd ed.). New York: Springer.

Kelly, J. A., Murphy, D. A., Bahr, G. R., Koob, J. J., Morgan, M. G., Kalichman, S. C., et al. (1993). Factors associated with severity of depression and high-risk sexual behavior among persons diagnosed with human immunodeficiency virus (HIV) infection. *Health Psychology, 12,* 215–219.

Kennamer, J. D., Honnold, J., Bradford, J., & Hendricks, M. (2000). Differences in disclosure of sexuality among African American and White gay/bisexual men: Implications for HIV/AIDS prevention. *AIDS Education & Prevention, 12,* 519–531.

Kilbourne, A. M., Justice, A. C., Rollman, B. L., McGinnis, K. A., Rabeneck, L., Weissman, S., et al. (2002). Clinical importance of HIV and depressive symptoms among veterans with HIV infection. *Journal of General Internal Medicine, 17,* 512–520.

King, M. B. (1989). Prejudice and AIDS: The views and experiences of people with HIV infection. *AIDS Care, 1,* 137–143.

Kinkel, R. J., Bailey, C. W., & Josef, N. C. (1989). Correlates of adolescent suicide attempts: Alienation, drugs and social background. *Journal of Alcohol & Drug Education, 34,* 85–96.

Kinnier, R. T., Metha, A. T., Keim, J. S., & Okey, J. L. (1994). Depression, meaninglessness, and substance abuse in "normal" and hospitalized adolescents. *Journal of Alcohol & Drug Education, 39,* 101–111.

Knox, M. D., Dow, M. G., & Cotton, D. A. (1989). Mental health care providers: The need for AIDS education. *AIDS Education & Prevention, 1,* 285–290.

Kopacz, D. R., Grossman, L. S., & Klamen, D. L. (1999). Medical students and AIDS: knowledge, attitudes and implications for education. *Health Education Research, 14,* 1–6.

Lawless, S., Kippax, S., & Crawford, J. (1996). Dirty, diseased and undeserving: The positioning of HIV positive women. *Social Science & Medicine, 43,* 1371–1377.

Leary, M. R., & Schreindorfer, L. S. (1998). The stigmatization of HIV and AIDS: Rubbing salt in the wound. In V. J. Derlega & A. P. Barbee (Eds.), *HIV and social interaction* (pp. 12–29). Thousand Oaks, CA: Sage.

Lehmann, L. P., Hubbard, J. R., & Martin, P. R. (2001). *Substance abuse and depression.* New York: Marcel Dekker.

LePoire, B. A. (1994). Attraction toward and nonverbal stigmatization of gay males and persons with AIDS: Evidence of symbolic over instrumental attitudinal structures. *Human Communication Research, 21,* 241–279.

LePoire, B. A., Ota, H., & Hajek, C. (1997). Self-disclosure responses to stigmatizing disclosures: Communicating with gays and potentially HIV+ individuals. *Journal of Language & Social Psychology, 16,* 159–190.

Lerner, M. J., & Miller, D. T. (1978). Just world research and the attribution process: Looking back and ahead. *Psychological Bulletin, 85,* 1030–1051.

Leslie, M. B., Stein, J. A., & Rotheram-Borus, M. J. (2002). The impact of coping strategies, personal relationships, and emotional distress on health-related outcomes of parents living with HIV or AIDS. *Journal of Social & Personal Relationships, 19,* 45–66.

Levin, B. W., Krantz, D. H., Driscoll, J. M., & Fleischman, A. R. (1995). The treatment of non-HIV-related conditions in newborns at risk for HIV: A survey of neonatologists. *American Journal of Public Health, 85,* 1507-1513.

Lewis, L. S., & Range, L. M. (1992). Do means of transmission, risk knowledge, and gender affect AIDS stigma and social interactions? *Journal of Social Behavior & Personality, 7,* 211–216.

Lewis, M. (1998). Shame and stigma. In P. Gilbert & B. Andrews (Eds.), *Shame: Interpersonal behavior, psychopathology, and culture* (pp. 126-140). New York: Oxford University Press.

Lichtenstein, B., Laska, M. K., & Clair, J. M. (2002). Chronic sorrow in the HIV-positive patient: Issues of race, gender, and social support. *AIDS Patient Care & STDs, 16,* 27–38.

Liebschutz, J. M., Geier, J. L., Horton, N. J., Chuang, C. H., & Samet, J. H. (2005). Physical and sexual violence and health care utilization in HIV-infected persons with alcohol problems. *AIDS Care, 17,* 566–578.

Limandri, B. J. (1989). Disclosure of stigmatizing conditions: The discloser's perspective. *Archives of Psychiatric Nursing, 3,* 69–78.

Link, B. G., & Phelan, J. C. (2001). Conceptualizing stigma. *Annual Review of Sociology, 27,* 363–385.

Littlefield, C. H., Rodin, G. M., Murray, M. A., & Craven, J. L. (1990). Influence of functional impairment and social support on depressive symptoms in persons with diabetes. *Health Psychology, 9,* 737–749.

Lyketsos, C. G., Hanson, A., Fishman, M., McHugh, P. R., & Treisman, G. J. (1994). Screening for psychiatric morbidity in a medical outpatient clinic for HIV infection: The need for a psychiatric presence. *International Journal of Psychiatry in Medicine, 24,* 103–113.

Major, B., & Crocker, J. (1993). Social stigma: The affective consequences of attributional ambiguity. In D. M. Mackie & D. L. Hamilton (Eds.), *Affect, cognition, and stereotyping: Interactive processes in intergroup perception* (pp. 345–370). New York: Academic Press.

Mancoske, R. J., Wadsworth, C. M., Dugas, D. S., & Hasney, J. A. (1995). Suicide risk among people living with AIDS. *Social Work, 40,* 783–787.

Marzuk, P. M., Tardiff, K., Leon, A. C., Hirsch, C. S., Hartwell, N., Portera, L., et al. (1997). HIV seroprevalence among suicide victims in New York City, 1991–1993. *American Journal of Psychiatry, 154,* 1720–1725.

Marzuk, P. M., Tierney, H., Tardiff, K., Gross., E. M., Morgan, E. B., Hsu, M. A., et al. (1988). Increased risk of suicide in persons with AIDS. *Journal of the American Medical Association, 259,* 1333–1337.

McCain, N. L., & Grambling, L. F. (1992). Living with dying: Coping with HIV disease. *Issues in Mental Health Nursing, 13,* 271–284.

McCann, T. V. (1997). Willingness to provide care and treatment for patients with HIV/AIDS. *Journal of Advanced Nursing, 25,* 1033–1039.

McCann, T. V. (1999). Reluctance amongst nurses and doctors to care for and treat patients with HIV/AIDS. *AIDS Care, 11,* 355–359.

McDonell, J. R., Abell, N., & Miller, J. (1991). Family members' willingness to care for people with AIDS: A psychosocial assessment model. *Social Work, 36,* 43–53.

Michels, R., & Marzuk, P. M. (1993). Progress in psychiatry: II. *New England Journal of Medicine, 329,* 628–638.

Miller, N., & Zimbardo, P. (1966). Motives for fear-induced affiliation: Emotional comparison or interpersonal similarity? *Journal of Personality, 34,* 481–503.

Moneyham, L., Seals, B., Demi, A., Sowell, R., Cohen, L., & Guillory, J. (1996). Perceptions of stigma in women infected with HIV. *AIDS Patient Care & STDs, 10,* 162–167.

Nemoto, T., Foster, K., & Brown, L. S. (1991). Effect of psychological factors on risk behavior of human immunodeficiency virus (HIV) infection among intravenous drug users (IVDUs). *International Journal of the Addictions, 26,* 441–456.

Norton, R., Schwartzbaum, J., & Wheat, J. (1990). Language discrimination of general physicians: AIDS metaphors used in the AIDS crisis. *Communication Research, 17,* 809–826.

Nyamathi, A. M., Bennett, C., & Leake, B. (1995). Predictors of maintained high-risk behaviors among impoverished women. *Public Health Reports, 110,* 600–606.

O'Dowd, M. A., Biderman, D. J., & McKegney, F. P. (1993). Incidence of suicidality in AIDS and HIV-positive patients attending a psychiatry outpatient program. *Psychosomatics, 34,* 33–40.

Orlander, J. D., Samet, J. H., Kazis, L., Freedberg, K. A., & Libman, H. (1994). Improving medical residents' attitudes toward HIV-infected persons through training in an HIV staging and triage clinic. *Academic Medicine, 69,* 1001–1003.

Ortloff, V. C. (1996). Perceptions of discrimination by AIDS patients in health care and employment (Doctoral dissertation, University of Alabama, 1996). *Dissertation Abstracts International, 57*(2A), 0860.

Parker, R., & Aggleton, P. (2003). HIV and AIDS-related stigma and discrimination: A conceptual framework and implications for action. *Social Science & Medicine, 57,* 13–24.

Parsons, T. (1951). *The social system*. Glencoe, IL: The Free Press.

Paxton, S. (2002). The paradox of public HIV disclosure. *AIDS Care, 14*, 559-567.

Peate, I. (1995). A question of prejudice. Stigma, homosexuality and HIV/AIDS. *Professional Nurse, 10*, 380-383.

Peters-Golden, H. (1982). Breast cancer: Varied perceptions of social support in the illness experience. *Social Science & Medicine, 16*, 483-491.

Petronio, S. (2000). The boundaries of privacy: Praxis of everyday life. In S. Petronio (Ed.), *Balancing the secrets of private disclosures* (pp. 37-49). Mahwah, NJ: Lawrence Erlbaum Associates.

Pittam, J., & Gallois, C. (1997). Language strategies in the attribution of blame for HIV and AIDS. *Communication Monographs, 64*, 201-218.

Pittam, J., & Gallois, C. (2000). Malevolence, stigma, and social distance: Maximizing intergroup differences in HIV/AIDS discourse. *Journal of Applied Communication Research, 28*, 24-43.

Pizzi, M. (1992). Women, HIV infection, and AIDS: Tapestries of life, death, and empowerment. *American Journal of Occupational Therapy, 46*, 1021-1027.

Price, V., & Hsu, M. (1992). Public opinion about AIDS policies: The role of misinformation and attitudes toward homosexuals. *Public Opinion Quarterly, 56*, 29-52.

Pryor, J. B., Reeder, G. D., & Landau, S. (1999). A social-psychological analysis of HIV-related stigma: A two-factor theory. *American Behavioral Scientist, 42*, 1193-1211.

Pryor, J. B., Reeder, G. D., & McManus, J. A. (1991). Fear and loathing in the workplace: Reactions to AIDS-infected co-workers. *Personality & Social Psychology Bulletin, 17*, 133-139.

Pryor, J. B., Reeder, G. D., Vinacco, R., & Kott, T. L. (1989). The instrumental and symbolic functions of attitudes toward persons with AIDS. *Journal of Applied Social Psychology, 19*, 377-404.

Quam, M. D. (1990). The sick role, stigma, and pollution: The case of AIDS. In D. A. Feldman (Ed.), *Culture and AIDS* (pp. 29-44). New York: Praeger.

Rashbaum, W. K. (2000, August 2). Silent fraternity: Police officers with HIV. *The New York Times*, p. B1.

Rehm, R. S., & Franck, L. S. (2000). Long-term goals and normalization strategies of children and families affected by HIV/AIDS. *Advances in Nursing Science, 23*, 69-82.

Rintamaki, L. S., Davis, T. C., Skripkauskas, S., Bennett, C. L., & Wolf, M. S. (2006). Stigma concern and HIV medication adherence. *AIDS Patient Care & STDs, 20*, 359-368.

Rintamaki, L. S., Hogan, T. P., & Weaver, F. M. (October, 2005). *Social stigma and the medication practices of U.S. military veterans living with HIV.* Paper presented at the International Conference on Communication in Healthcare, Chicago.

Rintamaki, L. S., Scott, A. M., Kosenko, K., Jensen, R., & Jordan, C. (2005, October). *HIV stigma in healthcare contexts.* Paper presented at the International Conference on Communication in Healthcare, Chicago.

Rose, L. (1994). Homophobia among doctors. *British Medical Journal, 308,* 586–587.

Roth, N. L., & Nelson, M. S. (1997). HIV diagnosis rituals and identity narratives. *AIDS Care, 9,* 161–179.

Rowland, P. A., Coe, N. P., Burchard, K. W., & Pricolo, V. E. (2005). Factors affecting the professional image of physicians. *Current Surgery, 62,* 214–219.

Rozin, P., Markwith, M., & Nemeroff, C. (1992). Magical contagion beliefs and fear of AIDS. *Journal of Applied Social Psychology, 22,* 1081–1092.

Rundell, J. R., Kyle, K. M., Brown, G. R., & Thomason, J. L. (1992). Risk factors for suicide attempts in a human immunodeficiency virus screening program. *Psychosomatics, 33,* 24–27.

Scambler, G., & Hopkins, A. (1990). Generating a model of epileptic stigma: The role of qualitative analysis. *Social Science & Medicine, 30,* 1187–1194.

Schacter, S. (1959). *The psychology of affiliation.* Stanford, CA: Stanford University Press.

Scheper-Hughes, N., & Lock, M. (1991). The message in the bottle: Illness and the micropolitics of resistance. *Journal of Psychohistory, 18,* 409–432.

Shenon, P. (1996, February 11). Reluctantly, Clinton signs defense bill. *The New York Times,* p. A12.

Siegel, K., & Krauss, B. J. (1991). Living with HIV infection: Adaptive tasks of seropositive gay men. *Journal of Health & Social Behavior, 32,* 17–32.

Simoni, J. M., Mason, H. R., Marks, G., Ruiz, M. S., Reed, D., & Richardson, J. L. (1995). Women's self-disclosure of HIV infection: Rates, reasons, and reactions. *Journal of Consulting & Clinical Psychology, 63,* 474–478.

Singh, N., Squier, C., Sivek, C., Wagener, M., Nguyen, M. H., & Yu, V. L. (1996). Determinants of compliance with antiretroviral therapy in patients with human immunodeficiency virus: prospective assessment with implications for enhancing compliance. *AIDS Care, 8,* 261–269.

Sontag, S. (1988). *AIDS and its metaphors.* New York: Farrar, Straus & Giroux.

Sowell, R. L., Lowenstein, A., Moneyham, L., Demi, A., Mizuno, Y., & Seals, B. F. (1997). Resources, stigma, and patterns of disclosure in rural women with HIV infection. *Public Health Nursing, 14,* 302–312.

Squire, C. (1999). "Neighbors who might become friends": Selves, genres, and citizenship in narratives of HIV. *Sociological Quarterly, 40,* 109–137.

Starace, F., & Sherr, L. (1998). Suicidal behaviours, euthanasia and AIDS. *AIDS, 12,* 339–347.

Steele, C. M., & Aronson, J. (1995). Stereotype threat and the intellectual test performance of African Americans. *Journal of Personality & Social Psychology, 69,* 797–811.

Stokes, J. P., & Peterson, J. L. (1998). Homophobia, self-esteem, and risk for HIV among African American men who have sex with men. *AIDS Education & Prevention, 10,* 278–292.

Suominen, K., Isometsa, E., Henriksson, M., Ostamo, A., & Lonnqvist, J. (1997). Hopelessness, impulsiveness and intent among suicide attempters with major depression, alcohol dependence, or both. *Acta Psychiatrica Scandinavica, 96,* 142–149.

Swain, K. A. (1999). Barriers and inroads to aids dialogue in the African-American church: Development of a strategic model and tool for network diffusion of abstinence-based HIV prevention advice (Doctoral dissertation, University of Florida, 1999). *Dissertation Abstracts International, 60*(6A), 1815.

Tang, A. M., Jacobson, D. L., Spiegelman, D., Knox, T. A., & Wanke, C. (2005). Increasing risk of 5% or greater unintentional weight loss in a cohort of HIV-infected patients, 1995 to 2003. *Journal of Acquired Immune Deficiency Syndrome, 40,* 70–76.

Taylor, S. E. (1995). *Health psychology.* New York: McGraw-Hill.

Topacoglu, H., Karcioglu, O., Ozucelik, N., Ozsarac, M., Degerli, V., Sarikaya, S., et al. (2004). Analysis of factors affecting satisfaction in the emergency department: a survey of 1019 patients. *Advances in Therapy, 21,* 380–388.

Vash, C. L. (1981). *The psychology of disability.* New York: Springer.

Wadland, W. C., & Gleeson, C. J. (1991). A model for psychosocial issues in HIV disease. *Journal of Family Practice, 33,* 82–86.

Weiner, B. (1993). AIDS from an attributional perspective. In J. B. Pryor & G. D. Reeder (Eds.), *The social psychology of HIV infection* (pp. 287–302). Hillsdale, NJ: Lawrence Erlbaum Associates.

Weitz, R. (1989). Uncertainty and the lives of persons with AIDS. *Journal of Health & Social Behavior, 30,* 270–281.

Weitz, R. (1993). Living with the stigma of AIDS. In M. Nagler (Ed.), *Perspectives on disability* (pp. 137–147). Palo Alto, CA: Health Markets Research.

Wiener, L. S., Battles, H. B., & Heilman, N. (2000). Public disclosure of a child's HIV infection: Impact on children and families. *AIDS Patient Care & STDs, 14,* 485–497.

Wolcott, D. L., Namir, S., Fawzy, F. I., Gottlieb, M. S., & Mitsuyasu, R. T. (1986). Illness concerns, attitudes towards homosexuality, and social support in gay men with AIDS. *General Hospital Psychiatry, 8,* 395–403.

Zierler, S., Cunningham, W. E., Andersen, R., Shapiro, M. F., Nakazono, T., Morton, S., et al. (2000). Violence victimization after HIV infection in a US probability sample of adult patients in primary care. *American Journal of Public Health, 90,* 208–215.

# 4

# Social Support and Living with HIV
## Findings From Qualitative Studies

*Daena J. Goldsmith*
Lewis and Clark College

*Dale E. Brashers*
University of Illinois at Urbana-Champaign

*Kami A. Kosenko*
University of Illinois at Urbana-Champaign

*Daniel J. O'Keefe*
Northwestern University

Due to improvements in anti-HIV medications (i.e., Highly Active Anti-Retroviral Therapy, or HAART) and in prophylaxis for opportunistic infections, HIV infection has been characterized as a chronic illness rather than a uniformly terminal disease (Siegel & Lekas, 2002). Improved treatments have increased life spans and heightened interest in how people manage the social and psychological effects of living with HIV or AIDS (Siegel & Schrimshaw, 2005). These individuals must cope with a number of illness-related stressors, including disruptions to identity, stigmatizing reactions of others, and uncertainty about the progression of their illness and the potential safety and efficacy of anti-HIV medication regimens (Brashers et al., 1999, 2003). The stress associated with HIV infection has been associated with depression (Porche & Willis, 2006), nonadherence to treatment regimens (Gebo, Keruly, & Moore, 2003), accelerated immune system decline (Kiecolt-Glaser, McGuire, Robles, & Glaser, 2002), and decreased health status (Evans et al., 1997).

Supportive interactions with family, friends, peers, and health care professionals can help develop skills and resources for coping with the stresses of an HIV infection. Theories of social support have long held that the caring and assistance exchanged in social and personal relationships can have a positive effect on the management of illness-related stress (e.g., Pierce, Sarason, & Sarason, 1996; Sarason, Sarason, & Gurung, 1997). Supportive relationships can be a source of positive meaning and affect (e.g., Serovich, Kimberly, Mosack, & Lewis, 2001) and can be a source of information, advice, modeling, encouragement, aid, and social comparison for how to make decisions about treatments and care, sustain one's personal relationships, find meaning in an uncertain future, and enact new identities (Brashers, Neidig, & Goldsmith, 2004). Support groups (e.g., Cawyer & Smith-Dupre, 1995; Sandstrom, 1996), residential facilities (e.g., Adelman & Frey, 1997), and community-based AIDS service organizations (ASOs) (e.g., Roy & Cain, 2001) can be particularly helpful settings for mutual assistance and support.

Social support has been linked to adaptation for individuals living with HIV (Gielen, McDonnell, Wu, O'Campo, & Faden, 2001). Supportive others can provide information, encouragement, and assistance for improving behavioral outcomes such as treatment decision making, treatment adherence, drug and alcohol management, or safer sexual behavior (e.g., Kimberly & Serovich, 1999). Sharing experiences and offering advice about treatments, financial and legal planning, and relational uncertainties can lead to improved physical and psychological management of the illness. For example, feedback and support from others may shape decisions about treatment adherence (Catz, Kelly, Bogart, Benotsch, & McAuliffe, 2000; Spire et al., 2002), which should, in turn, lead to better health outcomes.

In this chapter, we begin to assess the state of research on social support and HIV. As part of a larger project that involves meta-analysis (quantitative) and meta-synthesis (qualitative) procedures for examining patterns in that literature, we have developed a coding system for qualitative studies to capture and integrate findings. Synthesizing the literature is an important complement to future research and interventions involving social support. Only through a comprehensive and carefully implemented review of both quantitative and qualitative research can we find where we have consensus among studies, explanations for discrepancies between studies, and areas in which we need further research. In addition, determining what aspects of social support are most beneficial can lead to the development of interventions that highlight and reinforce those specific facets. Results of the meta-synthesis might lead to studies that target features of the support experience that have yet to be tested through interventions. As Campbell et al. (2003) noted, systematic understanding of qualitative research can "inform health policy and medical practice" (p. 671). For example, several studies described what support behaviors are helpful versus unhelpful (e.g., Barbee, Derlega, Sherburne, & Grimshaw, 1998; Hays, Magee, & Chauncey, 1994). Interventions for individuals living with HIV could help them develop support-seeking skills (see Cutrona & Cole, 2000), including how to ask for desired forms of support and how to handle well-meaning, but unhelpful support. Interventions also could be directed toward friends and family members of people living with HIV to help them understand what sorts of social support behaviors would be most helpful to their loved one who is living with an HIV infection.

This chapter summarizes themes that appear in qualitative studies of social support for people with HIV or AIDS. We describe the topics that have received attention, identify trends in qualitative research on these topics, and suggest directions for future research. Qualitative research is particularly useful for detecting meanings and patterns of communication. These findings are useful in their own right and can also complement quantitative research. For example, insights from qualitative research can help to explain patterns of association detected in quantitative studies, can point to additional processes or variables that have not previously been investigated through quantitative methods, and can juxtapose participant perceptions with researcher constructs. Thus, we begin our larger project by identifying the communication processes, challenges, and patterns that are described and conceptualized in qualitative studies. Meta-synthesis of findings on these various topics can eventually be compared to and integrated with results of meta-analysis of quantitative studies, which provides a summary of the statistical associations between social support and various behavioral, physical, and psychological outcomes.

Our notion of *qualitative methods* is broad, including, for example, narratives developed from case studies, ethnographic descriptions of communities, phenomenological interpretations of individual experiences, and grounded theories or typologies developed from in-depth interviews or focus groups (later, we describe trends we observed in the methodologies employed). We excluded from this review a genre of studies, which, although based on the author's contact with persons with HIV/AIDS, gave little or no description of participants, gave no description of a systematic form of data analysis, and used case material primarily to illustrate previous findings from research. We focused on studies from the United States, Canada, Britain, and Australia, reasoning that similarities in language and cultures made comparisons feasible.

Following Albrecht and Goldsmith (2003), we broadly viewed social support as a multifaceted construct that captures various health-related effects of involvement in a network of relationships as well as effects of conversations directed specifically toward coping with HIV and HIV-related stressors. We recognized that not all effects of relationships or interactions are positive. The source and type of support may influence whether relationships or interactions are beneficial. We considered studies not only of the social support desired, perceived to be available, and received by persons with HIV, but also support they provided to others, as well as the needs and experiences of persons who provide support to persons with HIV (e.g., caregivers). We differentiated social support received from one's network of social and personal relationships from formal support services (e.g., the receipt or availability of health care, disability benefits, housing); however, we also recognized that persons with HIV may develop ongoing supportive relationships with some service providers and may seek out those providers who not only give tangible aid but also do so in ways that are relationally meaningful. When a study (or, more often, a theme or concept within a larger study) reported how persons with HIV interpreted service providers as part of their support network, we included this in our corpus.

Our initial search of article databases used the key terms "social support" combined with "HIV or AIDS." After the development of our coding materials, we broadened the search using terms that we discovered often were used as markers or synonyms for social support (or, alternatively, for a lack of support). This new search included the terms "HIV or AIDS" combined with "social support," "support group," "social network," "social relations," "companion$," "relation$ quality," "social integration," "social capital," "caregiv$," "social interaction," "loneliness," "conflict," "withdrawal," and "criticism." Some terms were used with the wildcard ($) to capture variations on the term (e.g., a search with "caregiv$" would locate articles with caregiving or caregiver included in the study). We searched databases likely to include social and psychological research on HIV, including AIDS Search, CINAHL (Cumulative Index to Nursing and Allied Health Literature), Current Contents, Medline (1966–2006), ERIC, PsychInfo, Sociological Abstracts, and Dissertation Abstracts.

The topics and issues we report in this chapter were developed through a process of open coding and constant comparison (Strauss & Corbin, 1990). We began by creating for each article in the corpus a detailed abstract, including information about the participants, method, and main findings. We began with a subset of these abstracts and independently developed a set of topical themes observed in multiple articles. We met to compare and synthesize our topics, then independently examined another set of abstracts. Through this iterative and collaborative process, we developed the topics described next. We then tested our topical categories against the full articles to refine and modify the categories as needed and to select exemplary studies to illustrate each topic.

## Topics in Qualitative Studies of Social Support for Persons with HIV/AIDS

Table 4.1 provides an overview of the topics we identified. In what follows, we summarize the theoretical and practical significance of qualitative research on these topics and describe a few examples of studies in each category. A comprehensive review of research on all of these topics is beyond the scope of this chapter.

### Need for Support

One prominent theme in the study of social support focuses on how supportive actions and relationships assist in adaptation to stressful circumstances. An understanding of the particular needs of some population is important for determining what, how, and why social support might be beneficial because support that is not well adapted to particular needs may be irrelevant or even detrimental to recipients (Goldsmith, 2004). Qualitative research has yielded poignant descriptions of the challenges of living with HIV for which people

## TABLE 4.1

## Topical Categories of Qualitative Studies on HIV and Social Support

| Topical Category | Exemplars |
| --- | --- |
| Need for Support: Identifies challenges of living with HIV for which persons desire the support of others. Support is framed as a resource that enables (or would enable if available) people to more effectively meet the challenges of living with HIV. | Longo, Spross, & Locke (1990) Ciambrone (2001) |
| Functions and Processes of Support: Describes the various ways in which other people help someone cope with HIV (e.g., common types include emotional, informational, and tangible support). The focus is on provisions that address some problem or stress associated with living with HIV. | Miller & Zook (1997) Ka'opua (2001) |
| Sources of Support: Examines the different types of people, relationships, and/or social groups that provide social support to persons with HIV. The study identifies the attributes or qualities of people, relationships, or groups that are interpreted or experienced as supportive. | Cawyer & Smith-Dupre (1995) Ciambrone (2002) Haas (2002) Reeves (2000, 2001) |
| Positive and Negative Support Attempts: Identifies actions by others and/or relational dynamics that persons with HIV perceive as helpful or not helpful. | Brashers, Neidig, & Goldsmith (2004) Hays, Magee, & Chauncey (1994) |
| Managing Relationships: Describes how involvement in relationships and intimacy with others serve supportive functions and the effects of seropositivity on relationships. | Barroso (1997) Powell-Cope (1995) |
| Influences on Support: Describes social processes that, although not social support per se, are antecedent social processes. Describes the relationships between stigma, social isolation, disclosure, and support seeking. | Bennett (1990) Black & Miles (2002) Schrimshaw & Siegel (2003) Katz (1996) |
| Support Interventions: Describes how persons with HIV experience, evaluate, or respond to a program designed to improve social support. | Gifford & Sengupta (1999) Adelman & Frey (1997) Stewart et al. (2001) |
| Experience of Support Providers: Focuses on the rewards and/or challenges associated with providing support to persons with HIV and the experiences and perceptions of those providers. The study examines these issues from the perspective of the support provider. | Andrews, Williams, & Neil (1993) Kendall (1994) Hall (2001) Yallop, Lowth, Fitzgerald, Reid, & Morelli (2002) |

desire the support of others. In these studies, social support is framed as a resource that does enable (or would enable, if available) people with HIV to live with the illness. Some studies also provide insight into the reasons people seek support.

Longo, Spross, and Locke's (1990) examination of the adaptation problems and responses of 34 White gay men with AIDS serves as one exemplar of the need for support category. In this early study, the men reported uncertainty about the future, desires to maintain physical and psychological health, fears of becoming socially unacceptable, and concerns about fatigue and weight loss. Arranging for companionship with friends and family was a way to cope with feelings of uncertainty, vulnerability, isolation, and fear. Reconciliation with church or religion was another way some men dealt with HIV-related stressors. Openness with family members, friends, coworkers, and health care providers addressed the men's concerns about stigma, social isolation, and rejection. Tangible support with meals, transportation, and home care as well as help with entertaining at home were ways men dealt with fatigue and its impact on valued activities.

For some people living with the virus, HIV-related stressors are compounded by other negative life events. For example, Ciambrone (2001) interviewed 37 women about the meaning they attached to HIV/AIDS in the context of other life difficulties, including abusive relationships, separation from their children, and substance abuse. The women spoke of the intertwining of HIV with other difficult circumstances and the complex needs for support this created. Several women felt contracting HIV was related to their larger experience of social isolation and lack of esteem support in an environment of substance abuse and/or violent relationships. They also spoke of a desire to receive support for parts of their lives and identities that were not just HIV related, and they lamented how HIV interfered with being mothers and developing intimate relationships. Receiving positive reactions from others when they disclosed they had HIV, knowing other people with HIV, and having a spouse or significant other were among the social support–related factors that differentiated those women for whom HIV was the most disruptive life event from those who felt other difficult experiences had been or were more disruptive.

*Functions and Processes of Support*

Social–support theorists have called for differentiation among the functional types of support (e.g., emotional, informational, tangible, appraisal, esteem). For example, the provision of emotional support may have different benefits in different circumstances than the provision of informational or tangible support (Cutrona & Russell, 1990). There is also a need to move beyond simply showing positive effects of support to explaining the processes through which beneficial (and sometimes detrimental) effects occur (Cohen, Underwood, & Gottlieb, 2000). Qualitative research methods are particularly useful for developing concepts and probing the processes that link concepts. Accordingly, qualitative studies of social support for persons with HIV provide detailed descriptions of the functional types of support that help someone cope with HIV (e.g., how particular behaviors or relationships serve as emotional support or function to provide information or tangible assistance) and the processes through which supportive actions and relationships may result in positive outcomes (e.g., the way in which various supportive actions might enhance or detract from uncertainty management, personal control, or self-esteem).

Miller and Zook (1997) described the types of support for treatment given by informal care providers (including mothers, lovers, relatives, and friends) to people at various points on the HIV/AIDS trajectory. Care partners were involved in searching for information; assisting with medical appointments; providing companionship, comfort, and aid during hospitalizations; assisting with daily life at home; encouraging medical compliance; and helping to arrange for community services. Those partners who desired a high level of involvement in patient medical care were concerned about patient loss of function and/or wanted to be present when traumatic information was delivered. Care partners encountered barriers arising from traditional medical models that discouraged third-party involvement in direct medical care.

Ka'opua (2001) demonstrated how types of social support may take culturally specific forms. She interviewed six Native Hawaiian people with HIV and four *kokua* (people identified by participants as their primary support, including spouses or partners, an adult son, and a paraprofessional helper) to understand what role they played in adherence to HAART and how support for adherence was interpreted.

Participants reported many expected forms of tangible support for adherence, including reminders, behavioral cues, setting up calendars, and preparing pill boxes. In addition, participants valued *kokua* being able to detect a "bad day" and provide needed tangible support without having to be asked. Likewise, by unobtrusively ensuring the occurrence of everyday routines such as family mealtime, *kokua* made it easier to adhere to a medication schedule and provided culturally valued opportunities to socialize with family. Cultural palliation practices (e.g., applying ti leaf, giving lomilomi massage) were seen as supportive not only for physical relief from side effects and symptoms but also for the affection and identification with familiar cultural rituals that were conveyed. Informational and emotional support for other aspects of living with HIV were seen by participants to indirectly facilitate adherence to HAART because of the way they maintained a sense of well-being that contributed to motivation for self-care.

## Sources of Support

Social support occurs in a relational context, and it quite often matters who is providing support (e.g., Dakof & Taylor, 1990). It is often the diversity of relationships in one's support network, rather than sheer size alone, that is beneficial (Brissette, Cohen, & Seeman, 2000). Qualitative studies of support for people with HIV document the distinctive relational dynamics that occur when friends or family provide (or fail to provide) support and also point to a wide range of types of relationships from which people with HIV derive a sense of support. Qualitative studies are also particularly useful for illumining what attributes of people, relationships, or groups are supportive.

Support groups emerged as a main source of support mentioned in the literature. Cawyer and Smith-Dupre (1995) used ethnographic observations of a support group over a 3-month period to describe the types of episodes through which social support was communicated among 18 group members, including people with HIV as well as family, friends, lovers, and caregivers of people who had HIV or had died from AIDS. They described four interdependent kinds of interaction that had the overarching goal of providing social support. *Communicating to heal* involved disclosing concerns and frustrations and receiving responses of empathy, statements of similar experiences, and nonverbal expressions of comfort. Expressing feelings helped members work through difficult emotions and the sharing of similar feelings provided validation and social comparison. *Communicating to prepare* involved preparing members to live and die by providing information about services, medical care, treatment options, and opportunities to educate the public. These forms of informational support helped to offset the loss of control often experienced with HIV. *Communicating to vent emotions* gave participants a way to express anger at society, the government, and family and friends for unjust treatment and stigma. Although this may serve a useful cathartic function, it also can escalate hostility and create unfavorable comparisons between the support expressed in the group and the reactions of one's own network. *Communicating to change society* involved encouraging members to become involved in political and social causes related to HIV. Efforts to educate society enabled group members to show support for others affected by HIV and to take efforts to improve the social environment.

Not all supportive interactions among peers occur face-to-face; the Internet allows for mediated communication and support between fellow sufferers. Reeves (2000, 2001) interviewed six men and four women about their use of the Internet to cope with HIV. Her analysis revealed how the Internet serves as a source of social support. Respondents varied in the degree to which chat rooms and other forums for interaction were a primary source of the support they received or a supplement to support from the rest of their social network. Participants noted the Internet is available 24 hours a day and it was especially useful when physical limitations made it difficult to leave home. Participants said it was sometimes easier to address "heavy" or highly "personal" subjects in an electronic medium with others who shared these experiences. Internet interactions gave people with HIV an opportunity to engage in reciprocal support with others, not only through interactive media but also through creating and posting Web material. Internet connections created a sense of community with others.

Family emerged as a significant source of support for the 37 women interviewed by Ciambrone (2002), particularly for the women with a history of injection drug use and without a spouse or partner. Families were valued chiefly for the love and acceptance they expressed, and some women reported that their HIV diagnosis had brought them closer to their family. Some women said they tolerated family "fussing" or being overprotective because it was preferable to rejection and stigma. Family also provided tangible aid, including child care and financial support, but Ciambrone acknowledged that, due to the relatively good health of her sample, these women may have underestimated the importance of assistance with daily living.

Partners are also an important support resource for those living with HIV. Haas (2002) documented how partners in sero-discordant and -concordant gay couples supported one another and maintained their relationship. Partners provided various forms of support that appear in the broader literature, including emotional, informational, tangible, esteem, and network support. Partners especially valued love and companionship and a commitment to remain coupled in the face of a stigmatizing and life-threatening illness. Being in a committed relationship also affected participants' identities as gay. Haas's study is distinctive for examining not only support for coping with HIV but also support for maintaining a couple's relationship in the face of HIV. Friends and family can assist people with HIV directly by helping them with their illness but also indirectly, by helping to sustain a relationship with a supportive partner. A network of gay friends and couples validated a supportive couple relationship and helped prevent isolation. Some families were supportive of a significant relationship whereas others made the process of coping with HIV more difficult by opposing or simply denying a significant relationship.

### Positive and Negative Support Attempts

A considerable body of research shows that actions intended as supportive may be experienced as unhelpful or even harmful (for a review, see Goldsmith, 2004). Qualitative research has described dilemmas of support faced by people with HIV and has yielded insights into why some well-meaning support attempts are not experienced as helpful. Qualitative research is particularly important and appropriate for moving beyond measures of the sheer frequency of support that is received or available and developing explanations for the qualities that make support better or worse, more or less adapted to the needs of those with HIV.

Hays et al. (1994) explored specific helpful and unhelpful behaviors performed by friends and family in their interviews with 25 gay or bisexual men with AIDS. Helpful behaviors included both emotional and instrumental support. *Expressing love and concern* was one of the most valued behaviors. *Serving as a confidant* was appreciated, particularly from friends who also had AIDS. *Providing encouragement* for the men's coping abilities was desired, as was having access to a *positive role model.* Providing a *philosophical or spiritual perspective* was useful, so long as the perspective was one shared by both people. The men also found it helpful to be *treated normally* and to have opportunities to *reciprocate aid,* so that they felt esteemed and needed. Helpful instrumental support took the form of *providing information* or advice, not only about the illness but also about how to cope with social issues. *Practical assistance* with daily activities and *material aid* such as financial resources were also important. Opportunities to *provide tangible aid* to others and opportunities for *companionship* or enjoyment were valued.

The authors identified 11 categories of unhelpful behaviors. The most commonly reported complaint was being treated in a *patronizing or overprotective* manner. However, it was also unhelpful when network members made *unreasonable demands* without sensitivity to the limitations AIDS imposed. *Avoiding interaction, acting embarrassed or ashamed,* or *avoiding the expression of feelings* also were seen as unhelpful. The men resented unsolicited advice or *criticism* about how they were coping or acting in a *judgmental manner* that suggested they were at fault for their illness. The men were upset when others *violated confidentiality* by revealing their AIDS diagnosis to others without asking permission. The men found it unhelpful when others expressed a *pessimistic attitude* or *doubts about their medical care. Insensitive or inconsiderate behaviors* also were reported.

Brashers et al. (2004) described the benefits and costs of social support related to uncertainty management. Findings from focus group discussions among 29 men and 4 women paralleled previous work on the ways social support may *reduce* uncertainty (Albrecht & Adelman, 1987) and extended theory by showing how social support also may be used to *create or sustain* uncertainty. Family, friends, and peers assisted with both seeking and avoiding information, served as sources of stability and sounding boards for making sense of uncertainty, facilitated the development of skills needed for managing illness uncertainty, and provided acceptance and validation to create confidence in one's abilities and reduce relational uncertainty. Participants also reported costs and complications of support—for example, an increased need for support signaled a loss of control;

relational uncertainty (e.g., fear of rejection) complicated the experience of illness uncertainty; exchanging support with peers, who might be more ill, sometimes led to heightened fear of death or worsened illness; and coordinating preferences for seeking or avoiding information emerged as a challenge in utilizing social support. Participants reported managing these challenges by developing a self-advocacy orientation, reframing support attempts as beneficial to the support provider, accepting a lack of support, withdrawing from social situations, and maintaining boundaries.

## Managing Relationships

In contrast to a focus on how supportive relationships assist with coping, there is another tradition in the study of social support that focuses on the broader potentially positive effects of ongoing involvement in relationships (for a review, see Reis & Collins, 2000). This body of work focuses on how relationships meet fundamental human needs for connection and intimacy, how integration in a social network can provide behavioral regulation and meaning, and the ways in which fulfilling relational roles can be sustaining (for a review, see Brissette et al., 2000). Qualitative research demonstrates the difficulties and rewards of sustaining ongoing relationships and creating new relationships in the face of HIV. The narratives told by people with HIV reveal both positive and negative changes in relationships and underscore the dangers of social isolation.

Relationships affect and are affected by seropositivity. For example, Barroso (1997) described the relational implications of HIV infection in her interviews with 20 long-term survivors. The major theme of "being in relation to others" illustrated how participants needed to "establish new relationships and renegotiate old ones" (p. 561) as a consequence of life changes due to illness. For example, some participants who lacked support from their *families of origin* relied instead on *families of commitment* (e.g., close friends) for support. Relationships with families of origin often were complicated by the perceived obligation to reciprocate caregiving and by the stigma associated with the illness, leading some individuals to disassociate from their families. One participant who reported close relationships with his family of origin recognized that he was lucky to have that support available; others mentioned that family members (e.g., children) provided a reason for them to want to survive. Renegotiation of social networks also occurred when friends rejected them or died from AIDS. These new friendship networks, which often included others living with HIV, became families of commitment. Helping others with HIV, including serving as role models in support groups, became another form of relational negotiation.

Powell-Cope (1995) explored the relational context of HIV in an examination of nine gay couples in which at least one partner was HIV-positive. Her interviews revealed the process of *mutual protection,* which included the subprocesses and strategies of *maintaining, restoring,* and *preserving (a) relationship boundaries, (b) independence,* and *(c) intimacy.* Participants felt that establishing relationship boundaries was important to protect themselves from friends and family members who might threaten "the safe haven of their relationship" (p. 50). Maintaining relational boundaries became increasingly difficult as illness escalated, especially when social support from other network members was needed. Relationships with friends and family members often were strained, either because the couple distanced themselves from others (due to fear of negative reactions) or because they found that they had fewer common bonds once the illness became a focus of their lives. Another key factor in relationship negotiations was informal agreements about the level of independence and roles each partner was afforded. This became challenging as a partner became ill because caregiving could interfere with independence. Finally, maintaining intimacy was important to relational well-being, but was complicated by the desire to avoid HIV infection for an HIV-negative partner, or by the possibility of giving other infections to the person living with HIV.

## Influences on Support

The study of social support frequently has been concerned with predicting outcomes of supportive behaviors or relationships. Researchers have less often studied antecedents, such as barriers to seeking support or the role people play in mobilizing social support (Silver, Wortman, & Crofton, 1990). Qualitative research on social support for HIV yields insight into how stigma, social isolation, support seeking, and the experience of disclosing illness shape the social support that is available. These four subcategories of the influences on support category describe separate theoretical domains but are often experienced in tandem. Thus, considerable overlap exists in the four subcategories that describe the main influences on social support for those living with HIV.

The complex relationship between stigma and social support is nicely illustrated by an early study from Bennett (1990), who interviewed 10 gay men about their perception of AIDS-related stigma. The men described both direct and subtle forms of rejection from families, friends, roommates, employers, strangers, and society at large. Some perceived that others shied away from them, acting "cool," "standoffish," and reluctant to engage in physical or social contact. More obvious forms of rejection included staring, gossip, making fun, and displaying visible fear. Some men reported being cut off from employment, housing, and people and reported fears the public would resort to quarantines. These responses left them with few or no people with whom they could discuss their deaths. In contrast to rejection, the men also reported experiences of and strategies for stigma protection. Lovers, friends, and families might act as "bumper guards" who provided emotional, informational, and tangible support and warded off isolation and rejection by others. The men also reported psychological defenses against stigma, including directing anger at those who rejected them, being guarded about interactions with others, withholding information, concealing status, and comparing themselves to others less fortunate. Thus, stigma interfered with relationships, depriving men of social support and creating additional social stress. In contrast, social support was one resource for fighting stigma, but some of the men's strategies for coping (being angry or guarded, concealing status) might make it difficult to develop or sustain supportive relationships.

Black and Miles (2002) reported on disclosure from field notes taken by nurses during a 6-week intervention to promote self-care among 48 African-American women who were caring for young children. They described a *calculus of disclosure* by which women decided whether to disclose by weighing the risk of stigma against their needs for support. Having heard how others in their family, church, and community talked about people with HIV, the women feared gossip and stigma, felt personal shame, and worried about causing pain and shame to their families. At the same time, women experienced unmet needs to talk about HIV with a supportive listener. They also needed tangible help with child care and transportation when they needed to go to a clinic and with activities of daily life during illness. Most women carefully controlled what information they revealed, in order to protect themselves and loved ones. *Secretive disclosers* told only a few trusted individuals and some told no one outside the health care system. This protected fragile social ties but limited access to support, and some women acknowledged they would need to disclose later as illness or child-care needs required it. *Full disclosers* were completely open about their diagnosis with adults (they felt their children were too young to understand). Their reasons for disclosure varied, including wanting to support others with HIV, wanting to educate others about prevention, and deriving therapeutic benefit from being open. Most of the women were *selective disclosers* who told close family members (e.g., partners, mothers, or sisters) but few others outside their household. Having witnessed supportive reactions in the past and anticipating support in the future were among their reasons for disclosing. Reasons for not disclosing included deciding others did not need to know, protecting children from courtesy stigma, feeling children were too young to understand, and waiting for the right time to disclose.

In addition to stigma and disclosure, researchers have investigated the relationship between social isolation and support for seropositive individuals. For example, Schrimshaw and Siegel (2003) interviewed 63 adults over the age of 50 to understand their social-support deficits. Forty-two percent said they did not receive as much emotional support as they needed and 27% reported a lack of practical assistance. Those without satisfactory support had needs that went unmet and some reported feeling "profoundly lonely." Those who were satisfied with support often indicated that this was because they were currently doing well and did not need much support rather than saying that they had family and friends who gave support. Explanations for their lack of support were varied. Some went without support because they had not disclosed their status for fear of stigma or desire to protect their privacy. Some participants who had disclosed said friends and family were unable or unwilling to provide support because of fear, prejudice, or ignorance of the disease. Even when support was available from other sources (e.g., the gay community, HIV support groups), participants reported a sense of regret when family withheld their support. Those who valued self-reliance and independence were reluctant to ask for tangible help or for emotional support. Others were willing to admit they needed help but did not want to impose a burden on others or wanted to wait to ask for help until it was necessary. Some participants reported that family and friends had passed away, lived too far away, or had too many health problems and needs of their own. The networks of some older gay men in the sample had been decimated by HIV; supportive friends and partners had died and the living had withdrawn socially from the distress of repeated loss. Finally, some participants perceived that older infected adults received less compassion and sympathy because their situation was not so tragic as the untimely illness of younger people with HIV or because older adults were judged more harshly for having contracted the illness. Some of the gay participants felt their community emphasized youth and vitality so that those who were older and unhealthy were marginalized.

Researchers also have attended to support seeking by those living with HIV. Katz (1996) found that an HIV diagnosis profoundly altered the life perspectives of 10 interviewees. Participants reported that relationships took on new meaning after their diagnosis. Developing and maintaining this new life perspective took time, and the participants performed several actions to sustain this new view on life. It was maintained by surviving the diagnosis, taking care of themselves, living in the moment, emphasizing the positive, and seeking support. Participants took care of themselves by seeking information and medical advice. For example, asymptomatic patients saw physicians regularly in efforts to reduce their uncertainty. Support seeking proved to be somewhat problematic for participants who had to balance the need to disclose their status to access support with the desire to keep loved ones from the distressing information. Participants felt a need to control to whom and when they disclosed to assert some control over their situation. Those who decided to disclose found friends and family to be generally supportive. Some were rejected from family and friends, but those with supportive others felt closer after the disclosure. Asking for help from health professionals and other social-service providers and attending support groups also were mentioned as ways of seeking social support. Health care professionals and volunteers served as an important support resource, especially for those who did not live near their family or had few friends. Seeking informational, emotional, and tangible assistance from others helped the participants maintain their new life perspective and cope with the uncertainty of their illness.

*Support Interventions*

One impetus for the study of social support comes from a desire to develop interventions that can provide, improve, or facilitate support for people who need it. Unfortunately, much of the theoretical research on social support has not been tested by translation into intervention and too many interventions have proceeded without a strong theoretical basis or rigorous evaluation (Albrecht & Goldsmith, 2003; Cohen et al., 2000). Social-support interventions for people with HIV include programs designed to provide supportive links or resources (e.g., support groups, buddy programs, HIV residential facilities) as well as programs designed to improve the quality of naturally occurring support (e.g., patient education on how to utilize support, programs to enable family to better meet the needs of people with HIV). Qualitative studies of how these interventions are experienced by participants are especially useful for providing insight into how and why the intervention works (or does not work), providing a potential link between theory and practical intervention.

One theoretically based intervention that Gifford and Sengupta (1999) tested was the Positive Self-Management Program (PSMP). The authors used structured, open-ended telephone interviews with 24 of 71 participants in the seven-session peer-led intervention. The PSMP was based on a conceptual framework designed to increase self-efficacy, provide peer role models and a positive supportive environment, develop symptom management skills, and encourage goal setting. Themes from the interviews included the importance of contracts for committing to goals, connections that developed between group members, and the resource book (*Living Well with HIV & AIDS*; Gifford, Lorig, Laurent, & Gonzalez, 2005). Participants also described the possibility of having versions of PSMP for "beginners" (those who are newly diagnosed or have little information) and for the "experienced" (those who had previous knowledge of the disease). They also detailed behavioral and attitudinal changes that they attributed to the program, including making dietary changes, taking more responsibility for finding health information, and developing more positive attitudes about living with HIV.

Supportive links among individuals living with HIV and other potential support providers also may be fostered by AIDS services, like residential facilities. Adelman and Frey (1997) conducted an observational study of the Bonaventure House in Chicago, a residential facility for people living with HIV or AIDS founded by the Alexian Brothers of America. The researchers took different roles in relation to the study participants: Mara Adelman volunteered and conducted research in the house and Larry Frey served as an observer, allowing them to get insider and outsider perspectives. In their book *Fragile Community: Living Together with AIDS,* the authors described the development of community in the house and the rituals and routines that served to both reinforce and challenge relationships. House rules (no alcohol or drug use, required chores, signing out when leaving the house) and weekly house meetings served both as organizational devices and as sites of conflict. Staff and residents developed methods for easing entry into the house (which they called "parachutes") and building cohesion among the residents (including activities such as an annual Halloween party). Other activities were designed to help residents cope with the stresses of living in an environment in which many other residents died. One example was a ceremony in which a large collection of brightly colored helium-filled balloons was released to memorialize residents who had passed. Other activities that marked community included photographs and scrapbooks, which preserved memories and "symbolically assemble[d] and disassemble[d] social relationships" (p. 104). Overall, the authors concluded that community was both a source of support as well as tension for residents and staff at Bonaventure House.

Support groups designed to improve the quantity and quality of support are another type of intervention for people living with HIV. Stewart and colleagues (2001) evaluated the efficacy of a 12-week telephone support group intervention for people with hemophilia and HIV or AIDS and their family caregivers. Both groups of participants lived in geographically isolated areas, which made telephone-based support the most convenient mode of delivery. Data included transcripts of support group interactions, field notes from peer and professional group facilitators, and interviews with participants and facilitators. Support group sessions averaged 102 minutes (range 76–122) for the hemophilia/HIV group and 105 minutes (range 79–153) for the caregiver group. Both groups discussed some similar topics, including negative social attitudes, inadequate or inaccessible information, and dealing with the health system. Themes discussed mainly by the men living with hemophilia and HIV included illness treatment, financial strain, injustice, and advocacy. Themes discussed mainly by caregivers included monitoring the relative's health, dealing with relatives' reactions, impact on family, and personal needs. Each group described using problem-focused and emotion-focused coping strategies, and discussed various types and sources of social support. The discussions also revealed that participants felt that the group helped satisfy their support needs, mobilize their coping strategies, diminish feelings of loneliness and isolation, enhance communication and their relationships, and increase their confidence. All participants reported disappointment that the intervention ended after 12 sessions—the caregivers even exchanged numbers to arrange a later face-to-face meeting.

## Experience of Support Providers

Providing social support can be both rewarding and costly (sometimes simultaneously), and when family, friends, and significant others are support providers, their experience is also influenced by their own coming to grips with the stressful circumstances of a loved one (Coyne, Ellard, & Smith, 1990; Goldsmith, 2004). Although the prognosis for people with HIV has improved dramatically, it is still a life-threatening illness whose later stages can require heroic emotional and tangible care. Even before the end stages, support providers and those for whom they care face the documented challenges of coping together with chronic illness, such as managing illness uncertainty (Brashers, Neidig et al., 2000) and remaking biography and identity (Ezzy, 2000). Qualitative research has begun to explore the experiences of those who give care and provide support to people with HIV. HIV support providers fall into two general categories: informal care providers who are HIV-positive themselves and professional HIV caregivers.

Those living with HIV are not always just the recipients of support from others; some provide care for children or others living with the virus. In interviews with 80 mothers living with HIV, Andrews, Williams, and Neil (1993) found that they frequently listed their children (even those 8 years old or younger) as sources of support. Having children in their lives helped reduce the mothers' feelings of isolation and provided affection. Attachment to children helped offset the stigma and detachment women experienced in other parts of their social world. Commitment to their children also prevented women from running away from their lives and gave an incentive for positive coping and healthful behavior. Caring for children was a source of self-esteem and helped distract mothers from dwelling on their own vulnerability and fears. At the same time, motherhood entailed burdens and stresses. Women reported anxiety about where their children would go if they died before their children reached adulthood, particularly when children were also seropositive and might require special care. Women also worried about the health of seropositive children and the prospect of long hospitalizations and eventual death. Having children also decreased mothers' privacy and, for those mothers who had not disclosed their status to their children, created a burden of secrecy. Finally, some children reacted to their mother's diagnosis with anger and hostility.

Reciprocal support, or giving *and* receiving help, is also an important component of HIV support provision. Based on interviews with 29 gay men, Kendall (1994) developed a concept of *wellness spirituality* grounded in human connectedness, meaning, and self-acceptance. Several components of wellness spirituality entailed the ability to *give* as well as receive support. Belonging to a community in which members cared for one another was one component of spiritual well-being. Sharing information, emotions, and activities and engaging in reciprocal social support were also components. Connecting with other gay men in nonsexual ways and engaging in physical nonsexual touch helped to overcome feelings of rejection and provided affirmation for identity. Expressing honest criticisms or disagreements in supportive and caring ways were also part of the men's understanding of wellness. These social processes were linked to the men's abilities to find meaning and self-acceptance.

Those living with HIV benefit from the care provided by professional caregivers, including health care providers and trained volunteers who may or may not be HIV-positive themselves. For example, Hall (2001) interviewed 17 volunteers (some HIV-positive, some HIV-negative) in community-based AIDS service organizations (ASOs) about the purpose and meaning of volunteering. He identified "bearing witness to suffering" as a core process of constructing meaning and described three interrelated stages. *Experiencing suffering* involved suffering, loss, and despair that resulted in coming in contact with an ASO. People with HIV and those close to them lost autonomy, relationships, and self. These cumulative losses contributed to a larger loss of control and a desire to act, to reestablish order and regain a sense of purpose. ASOs met needs for services and also provided opportunities to volunteer. *Containing suffering* occurred through performing acts of witness and fulfilling roles in the ASO that resulted in hope. Acts of witness included public speaking to educate others, caregiving, and political advocacy. Roles of witness included acting as an eyewitness who can speak out about suffering observed, acting as an expert with direct knowledge of suffering, acting as an advocate who challenges indifference and intolerance, and acting as a visionary who expresses concern for the future consequences of stigma. Mastery of words and action and enactment of roles had intrapersonal effects (feelings of hope, insight to self, self-efficacy, liberation from stigma) and interpersonal effects (providing new supportive relationships, leaving a legacy, gaining connections with others, developing greater acceptance of others) that enabled volunteers to contain suffering. *Transforming suffering* occurred as participants experienced unforeseen gains that allowed them to come to terms with loss and give meaning to suffering. Volunteers regained a sense of control, felt enhanced self-worth from expressing their values and beliefs, and developed a sense of purpose through connection to others, helping, and advocacy.

Providing care for patients or clients affected by HIV creates support needs for professional support providers. Yallop, Lowth, Fitzgerald, Reid, and Morelli (2002) compared the uncertainty described by HIV survivors in Brashers and colleagues (1999) to similar feelings reported by 48 health care providers who participated in focus group discussion and/or interviews. Brashers and colleagues found that when life expectancy improved with the advent of new medications, some people with HIV experienced challenges related to the uncertainty of their "revival." Similarly, Yallop and colleagues found that health care providers experienced a shift *from fear to optimism and hope* while simultaneously holding concerns about the long-term effects of new drugs and their patients' sustained adherence. Health care providers felt obligated to reassure clients even as they experienced their own uncertainty. Some reported that overcoming their fears of telling clients "I don't know" provided a basis for creating empathy, empowering patients, and developing collaborative relationships. Health care providers reported *changes in their role* to include not only "caring professional" but also friend, advocate, or radical. Roles for nurses, social workers, and occupational therapists changed as their focus shifted from care for the dying to assistance for those living with a chronic illness. Some physicians observed that more effective medications had shifted their focus from dying and caring to prescribing, a shift they felt had remedicalized and depersonalized care for people with HIV. Participants agreed that they had experienced *changes in relationships* with their HIV patients, but disagreed about whether relationships were more emotionally intense when the focus was on dying or more intimate as they had longer term contact with patients. Developing trust and honesty about noncompliance and keeping patients from becoming too dependent on services were new relational issues. Physicians reported a greater sense of responsibility for prescribing effective treatments (and a corresponding feeling of failure when treatments were unsuccessful).

In summary, qualitative studies on social support for people living with HIV have addressed eight core topics. Although the HIV diagnosis and the resulting life changes can have positive consequences for those infected, difficult life circumstances and HIV-related stressors create unique support needs for this population. Whereas the need for support category describes studies that emphasize the stressors associated with living with HIV and the role of social support in mitigating the negative effects of the virus, the functions/processes category focuses on how support can achieve positive outcomes and the functions of various types of support. Support groups, the Internet, friends, peers, family, and partners are all potential support sources for individuals living with HIV. The support provided by these sources can go astray, leading some researchers to explore both positive and negative support attempts. In contrast to studies that focus on specific supportive acts by others, studies that attend to the broader relational context in which social support occurs fall into the managing relationships category. Several influences on social support, including stigma, disclosure, social isolation, and support seeking, affect the ability of those living with HIV to mobilize their support resources. Interventions designed to foster new ties through support groups and residential facilities as well as those created to meet the informational needs of sufferers all fall into the support intervention category. Finally, studies that delve into the role of support provision in the context of HIV and the unique needs of the support provider round out the final category—the experience of support providers.

## Trends in Qualitative Studies of Social
## Support for People With HIV/AIDS

Qualitative investigations utilized a range of data collection methods and analytic strategies (for discussions and comparisons of the different qualitative methods, see Creswell, 1998; Morse & Field, 1995). Qualitative methods used in these studies included *ethnography* (e.g., Carr, 1996), *observations* (e.g., Black & Miles, 2002), and *case studies* (e.g., Williams, 1995). The most commonly described technique for data collection was *interviews,* including those described as *in-depth* (e.g., Powell-Cope, 1995), *longitudinal* (e.g., Andrews et al., 1993), *semistructured* (e.g., Reeves, 2000, 2001), *ethnographic* (e.g., Barroso, 1997), and *focus group* (e.g., Brashers et al., 2004). Data collection that involved recording supportive interactions occurred relatively infrequently; however, a few studies used conversational data from the interactions of HIV support groups for analysis (e.g., Stewart et al., 2001). *Constant comparative analysis* based on grounded theory was the analytic method used in many of these qualitative studies (e.g., Cawyer & Smith-Dupre, 1995) sometimes combined with *content analysis* (e.g., Barroso, 1997). Others described their analyses as *thematic* (e.g., Schrimshaw & Siegel, 2003), *content-analytic* (e.g., Longo et al., 1990), *hermeneutic* (e.g., Bunting & Seaton, 1999), *inductive* (e.g., Adam & Sears, 1994), *narrative* (e.g., Cherry & Smith, 1993), *phenomenological* (Bennett, 1990), and *interpretive interactionism* (Hall, 1994). Several researchers reported using computer software to assist in data analysis, including QSR Nvivo (e.g., Bontempi, Burleson, & Lopez, 2004), Nudist (e.g., Parsons, VanOra, Missildine, Purcell, & Gomez, 2004), and The Ethnograph (e.g., Ueno & Adams, 2001).

Few studies had more than 25 participants. This is not particularly surprising in qualitative research and not necessarily problematic. What was troubling, however, was the frequent lack of explanation and justification for sample size and selection. The composition of samples appeared to parallel the distribution of HIV and AIDS across populations over time. For example, studies published prior to 1995 had samples that were all or mostly men. From 1995 to the present, there were about as many samples composed of all or mostly women as there were samples of all or mostly men. Studies rarely reported roughly equal representation of men and women, making it difficult to engage in systematic gender-based comparisons. Prior to 1995, most samples were all or mostly White. Over time (and paralleling the spread of HIV), samples became more diverse. Of studies published since 2000, more samples include multiple racial and ethnic groups with no one group making up more than 75% of the sample. Early studies were more likely than later studies to focus exclusively on gay samples. Many studies did not provide information about participants' sexual orientation or risk factors. This may have been intentional, motivated by a desire to resist stigma and popular misconceptions about who contracts HIV. Nonetheless, omission of information about sexual orientation and risk factors undermines scholarly attempts to compare the experience of HIV and social support for homosexual and heterosexual people or for groups with different risk factors.

A final trend we observed was the recognition of support providers' perspectives and examination of how HIV and social support operate within a social system (e.g., couples, families, communities). Although most studies identified through our search focused on the experience of social support for people with HIV, studies increasingly have examined the experience of partners, families, caregivers, and support providers for people with HIV. A number of studies have begun to explore the experience of mothers who are HIV-positive and their relationships with their children. A few studies examined how couples cope together with one or both partners' HIV.

## Directions for Future Research

Qualitative research on social support for people with HIV has provided many useful insights and holds great future potential. We comment here on how extant and future research can enrich our understanding of the experiences of people with HIV and can serve as a foundation for efforts to assist them. In addition, we discuss the significance of studying social support for people with HIV within the broader context of theories of social support and interventions to improve social support.

### Enriching Understanding of the HIV Experience

Qualitative research on social support can help us more broadly understand the nuanced and multifaceted experience of living with

HIV and AIDS. As we noted at the beginning of the chapter, people infected with HIV are living longer today than those facing the illness even 10 years ago, largely due to improvements in medications. Thus, it has become increasingly important to understand the holistic experience of living with HIV as a chronic condition (Siegel & Lekas, 2002). Studies of the need for support, for example, reveal that stress associated with HIV has a major impact on the lives of people with the illness. Many concerns that might have diminished over time (e.g., with improved medications, increased education and public awareness, etc.) seem to persist, including stigma, social isolation, and uncertainty about the illness (Siegel & Schrimshaw, 2005). Studies of sources of support reveal the complexity of social networks that may (or may not) include supportive family, friends, and peers living with HIV. Studies of managing relationships reveal that living with HIV illness can lead to a need to develop new relationships and to finds ways to renegotiate and maintain old ones. Taken together, the research to date reveals the complexity of managing an illness while managing one's relationships, identity, and emotional well-being. Continued research is needed to understand how people manage the social and relational pressures associated with illness and how those pressures affect psychological and physical health management. Because of the chronic nature of HIV infection today, increased attention to how coping strategies develop and change over time is an important direction for future research (e.g., Reeves, Merriam, & Courtenay, 1999).

Qualitative research on HIV shows how people meet the challenges of HIV, both individually and with the support of others. The literature portrays the potential for people with HIV to live as empowered agents who reason carefully about how to present themselves, manage information, avoid or fight stigma; as people who learn to build and strategically use networks; as relational partners who work to balance their own needs with those of others; and as individuals who find meaning and growth in difficult circumstances. Hearing their voices, discerning their reasoning processes, and identifying their skills and strategies are important for representing not only their risks and needs but also their strengths and abilities. The extant research suggests variation among groups: older versus younger, parents versus those without children, people who are still quite healthy versus those whose health is in decline, those who contract the disease from an infected partner or blood versus from injection drug use, those for whom HIV occurs in the context of other, perhaps more intrusive, traumatic life conditions versus those for whom HIV is the most traumatic life event. Understanding these different lives and life circumstances can help us better explain the processes through which these individuals learn to cope with their illness. Understanding how individuals manage HIV illness with many varied comorbid conditions (e.g., homelessness, mental illness, drug and alcohol addiction, other infections such as hepatitis C, and so on) is increasingly important.

Qualitative research on HIV also points to the challenges and rewards of those who provide support and care for individuals living with HIV. Research on communal coping, for example, reveals that relational partners sometimes perceive a stressor as "our problem" (see Lyons, Mickelson, Sullivan, & Coyne, 1998). As tensions in the family and friendship system occur, it is important to understand the support providers' perspectives, especially as HIV becomes a chronic illness requiring longer periods of informal and formal care. Knowing about the dilemmas, rewards, and drawbacks of AIDS care can enrich our understanding of care provision and of caregivers' own needs for social support. Reducing burnout, retaining experienced care providers, and sustaining informal caregivers has implications for the quality of care received by those living with HIV. Research attention to those who are providing care for others living with HIV and who themselves also are infected (e.g., partners in a sero-concordant relationship, HIV-infected mothers who have children who are also infected) should continue.

Qualitative methods have been underutilized for the evaluation of intervention programs. Quantitative data can help us assess the average effect of intervention studies (e.g., "Does the intervention group experience less depression, better quality of life, or better physical health than the control group?"), but qualitative data can help us examine what components of the intervention contribute to the strength of the effect (e.g., "Do some parts of the intervention seem the most popular or useful?"), as well as examining variability in the effect (e.g., "Are there discernable features of the intervention that work better for some people than for others?"). By asking questions in interviews or observing intervention sessions, we can attempt to find out whether participants understand or embrace our recommendations, or whether they actually can and will implement those suggestions.

## Informing Social-Support Theory and Practice

Studying social support in the context of HIV, and using qualitative methodologies to do so, holds great potential for developing theories of social-support processes. HIV is an illness marked by high levels and multiple types of uncertainty, including uncertainty about the illness and its trajectory, treatments and their efficacy, one's identity, and social reactions. Studies of how people with HIV utilize support to manage HIV can contribute to theories of illness uncertainty and uncertainty management (Brashers et al., 2003). Likewise, the stigma and isolation that all too often accompany HIV make this an important context for understanding the ways in which social support operates by conveying acceptance, affiliation, and identity support. Description of the processes by which support achieves beneficial effects is an essential foundation to the development of theories to explain and interventions to reliably produce those benefits (Cohen et al., 2000).

Qualitative studies give insight to the meaning and communication of social support, such as the reasons behind an amount of support available or received, why people choose not to disclose or to seek support, what they perceive as supportive, or what different sources have to offer. We can also learn more about communication strategies that parallel these concerns—how to provide support in ways that satisfy needs, but that are minimally intrusive or resource dependent; how to assist with disclosure or support-seeking requests; how to craft or interpret messages so that they will be perceived as supportive; and how to target support seeking to different sources of support for different needs. These ways of thinking about supportive interactions can be valuable for designing services and for explaining conditions under which support occurs and how and why it is beneficial.

Because of the stigma associated with HIV and the need to manage relationships, studies in this context direct attention to precursors to social-support provision. For example, studies of HIV have pointed to stigma and isolation as barriers to support and have begun to describe how patterns of disclosure, self-presentation, and support seeking can influence support availability. Future studies that focus not only on *whether* disclosure occurs but also on *how* individuals strategically manage disclosures would be useful (Donovan-Kicken et al., 2006). The HIV context also reminds us that a social network that has been supportive for other needs might not be available for a stigmatizing condition or for the long-term demands of a chronic illness. This is a useful context in which to study how individuals not only mobilize and utilize their social networks but also reconfigure them over the course of an illness trajectory. Future interventions may profitably focus on assisting people with HIV in developing communicative strategies for disclosing, confronting stigma, seeking support, and managing relationships.

Studies of social support for HIV also document the relational (e.g., Coyne et al., 1990) and communal (e.g., Lyons et al., 1998) nature of support. Because of the ways that HIV may be transmitted, it may be more likely that people with this illness rather than other illnesses will cope together in the context of a sero-concordant relationship (e.g., sexual partners), a community that shares risk factors (e.g., networks of ID users, the gay community), or a family in which multiple members are infected (e.g., mothers and children infected perinatally). These particular contexts draw attention to the ways relational partners may be both providers and recipients of support. In fact, the distinction between provider and recipient may break down as we consider how people coordinate needs, support, and coping (cf. Goldsmith, 2004). The HIV context also demonstrates how obtaining support is intertwined with managing relationships (Haas, 2002). For some individuals, this entails negotiating acceptance of lifestyle and stigma so that support for illness can occur. For others, rejection may mean they need to rebuild their network, developing new relationships and community identities while withdrawing from or breaking off other relationships.

Studying social support in the HIV context draws attention to sources of support that have not been so well researched in other contexts. As studies of women's experience of HIV have begun to appear, the potential for children to serve as support providers has emerged. Because of the stigma associated with HIV and also the rapidly changing nature of treatments, peers are an especially important source of emotional and informational support for people with HIV. Continued study of how people with HIV develop and sustain a peer network and how peer support interventions can be developed is warranted. Similarly, viewing service organizations and health care providers as sources of support may be somewhat distinctive to people with HIV because of the ongoing and collaborative relationships that may develop with formal care providers. The ways that social support may be derived from participation in advocacy and activism (Brashers, Haas, Klingle, & Neidig, 2000) or living in residential facilities for people living with AIDS (Adelman & Frey, 1997) have seldom been explored in the larger social support literature but could have useful implications for other kinds of life transitions, stressors, or illnesses.

Finally, because HIV so often has affected marginalized populations, study of support for people with HIV draws our attention to social groups that are not well represented in the larger social-support literature. People of color, people with various sexual orientations, and diverse configurations of couples and families are represented in research on HIV to a greater degree than is usually the case in studies of social support. This holds potential for examining cultural and socioeconomic variability in social-support availability, meaning, and process. Systematic comparisons of social groups and exploration of socioculturally distinctive meanings of social support are needed. Future research might profitably explore the experiences of HIV for older adults and for transgendered people.


## Conclusion

A growing and vibrant literature has emerged that employs qualitative methods to explore the experience of social support for people with HIV. To date, studies have illumined needs for social support, functions and processes of support, sources of support, helpful and unhelpful attributes of support attempts, ways of managing relationships, influences on social support, interventions to improve support, and experiences of support providers. Many different data collection and analytic strategies have been employed and samples have increasingly reflected the diversity of social groups affected by HIV. This continues to be an area ripe with potential for enriching our understanding of HIV and for improving social-support theory and intervention.


## Acknowledgment

We thank the National Institutes of Health for supporting this project through grant number R01MH 67511.

# References

Adam, B. D., & Sears, A. (1994). Negotiating sexual relationships after testing HIV-positive. *Medical Anthropology, 16,* 63–77.

Adelman, M. B., & Frey, L. R. (1997). *The fragile community: Living together with AIDS.* Mahwah, NJ: Lawrence Erlbaum Associates.

Albrecht, T. L., & Adelman, M. B. (1987). Communicating social support: A theoretical perspective. In T. L. Albrecht & M. B. Adelman (Eds.), *Communicating social support* (pp. 18–39). Newbury Park, CA: Sage.

Albrecht, T. L., & Goldsmith, D.J. (2003). Social support, social networks, and health. In T. Thompson, A. Dorsey, K. Miller, & R. Parrott (Eds.), *Handbook of health communication* (pp. 263–284). Mahwah, NJ: Lawrence Erlbaum.

Andrews, S., Williams, A. B., & Neil, K. (1993). The mother–child relationship in the HIV-1 positive family. *Image—The Journal of Nursing Scholarship, 25,* 193–198.

Barbee, A. P., Derlega, V. J., Sherburne, S. P., & Grimshaw, A. (1998). Helpful and unhelpful forms of social support for HIV-positive individuals. In V. J. Derlega & A. P. Barbee (Eds.), *HIV and social interaction* (pp. 83–105). Thousand Oaks, CA: Sage.

Barroso, J. (1997). Social support and long-term survivors of AIDS. *Western Journal of Nursing Research, 19,* 554–573.

Bennett, M. J. (1990). Stigmatization: Experiences of persons with acquired immune deficiency syndrome. *Issues in Mental Health Nursing, 11,* 141–154.

Black, B. P., & Miles, M. S. (2002). Calculating the risks and benefits of disclosure in African American women who have HIV. *Journal of Obstetric, Gynecologic, & Neonatal Nursing, 31,* 688–697.

Bontempi, J. M., Burleson, L., & Lopez, M. H. (2004). HIV medication adherence programs: The importance of social support. *Journal of Community Health Nursing, 21,* 111–122.

Brashers, D. E., Haas, S. M., Klingle, R. S., & Neidig, J. L. (2000). Collective AIDS activism and individual's perceived self-advocacy in physician–patient communication. *Human Communication Research, 26,* 372–402.

Brashers, D. E., Neidig, J. L., Cardillo, L. W., Dobbs, L. K., Russell, J. A., & Haas, S. M. (1999). "In an important way I did die." Uncertainty and revival for persons living with HIV or AIDS. *AIDS Care, 11,* 201–219.

Brashers, D. E., Neidig, J. L., & Goldsmith, D. J. (2004). Social support and the management of uncertainty for people living with HIV or AIDS. *Health Communication, 16,* 305–331.

Brashers, D. E., Neidig, J. L., Haas, S. M, Dobbs, L. K., Cardillo, L. W., & Russell, J. A. (2000). Communication in the management of uncertainty: The case of persons living with HIV or AIDS. *Communication Monographs, 67,* 63–84.

Brashers, D. E., Neidig, J. L., Russell, J. A., Cardillo, L. W., Haas, S. M., Dobbs, L. K., et al. (2003). The medical, personal, and social causes of uncertainty in HIV illness. *Issues in Mental Health Nursing, 24,* 497–522.

Brissette, I., Cohen, S., & Seeman, T. E. (2000). Measuring social integration and social networks. In S. Cohen, L. Underwood, & B. H. Gottlieb (Eds.), *Social support measurements and intervention* (pp. 53–85). New York: Oxford University Press.

Bunting, S. M., & Seaton, R. (1999). Health care participation of perinatal women with HIV: What helps and what gets in the way? *Health Care for Women International, 20,* 563–578.

Campbell, R., Pound, P., Pope, C., Britten, N., Pill, R., Morgan, M., et al. (2003). Evaluating meta-ethnography: A synthesis of qualitative research on lay experiences of diabetes and diabetes care. *Social Science & Medicine, 56,* 671–684.

Carr, G. (1996). Ethnography of an HIV hotel. *Journal of the Association of Nurses in AIDS Care, 7,* 35–42.

Catz, S. L., Kelly, J. A., Bogart, L. M., Benotsch, E. G., & McAuliffe, T. L. (2000). Patterns, correlates, and barriers to medication adherence among persons prescribed new treatments for HIV disease. *Health Psychology, 19,* 124–133.

Cawyer, C. S., & Smith-Dupre, A. (1995). Communicating social support: Identifying supportive episodes in an HIV/AIDS support group. *Communication Quarterly, 43,* 243–358.

Cherry, K., & Smith, D. H. (1993). Sometimes I cry: The experience of loneliness for men with AIDS. *Health Communication, 5,* 181–208.

Ciambrone, D. (2001). Illness and other assaults on self: The relative impact of HIV/AIDS on women's lives. *Sociology of Health & Illness, 23,* 517–540.

Ciambrone, D. (2002). Informal networks among women with HIV/AIDS: Present support and future prospects. *Qualitative Health Research, 12,* 876–896.

Cohen, S., Underwood, L., & Gottlieb, B. (Eds.). (2000). *Social support measurement and interventions: A guide for health and social scientists.* New York: Oxford University Press.

Coyne, J. C., Ellard, J. H., & Smith, D.A.F. (1990). Social support, interdependence, and the dilemmas of helping. In B. R. Sarason, I. G. Sarason, & C.R. Pierce (Eds.), *Social support: An interactional view* (pp. 129–149). New York: Wiley.

Creswell, J.W. (1998). *Qualitative inquiry and research design: Choosing among five traditions.* Thousand Oaks, CA: Sage.

Cutrona, C. E., & Cole, V. (2000). Optimizing support in the natural network. In S. Cohen, L. G. Underwood, & B. H. Gottlieb (Eds.), *Social support measurement and intervention* (pp. 278–308). New York: Oxford University Press.

Cutrona, C. E., & Russell, D. (1990). Type of social support and specific stress: Toward a theory of optimal matching. In B. R. Sarason, I. G. Sarason, & C. R. Pierce (Eds.), *Social support: An interactional view* (pp. 319–366). New York: Wiley.

Dakof, G. A., & Taylor, S. E. (1990). Victim's perceptions of social support: What is helpful from whom? *Journal of Personality and Social Psychology, 58,* 80–89.

Donovan-Kicken, E., Ramey, M., Kosenko, K., Bute, J., Caughlin, J. P., & Brashers, D. E. (2006, July). *Message features as predictors of reactions to HIV disclosures.* Paper presented at the annual meeting of the International Association of Relationship Researchers, Crete, Greece.

Evans, D. L., Leserman, J., Perkins, D. O., Stern, R. A., Murphy, C., Zheng, B., et al. (1997). Severe life stress as a predictor of early disease progression in HIV infection. *American Journal of Psychiatry, 154,* 630–634.

Ezzy, D. (2000). Illness narratives: Time, hope, and HIV. *Social Science & Medicine, 50,* 605–617.

Gebo, K. A., Keruly, J., & Moore, R. D. (2003). Association of social stress, illicit drug use, and health beliefs with nonadherence to antiretroviral therapy. *Journal of General Internal Medicine, 18,* 104–111.

Gielen, A. C., McDonnell, K.A., Wu, A., O'Campo, P., & Faden, R. (2001). Quality of life among women living with HIV: The importance of violence, social support, and self care behaviors. *Social Science and Medicine, 52,* 315–322.

Gifford, A. L., Lorig, K., Laurent, D., & Gonzalez, V. (2005). *Living well with HIV & AIDS* (3rd ed.). Boulder, CO: Bull.

Gifford, A. L., & Sengupta, S. (1999). Self-management health education for chronic HIV infection. *AIDS Care, 11,* 115–130.

Goldsmith, D. J. (2004). *Communicating social support.* New York: Cambridge University Press.

Haas, S. M. (2002). Social support as relationship maintenance in gay male couples coping with HIV or AIDS. *Journal of Social & Personal Relationships, 19,* 87–111.

Hall, B.A. (1994). Ways of maintaining hope in HIV disease. *Research in Nursing and Health, 17,* 283–293.

Hall, V. P. (2001). Bearing witness to suffering in AIDS: Constructing meaning from loss. *Journal of the Association of Nurses in AIDS Care, 12,* 44–55.

Hays, R. B., Magee, R. H., & Chauncey, S. (1994). Identifying helpful and unhelpful behaviours of loved ones: The PWA perspective. *AIDS Care, 6,* 379–392.

Ka'opua, L. (2001). Treatment adherence to an antiretroviral regime: The lived experience of Native Hawaiians and kokua. *Pacific Health Dialog, 8,* 290–298.

Katz, A. (1996). Gaining a new perspective on life as a consequence of uncertainty in HIV infection. *Journal of the Association of Nurses in AIDS Care, 7,* 51–60.

Kendall, J. (1994). Wellness spirituality in homosexual men with HIV infection. *Journal of the Association of Nurses in AIDS Care, 5,* 28–34.

Kiecolt-Glaser, J. K., McGuire, L., Robles, T. F., & Glaser, R. (2002). Psychoneuroimmunology: Psychological influences on immune function and health. *Journal of Consulting and Clinical Psychology, 70,* 537–547.

Kimberly, J. A., & Serovich, J. M. (1999). The role of family and friend social support in reducing risk behaviors among HIV-positive gay men. *AIDS Education and Prevention, 11,* 465–475.

Longo, M. B., Spross, J. A., & Locke, A. M. (1990). Identifying major concerns of persons with acquired immunodeficiency syndrome: A replication. *Clinical Nurse Specialist, 4,* 21–26.

Lyons, R., Mickelson, K., Sullivan, M., & Coyne, J. (1998). Coping as a communal process. *Journal of Social & Personal Relationships, 15,* 570–605.

Miller, K., & Zook, E. G. (1997). Care partners for persons with AIDS: Implications for health communication. *Journal of Applied Communication Research, 25,* 57–74.

Morse, J. M., & Field, P. A. (1995). *Qualitative research methods for health professionals.* Thousand Oaks, CA: Sage.

Parsons, J. T., VanOra, J., Missildine, W., Purcell, D. W., & Gomez, C. A. (2004). Positive and negative consequences of HIV disclosure among seropositive injection drug users. *AIDS Education & Prevention, 16,* 459–475.

Pierce, G. R., Sarason, I. G., & Sarason, B. R. (1996). Coping and social support. In M. Zeidner & N. S. Endler (Eds.), *Handbook of coping* (pp. 434–451). New York: Wiley.

Porche, D., & Willis, D. (2006). Depression in HIV-infected men. *Issues in Mental Health Nursing, 27,* 391–401.

Powell-Cope, G. M. (1995). The experiences of gay couples affected by HIV infection. *Qualitative Health Research, 5,* 36–62.

Reeves, P. M. (2000). Coping in cyberspace: The impact of Internet use on the ability of HIV-positive individuals to deal with their illness. *Journal of Health Communication, 5*(Suppl. S), 47–59.

Reeves, P. M. (2001). How individuals coping with HIV/AIDS use the Internet. *Health Education Research, 16,* 709–719.

Reeves, P. M., Merriam, S. B., & Courtenay, B. C. (1999). Adaptation to HIV infection: The development of coping strategies over time. *Qualitative Health Research, 9,* 344–361.

Reis, H. T., & Collins, N. (2000). Measuring relationship properties and interactions relevant to social support. In S. Cohen, L. Underwood, & B. H. Gottlieb (Eds.), *Social support measurements and intervention* (pp. 136–192). New York: Oxford University Press.

Roy, C. M., & Cain, R. (2001). The involvement of people living with HIV/AIDS in community-based organizations: Contributions and constraints. *AIDS Care, 13,* 421–432.

Sandstrom, K. L. (1996). Searching for information, understanding and self-value: The utilization of peer support groups by gay men with HIV/AIDS. *Social Work in Health Care, 23,* 51–74.

Sarason, B. R., Sarason, I. G., & Gurung, R. A. R. (1997). Close personal relationships and health outcomes: A key to the role of social support. In S. Duck (Ed.), *Handbook of personal relationships* (pp. 547–573). New York: Wiley.

Schrimshaw, E. W., & Siegel, K. (2003). Perceived barriers to social support from family and friends among older adults with HIV/AIDS. *Journal of Health Psychology, 8,* 738–752.

Serovich, J. M., Kimberly, J. A., Mosack, K. E., & Lewis, T. L. (2001). The role of family and friend social support in reducing emotional distress among HIV-positive women. *AIDS Care, 13,* 335–341.

Siegel, K., & Lekas, H. M. (2002). AIDS as a chronic illness: Psychosocial implications. *AIDS, 16* (Suppl. 4), S69–S76.

Siegel, K., & Schrimshaw, E. W. (2005). Stress, appraisal, and coping: A comparison of HIV-infected women in the pre-HAART and HAART eras. *Journal of Psychosomatic Research, 58,* 225–233.

Silver, R. C., Wortman, C. B., & Crofton, C. (1990). The role of coping in support provision: The self-presentational dilemma of victims of life crises. In B. R. Sarason, I. G. Sarason, & C. R. Pierce (Eds.), *Social support: An interactional view* (pp. 397–426). New York: Wiley.

Spire, B., Duran, S., Souville, M., Leport, C., Raffi, F., Maotti, J. P., et al. (2002). Adherence to highly active antiretroviral therapies (HAART) in HIV-infected patients: From a predictive to a dynamic approach. *Social Science & Medicine, 54,* 1481–1496.

Stewart, M. J., Hart, G., Mann, K., Jackson, S., Langille, L., & Reidy, M. (2001). Telephone support group intervention for persons with hemophilia and HIV/AIDS and family caregivers. *International Journal of Nursing Studies, 38,* 209–225.

Strauss, A., & Corbin, J. (1990). *Basics of qualitative research: Grounded theory procedures and techniques.* Thousand Oaks, CA: Sage.

Ueno, K., & Adams, R. G. (2001). Perceptions of social support availability and coping behaviors among gay men with HIV. *Sociological Quarterly, 42,* 303–324.

Williams, J. K. (1995). Afro-American women living with HIV infection: Special therapeutic interventions for a growing population. *Social Work in Health Care, 21,* 41–53.

Yallop, S., Lowth, A., Fitzgerald, M. H., Reid, J., & Morelli, A. (2002). The changing world of HIV care: The impact on health professionals. *Culture, Health & Sexuality, 4,* 431–441.

# 5

# Infusing HIV Test Counseling Practice with Harm Reduction Theory
## An Integrated Model for Voluntary Counseling and Testing

*Marifran Mattson*

*Iccha Basnyat*
Purdue University

The threat of HIV/AIDS has become a familiar aspect of our national and international social and health care milieu. The familiarity for many people manifests in a daunting daily grind of interaction with health care providers as they and their fellow patients, significant others, friends, and family attempt to attend to the devastating effects of a disease that still results in certain, although increasingly prolonged, death. For others, HIV/AIDS is a common phrase but is perceived as a distant threat even though statistics suggest a resurgence of HIV/AIDS in the United States since 2001. People of color, women, and young people have been especially hard hit by the HIV/AIDS epidemic in recent years (Centers for Disease Control and Prevention [CDC], 2005b). New cases are highest among both heterosexual and homosexual young people aged 15 to 29 (CDC, 2005a) who either do not consider their sexual behavior risky or acknowledge their risky behavior but may maintain a fatalistic attitude. In addition, as part of a major HIV prevention policy shift the CDC has begun focusing on "positive prevention" out of concern for reaching those who test positive for HIV/AIDS so they do not infect others (CDC, 2003a; Kalichman, 2005; see also chap. 11, this volume). It is with these diverse at-risk populations that HIV test counseling may hold the most promise. And it is through a philosophy known as harm reduction theory (HRT), already used in successful interven-tion programs targeting injection drug users (IDUs) and to frame HIV test counseling in other countries ravaged by HIV/AIDS, that these prevention education opportunities can be best realized to promote safer sex and other harm-reducing behaviors.

In this chapter, we argue that a critical HIV/AIDS prevention oppor-tunity is being squandered by a relatively conservative and overly standardized approach to HIV test counseling. Two brief excerpts from actual HIV test counseling sessions that used the CDC's coun-seling and testing protocol illustrate the tenor of current practice.[1]

## Excerpt 1

*Health Care Provider (HP):* OK, looking back now are you comfortable with the choices you made?

*Client (C):* Pregnancy is big deal, it changes your life but AIDS pretty much kills you, so no, I guess I was focusing on the wrong thing.

*HP:* So, what will happen if this comes up again, you meet someone you are attractive to him and he is attracted to you?

*C:* No, I wouldn't sleep with him unless I was in a relationship.

*HP:* He offers a relationship and things are going well, so do you have unprotected sex with him?

*C:* Yeah, well, I don't know. I wouldn't have unprotected sex unless I knew. First of all I would still be on birth control but that doesn't affect AIDS, hmm. I would want to know if he has been tested.

*HP:* OK, so he shows you a piece of paper and oh he's everything, totally groovy, he shows you the lab result and has been tested nega-tive, he tells you he has only been with few other women in his life and that you are so beautiful. That's all going great and you know you have been tested negative. Do you have unprotected sex with him?

*C:* I mean I guess I would, I would feel guilty if I didn't.

*HP:* Are you telling me what you think I want to hear or what you believe?

*C:* Obviously, unless I didn't trust him.

*HP:* OK, let's talk about the holes in that particular process. It would seem from the outside that it wasn't necessarily a bad thing. You are entering into a relationship, you are monogamous, he's tested, you are tested, you talk about the past and he admits about the people he has been with in the past and the people you have been with and you do all that stuff, so what's the problem?

*Excerpt 2*

HP: OK, so when you guys are off and on and you are off and he normally does things and sees other people and when it's on hmm, you guys go six months no sex or safe sex and then he takes a test and after the test you go back to not using protection.

C: (interrupting) Oh now, it's not like we have a set pattern or this calendar here. No. It's not like that OK. We were monogamous for 2½ years and then we didn't see each other for two years and he had a girlfriend in that period of time and was monogamous with her and we just got back together since like January.

HP: OK, and after the breakup with his girlfriend he waited six months and took the HIV test.

C: No, he's taken them in between.

HP: So he waited less than six months and so it's been less than six months since the last time he has been with his ex-girlfriend, right?

C: Just about.

HP: Yeah, so just about but not totally.

C: Well, in December.

HP: Which means the test he took is totally inaccurate.

C: But if he has been with the same girl.

HP: It doesn't matter. And if she never got tested. Do you know if she got tested?

C: I believe so, but I wouldn't say I am positive on that.

HP: Well, if she never got tested and she did things you know during the time of the breakup, it doesn't mean a thing.

C: But they weren't together after the breakup.

HP: Even before they got together and if she didn't get tested before that and she did and it was less than six months, then it's inaccurate test. You have to remember what the person does six months before the test or after does not make that test accurate. So, even though you might feel that you are safe, think about it, you may not be.

These representative excerpts highlight the lack of a genuine, personalized approach to HIV test counseling sessions and the parental and assuming tone often heard in the dialogue that may explain why HIV test counseling has been criticized as ineffective for encouraging clients to practice safer sex (Mattson, 2000; Weinhardt, Carey, Johnson, & Bickham, 1999). Instead, a more agency-promoting, truly client-centered approach to HIV test counseling and training that adapts to the unique needs and challenges faced by each client is recommended. This approach could be framed by HRT, which when applied to disease prevention practice suggests movement away from traditional, one-way medical approaches of counselor-to-client interviewing in favor of more realistic, nonjudgmental, client-involved, collaborative sessions promoting sexual health and HIV/AIDS prevention for the client and others.

The goals of this chapter, then, are to review and critique current HIV test counseling research and practice and propose a reframing of the HIV test counseling model using an HRT perspective in the hopes of addressing the unique needs of those potentially affected by the resurgence of HIV/AIDS. To accomplish these goals, this chapter is organized into four sections. First, HIV test counseling studies that consider the merits and drawbacks of mandatory and voluntary testing are reviewed, emphasizing the opportunity to capitalize on these sessions as a tool for HIV/AIDS prevention. Second, the current CDC protocol for HIV test counseling is reviewed to expose the underpinnings of current practice and seek areas ripe for reframing. Third, the tenets of HRT are considered with attention to the proponents of the theory, the political criticisms associated with this controversial approach, and ideas for why these criticisms may be overshadowing its practicality in promoting safer sex through HIV test counseling. Fourth, an integrated HIV test counseling model framed by HRT is proposed that infuses the current protocol with HRT philosophy and revisits the previous excerpts to illustrate how this model could be accomplished in practice. The chapter concludes with a discussion of the limitations for this extension of HRT into HIV test counseling practice and suggests future directions for implementation and evaluation.

## Debating the Effectiveness of Mandatory and Voluntary HIV Testing

HIV testing occurs in one of two ways: either by mandatory testing or through voluntary counseling and testing (VCT). Mandatory testing most often takes place when an HIV test is included within a battery of tests for which a patient's blood has been drawn (American Medical Association, 2002; CDC, 2001a, 2003a, 2003b). Although even in these situations counseling is recommended, often it does not occur because of the extenuating circumstances surrounding the initial need for tests. In the most controversial situations, mandatory HIV-testing programs have been used to test couples planning to marry, pregnant women, and prisoners. Although these programs are generally considered an infringement on human rights, they still exist in some places as relatively desperate measures in response to the persistence of HIV/AIDS (Luginaah, Yiridoe, & Taabazuing, 2005).

In contrast, VCT occurs when a person seeks out an otherwise unsolicited HIV test. In most cases, the blood test is supposed to be accompanied by a pretest and posttest counseling session designed to determine why the person is being tested and to encourage adoption and maintenance of safer behaviors (e.g., safer sex, clean needles for drug use) so as not to risk contracting and/or spreading HIV/AIDS (CDC, 2003b; Weinhardt et al., 1999). Because VCT most often involves an interpersonal counseling session, it is at the center of this discussion.

Despite the seriousness of the HIV/AIDS epidemic, the emphasis on prevention strategies, and the concomitant factors that have influenced the spread of the disease, especially the resurgence of the epidemic in recent years (CDC, 2005a), HIV test counseling continues to receive relatively scant research attention (McKee, Bertrand, & Becker-Benton, 2004). Based on reports published in the early 2000s about the changing nature of the HIV/AIDS epidemic (Institute of Medicine, 2000; Janssen et al., 2001; Schiltz & Sandfort, 2000), the CDC published a series of new strategies for adapting to the trajectory of the HIV/AIDS epidemic. As part of its strategic plan to advance HIV prevention by increasing the percentage of people who know they are infected from 70% to 95%, CDC recognized the need to expand VCT efforts (CDC, 2003a, 2003b). Furthermore, a new emphasis was placed on "positive prevention" or reaching out to people living with HIV/AIDS so they do not transmit HIV to others. These prevention strategies target those who may not know they are HIV-positive and those who are aware of their positive serostatus but may practice risky behaviors anyway.

Kalichman and his colleagues are developing a distinct body of literature that addresses the complex predictors of the one in three individuals who practice risky behaviors in light of their positive HIV status (Kalichman, 2000). Reasons for continued risky behaviors include emotional and personality states (Kalichman et al., 2001), confidence in AIDS therapies (Kelly, Hoffmann, Rompa, & Gray, 1998), substance abuse (Kalichman, Rompa, & Cage, 2000; Strathdee & Patterson, 2005), relationship factors (Aidala, Lee, Garbers,

& Chiasson, 2006; Kalichman, 2000), and adverse economic conditions (Kalichman, 2000). To address this uniquely at-risk audience, CDC dedicated resources to increasing the number of individuals who know they are infected with HIV in order to protect against naive transmissions and to blend prevention habits with HIV/AIDS care services (CDC, 2003a). HIV test counseling could serve an even larger role in achieving these goals.

Recent studies suggested that VCT can be a successful and efficient way to reduce risky behaviors (Mattson, 2000; Sweat et al., 2000; Voluntary HIV-1 Counseling and Testing Efficacy Study Group, 2000); however, some early studies questioned the effectiveness of HIV test counseling as a prevention strategy (Ickovics, Morrill, Beren, Walsh, & Rodin, 1994; Weinhardt et al., 1999). Research conducted both internationally and domestically has indicated that HIV test counseling can be an important prevention tool in the fight against the spread of HIV/AIDS. Although research on HIV test counseling is minimal, a few studies have implicated the role of HIV test counseling in encouraging people to practice safer sex and other harm-reducing behaviors to protect themselves and/or others from HIV/AIDS (Rosenberg, 2003). Mattson (1999) reported that certain persuasive strategies used by HIV test counselors resulted in short-term adoption of safer-sex behaviors. In a subsequent study, Mattson (2000) argued that if HIV test counseling protocols encouraged agency-promoting and empowering dialogue, the inherently interpersonal and persuasive nature of HIV test counseling sessions could be even more effective in promoting harm reduction relative to HIV/AIDS. Furthermore, citing cross-cultural data collected from individuals and couples who filled out a survey about their sexual behaviors, were then enrolled in either individual HIV test counseling or a group intervention, and a few months later participated in follow-up interviews, Hollander (2001) reiterated that personalized HIV counseling and testing showed the most promise in reducing risky sexual behaviors.

In addition, mounting literature from around the world emphasizes the benefits over the barriers to VCT. As Van de Perre (2000) noted, "The challenge is no longer the need to show the efficacy of VCT but to make it accessible to those who desperately need it and to expand it and render it more acceptable, innocuous, and less expensive" (p. 86). For example, Fylkesnes and Siziya (2004) found that although respondents reported being ready to access VCT, they experienced a number of barriers to being tested including perceptions of low personal risk

(Hopkins et al., 2005), concerns about confidentiality (Hopkins et al., 2005; Judson & Vernon, 1988), waiting period before results, and fear of being HIV-positive (Hopkins et al., 2005). In another study, Pronyk et al. (2002) determined through archival data, interviews, and mock HIV test counseling sessions that improving access to high-quality VCT is desirable and achievable. When barriers to receiving VCT, such as user fees, transportation costs, privacy protection, and low-quality counseling were removed, participants were more likely to acknowledge the value of knowing their HIV status, take advantage of testing services, and report satisfaction with the testing and counseling experience.

In other studies, although the effects of HIV testing and counseling were limited, positive outcomes were reported. Ickovics et al. (1994) found that level of sexual risk was lower for women who participated in VCT than for women who did not seek testing but there was no significant change in sexual risk from prior to VCT to the 3-month follow-up interview. Women who tested and were counseled, though, did have fewer intrusive thoughts about HIV/AIDS and they had a decreased chance of contracting HIV/AIDS. In a study grounded in the transtheoretical model (Prochaska, Redding, Harlow, Rossi, & Velicer, 1994), Amaro, Morrill, Dai, Cabral, and Raj (2005) investigated the risk behaviors of heterosexually active participants in VCT relative to their stage of change for safer sex. Positive HIV status was the most significant predictor of safer behavior after VCT. However, many participants who tested negative for HIV stopped having sex with nonprimary partners whereas behaviors with primary partners were particularly resistant to change. The researchers concluded that VCT needed to be more closely tailored to the client's stage of change.

Upon conducting a meta-analysis of HIV counseling and testing studies and reporting that this "is not an effective primary prevention strategy for uninfected participants" (p. 1397), Weinhardt et al. (1999) also recognized the complexity of the HIV/AIDS prevention context and suggested that more theory-driven behavior change research be undertaken to determine effective approaches that HIV test counselors will commit to and utilize. Our integrated model of HIV test counseling begins to address this challenge.

Although not all researchers and practitioners agree, there seems to be ample evidence to support the effectiveness of HIV test counseling as an HIV/AIDS prevention strategy that reduces risky behaviors and to justify continued efforts to improve the HIV test counseling process. The next section reviews the existing CDC HIV test counseling protocol and offers examples to suggest that this protocol needs to be framed in order to encourage a more personally tailored, harm reduction approach.

## HIV Test Counseling Protocol

In 2001, CDC published "Revised Guidelines for HIV Counseling, Testing, and Referral" (CTR) to replace the HIV test counseling standards issued in 1994. The new guidelines emphasized evidence-based and best-practice approaches for all health care providers of VCT (CDC, 2001c). To train new HIV test counselors for state-funded and private programs, state departments of health offer 2- to 4-day workshops based on the CDC guidelines. Following is an outline of the goals, principles, and tenets of the revised CTR protocol (CDC, 2001b).

### Goals

The broad goals for VCT include:

1. Promote knowledge by:
    - Promoting early recognition of HIV status through HIV testing.
    - Providing information about transmission, prevention, and the meaning of HIV test results.

2. Ensure that people at increased risk for acquiring HIV and HIV-infected people:
    - Have access to HIV testing to promote early knowledge of their HIV status.
    - Receive high-quality HIV prevention counseling to reduce the risk for acquiring and/or transmitting HIV.
    - Have access to appropriate medical, preventive, and psychosocial support services.

### Principles

Based on these goals, the following principles have been created for effective HIV CTR:

- Protect confidentiality of clients who receive HIV CTR services.
- Obtain informed consent before HIV testing.
- Provide clients the option of anonymous HIV testing.
- Provide information regarding the HIV test to all who are recommended the test and to all who receive the test, regardless of whether prevention counseling is provided.
- Adhere to local, state, and federal regulations and policies that govern provision of HIV services.
- Provide services that are responsive to client and community needs and priorities.
- Provide services that are appropriate to the client's culture, language, sex, sexual orientation, age, and developmental level.

## Guidelines

Grounded in the aforementioned goals and principles, CDC recommended the following guidelines for implementing HIV CTR.

Information.    For those clients who are recommended for testing, regardless of whether they get tested, CDC recommends they receive the following information: (a) information regarding the HIV test and its benefits and consequences; (b) risks for transmission and how HIV can be prevented; (c) the importance of obtaining test results and explicit procedures for doing so; (d) the meaning of the test results in explicit, understandable language; (e) where to obtain further information or, if applicable, HIV prevention counseling; and (f) where to obtain other services.

HIV Prevention Counseling.    CDC notes that regardless of the HIV prevention counseling model used, the "counselor should focus on assessing the client's personal risk or circumstances and helping the client set and reach a specific, realistic, risk-reduction goal" (CDC, 2001b, p. 14). Furthermore, regardless of the model used, CDC notes that the following elements for HIV prevention counseling have been shown to be most effective:

- Keep the session focused on HIV risk reduction. Each counseling session should be tailored to address the personal HIV risk of the client rather than providing a predetermined set of information.

- Include an in-depth, personalized risk assessment. The assessment should explore previous risk reduction efforts and identify successes and challenges in those efforts.
- Acknowledge and provide support for positive steps already made. Support for positive steps already taken increases clients' beliefs that they can successfully take further HIV risk reduction steps.
- Clarify critical rather than general misconceptions.
- Negotiate a concrete, achievable behavior change step that will reduce HIV risk. Behavioral risk reduction steps should be acceptable to the client and appropriate to the client's situation.
- Seek flexibility in the prevention approach and counseling process. Counselors should avoid a "one-size-fits-all" prevention message.
- Provide skill-building opportunities.
- Use explicit language when providing test results. Test results should be provided at the beginning of the follow-up session.

The revised HIV test counseling protocol provides goals, principles, and guidelines that were evidence-based and emphasized client-centered interaction. However, as the excerpts presented earlier and continued next illustrate, the way these rather vague statements are enacted in practice is problematic and may be decreasing the effectiveness of HIV test counseling (Mattson, 1999, 2000).

## Excerpt 1

HP: Assuming the test is correct, the next problem that you mentioned what if he is not faithful to you. That is a very strong possibility. We know that in relationships there are a lot of infidelities going on and I talk to people all the time who are cheating on or being cheated on by a partner. Relationships start out and they are very romantic and very passionate that it's hard to imagine that this person would be anything but faithful and honest with you. What about a year, two, or five years down the road because you know relationships peak and valley that's very normal and you guys are on a rough spot and you are starting a career, working long hours and you are just trying hard to make your life and build up your career but he's feeling neglected and this goes on for months and months and he is really getting to the point where he feels obviously she doesn't love me because she is not giving me the energy that she was giving me at the beginning of the relationship. So he goes out with his friends, happy hour one day after work, so he's kinda feeling sorry for himself and had a couple beers and this woman he works with has just been very very nice to him. They have lunch a couple times a week and she's just very sweet and understanding and one thing leads to another and they sleep together. Does he come back and tell you, honey we need to wear condoms because at lunch today I slept with someone or after work. Does that sound unrealistic?

C: No, it does sound unrealistic of the guy I am dating. But in a way, you can say that to every married couple so every person who is married should ...

HP: And I do. I recommend to every person who comes in here that they practice protected sex. Now whether they go out and do it or not is another matter but I try to show every person where the potential risks could come in. Let me tell you how I explain HIV disease to the people. HIV disease is very much like a car accident in the way that it occurs. If you are in a car accident then you are within 5 miles of your home and it's not when you are driving down to Tucson and it's not when you are driving down for spring break, it's when you are within a few miles of your home. And if you get infected with HIV disease it's not going to be from the guy you slept with one time that you picked up at the bar one day after finals, it's the guy you are with, the one you are in love with because that is when you are letting your guard down and place yourself at risk. Most women get infected from their husband or primary partners.

## Excerpt 2

HP: What are you going to do, if you test positive? How are you going to react?

C: Well, probably badly, that would be the normal reaction.

HP: You would be really surprised wouldn't you?

C: Well, yeah.

HP: Remember one thing, there is no high, there is no low and there is no in between in this. Anytime you put yourself at risk, anytime you have unprotected sex, anytime you use a needle, anytime you do anything—all it takes is one time and one time only.

C: Yes, but there is a high-risk group.

HP: Not anymore, in my opinion there isn't. Yeah, one sex one time, unprotected. All it takes is one time, OK. One time and one time only. You should never feel that you are high, middle, or low. There is always that risk. There is always that possibility. Yes, it's true the more things you do, the odds are not in your favor, OK. But it doesn't matter all it takes is once.

*C:* But I really feel ...

*HP:* (interrupting) OK, so what you feel is normal. Well, his ex-girlfriend didn't do nothing and they were committed for two years but think about it they were together, they broke up, you were together, you broke up, he went back. I mean OK, always better to be safe than sorry, always. You don't want to be that one person who has to tell people, you know what I thought I was low risk and my boyfriend and I didn't do anything risky together.

*C:* Well, that's why I am here.

*HP:* You don't want to do that, OK. Now, ask yourself why you prefer to use a condom, have you shared that with him? That I prefer to use a condom until the day you and I get married or until the day I decide to become a mother. Have you expressed those feelings towards him?

Despite CDC's recommendation of a client-centered counseling approach, including a personalized risk assessment, neither of these counselors tailored their sessions to the needs and behaviors of their clients. For example, each counseling session began with the exact same battery of risk assessment questions (Table 5.1).

**TABLE 5.1**

**Typical Risk Assessment Questions**

### Questions about Sex

In the last year how many men have you had sex with?
Have you ever had sex with a man who had sex with other men?
Have you ever paid for sex?
Have you ever been paid for sex?
Have you ever had sex with a person who you knew had HIV or AIDS?
Have you ever been sexually assaulted?

### Questions about Drugs

Have you ever used injectable drugs?
How about noninjectable drugs like marijuana, cocaine, crystal?
Have you ever had sex with an injectable drug user?

### Questions about Health

Have you ever had any sexually transmitted diseases?
Have you ever been tested for sexually transmitted diseases?
Have you ever had a blood transfusion?
Have you ever worked in the health care field?

The questions in Table 5.1 may have only succeeded in creating a false sense of safety because clients answered "No" to most of the questions and the list was accomplished quickly without much personalized attention to individual risk behaviors. Many counselors may even disregard the CDC technical guidelines for HIV CTR, believing that risk reduction counseling is ineffective. Also apparent in the HIV test counseling approaches illustrated in these excerpts is a lack of acceptance and respect for individual behavioral choices, regardless of risk. Instead, the assumption is that if clients are testing, they must have done something wrong placing themselves and/or others at risk for HIV/AIDS and subsequently a very paternalistic approach is undertaken with a tone of reprimand for clients' personal choices. Although a variety of factors likely contributed to the progression of communication in these excerpts and the general content and demeanor of many HIV test counseling sessions (Kamb, Dillon, Fishbein, & Willis, 1996; Kamb et al., 1998; Mattson, 1999, 2000; Mattson & Roberts, 2001; Weinhardt et al., 1999), the rather general, sweeping statements of the revised guidelines without an underlying theoretical model or concrete examples likely decreased the influence of these HIV test counseling interventions (Aidala et al., 2006). The next section considers HRT as a guiding framework for revisiting the predominant HIV test counsel protocol in an effort to make these sessions more personalized, respectful, agency-promoting, and effective for HIV/AIDS prevention.

## Harm Reduction Theory as a Complementary Approach

Harm reduction is not a new public health phenomenon and though traditionally applied to preventing the tangential harms of illicit drug use through needle exchange programs, it can be extended to other health behaviors. Quintessentially, HRT improves public health strategies that previously have had limited effects (McHale, 1996). As noted by Hilton, Thompson, Moore-Dempser, and Janzen (2001), HRT is frequently operationalized within a comprehensive health promotion agenda, making it compatible with evolving public health, epidemiology, and population health strategies like HIV/AIDS prevention.

*Proponents of Harm Reduction*

Proponents of HRT accept that some harm is inevitable, but believe that the ideal of zero tolerance excludes compromise and sets goals that are impossible to attain (Riley, 1993). Instead, HRT proposes minimizing the negative consequences of a phenomenon for the members of a society without necessarily eliminating the phenomenon (Des Jarlais, 1995). Consequently, health services become an important determinant of health and can greatly influence the outcomes associated with client contact because of the positive nature of interaction with health professionals (Hilton et al., 2001). When applied to HIV test counseling, HRT suggests movement away from traditional, one-way medical approaches of practitioner-to-client interviewing in favor of more realistic, nonjudgmental, client-involved, collaborative approaches to promoting sexual health (Bradley-Springer, 1996; Mattson, 2000; Miller & Rollnick, 1991).

*Tenets of HRT*

Currently there is no specific formula for implementing HRT in practice; however, harm reduction coalitions such as the World Health Organization (www.who.int), the worldwide Harm Reduction Network,[2] and the Canadian Centre on Substance Abuse (http://www.ccsa.ca) consider the following central tenets of an HRT perspective. Implications for HIV test counseling are also considered.

Humanistic Value.   HRT endorses recognition of individuals' decisions about their health and respecting individuals' rights to make their own choices. In practice, this is accomplished by accepting another's behavior without attaching moral judgment to either agree with or condemn that behavior. For HIV test counseling, a harm reduction perspective means that the counselor would accept the client's situation and behaviors without attaching judgment, regardless of whether or not the counselor approves of the situation or the behavior.

Pragmatism.   HRT promotes accepting both the positive and negative consequences of a behavior without necessarily eliminating the behavior altogether. Harm reduction accepts individuals' engagement in risky behaviors as fact and focuses on risk minimization (Reid,

2002). During HIV test counseling, a harm reduction approach would mean counselors accepting unconditionally that individuals engage in risky behaviors and rather than eliminating the cause (i.e., unsafe sex), they would focus on minimizing the negative effects of that risk.

Focus on Harm.    From an HRT perspective, the extent of individuals' engagement in risky behavior is secondary to the immediate harms of that risky behavior. Reid (2002) emphasized that harm reduction neither excludes nor presumes the long-term treatment goal of abstinence; instead, it focuses on the consequences of the immediate harms. The harms addressed can relate to factors including individuals' physical and psychological health, social environment, economic outlook, or a multitude of other factors. For HIV test counseling, the focus of the discussion would not be on how individuals placed themselves at risk for HIV but rather how to cope with the outcome of that behavior because of the understanding that behavior is a multifaceted phenomenon and impacts the community within which it is embedded.

Priority of Immediate Goals.    HRT focuses attention on immediate concerns and offers choices in addressing those concerns. Most harm reduction programs have a hierarchy of goals, with an emphasis on proactively engaging individuals, target groups, and communities to address their most pressing needs. During HIV test counseling sessions this translates into the client, rather than the counselor, being the primary agent for reducing the harm of risky behaviors to self and others. The counselor mostly listens and offers healthier options for consideration by the client.

Balancing Costs and Benefits.    HRT encourages a utilitarian cost–benefit analysis that extends beyond the immediate interests of individuals to include broader community and societal interests—such that the harmful costs of risky behaviors are recognized and reduced while maximizing the benefits of healthy behaviors for all. For HIV test counseling, this means providing immediate, personalized care to individuals that would help curb the long-term use of community resources such as mental health and other health care services.

Reid (2002) summarized that harm reduction seeks to remedy problems through pragmatic, nonjudgmental interventions and policies. The tenets of HRT thus encompass a pragmatic, nonjudgmental focus on harm, costs, and benefits; and rather than striving to understand how and why individuals placed themselves at risk for HIV/AIDS, the focus is on the current and immediate future goals of individuals for reducing the risk of harms for themselves and others in their community.


## Criticisms of Harm Reduction

HRT is not without strong political critics. Arguments against HRT stem from its historical roots in drug abuse prevention, the difficulties evaluating the philosophy of harm reduction except through specific activities or programs, and the potential for conflicts of interest by harm reduction staff. In the United States, in particular, there is grave concern that harm reduction strategies, such as needle exchange programs for IDUs, actually condone drug use and may serve as masks worn by the drug legalization movement. Accordingly, public health efforts tend to focus on use reduction rather than harm reduction (MacCoun, 1998).

Another major criticism is that harm reduction programs are difficult, if not impossible, to measure and evaluate unlike programs aimed at reducing prevalence (MacCoun, 1998). Hilton et al. (2001) noted that doing harm reduction can be "costly, hard to contain, hard to control and requires observation and action at times and in a manner that is unusual for many researchers, such as collecting information that can be ethically and legally problematic" (p. 266). Ironically, the key reason for the failure to effectively evaluate harm reduction programs may stem from the political opposition to allowing this approach to cultivate.

A related problem of conflict of personal and professional interests may be inherent within staff. If a staff member is trained and/or believes in abstinence, for example, a conflict of interest can arise because HRT requires that staff members be open, nonjudgmental, and accepting of all behaviors, even risk-taking and risk-causing behaviors. In addition, Conley et al. (1998) suggest that because HRT is often applied to marginalized behaviors, practitioners must be careful not to get too caught up in related-issue advocacy such as poverty, racism, and human rights because their primary focus should be reducing immediate harm to the individuals and their community. Despite these criticisms, HRT holds great promise for reinvigorating HIV test counseling as an HIV prevention tool.

*Reframing HRT Tenets for Application to HIV/AIDS Prevention*

According to Mattson (2000), when applied to HIV/AIDS and safer sex, the tenets of HRT can be modified to include the following:

- Individuals deserve to be treated with respect, dignity, and compassion.
- Inevitably most people will practice unsafe sex.
- Unsafe sex is not necessarily the problem but likely is a symptom or a coping mechanism for dealing with other complex issues (e.g., low self-esteem, abuse, relationship problems).
- Unsafe sex can result in harm to individuals who practice unsafe sex, their loved ones, and their communities.
- This harm can result in personal, social, political, and economic hardship.
- Individuals can make reasonable, informed choices to reduce harm to themselves and others.
- HIV/AIDS interventionists need to recognize, through training and self-reflexivity, that they may have personal biases and make judgments about individuals who practice unsafe sex. After recognizing these biases, they need to consciously alleviate their impact on counseling these individuals.
- HIV/AIDS prevention strategies must be relevant to and practical for individuals.
- The emphasis of HIV/AIDS prevention needs to be on attainable, short-term, personalized results over idealistic and often impractical long-term goals.

Consistent with Mattson's reframing of HRT for HIV test counseling, MacCoun (1998) and Roche, Evans, and Staton (2001) have suggested integrative or complementary frameworks for approaching drug use and other risky health behaviors. These frameworks recognize that continued use of unhealthy behaviors, abstinence, and harm reduction need to be conceptualized and practiced as overlapping strategies embedded within societal, community, and individual environments. The application-driven HIV test counseling model we propose in the next section is grounded in HRT and a constellation of ideas about integrated approaches to risk reduction.

Toward a Reconceptualized HIV Test
Counseling Model Framed by HRT

Like other difficult and controversial health issues that have been considered from a harm reduction perspective including abuse of drugs
and alcohol, persuading individuals to practice safer sex is a complicated issue that will likely require a contextualized, integrated model
that respects challenges to the individual but also respects community-level needs. Roche et al. (2001) forwarded a two-level model of
integrated drug strategy. The micro level consists of four intersecting
rings representing the nonjudgmental yet understandably contested
integration of current operational approaches to decreasing drug
abuse including harm reduction, use reduction, nonuse, and abstinence. Areas of overlap among these approaches, no matter how small,
are emphasized as places to build common ground for individual and
community health. These concentric circles are located within a wider
context consisting of macrolevel forces such as equity, culture, and
gender. Health care and other organizations must take these factors
into consideration as they respond to health issues that threaten their
community. We were drawn to this model because it embraces integration allowing the scope and latitude for various approaches to operate in concert. Similarly, we acknowledge the benefits of the current
CDC protocol for CTR, especially its client-centered design, but we
suggest that infusing the tenets of HRT will provide a more integrated
approach to addressing the complex issue of preventing HIV/AIDS.

MacCoun (1998) also proposes an integrated model of use reduction
and harm reduction interventions for drug abuse. This model emphasizes the importance of specifying levels of analysis and incorporates
three approaches to reducing the harms associated with drug use
including prevalence reduction, quantity reduction, and harm reduction. Basically, this framework proposes a causal path model including
a formula for determining the total harm of drug use as equaling average harm per use (i.e., harms to users and nonusers) multiplied by total
use (i.e., number of users and quantity each user consumes). Although
we shy away from linear approaches to VCT, MacCoun's attention to
the links between personal-level and community-level harms and the
implications for harm reduction interventions is instructive for our
proposed harm reduction framework for VCT.

Informed by the integrative harm reduction models proposed by
Roche et al. (2001) and MacCoun (1998), Figure 5.1 depicts an integrative

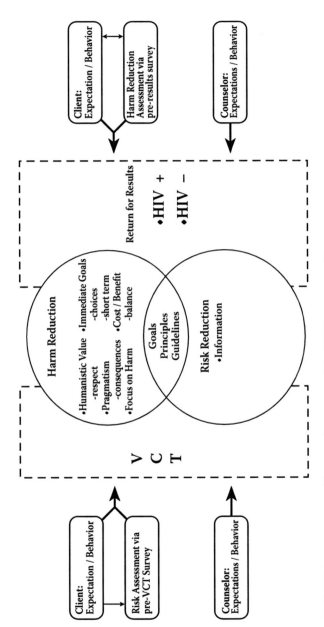

**FIGURE 5.1.** Integrated harm reduction model of HIV test counseling.

model for HIV test counseling that blends the tenets of HRT with the current CDC protocol for CTR. The VCT session is represented by the two rectangular boxes outlined with dashes—that is, the initial HIV test counseling session and the return-for-results session. Each of these sessions is influenced by the client's and the counselor's pre-existing expectations about the session. For example, clients come to the HIV test counseling session with a set of expectations about how the session will be conducted and what they will talk about with the counselor. Realizing that in most cases clients make an appointment for VCT because they have practiced risky behaviors, an important revision within this integrated approach would be for clients to fill out a risk assessment survey about their attitudes and safer-sex behaviors prior to the beginning of the counseling session (i.e., while in the waiting room). In preparation for the session, the counselor would review the survey responses. This would assist the counselor in understanding the perspective of the client and would give the counselor clues about how to approach the session in an individualized and tailored way with the goal of harm reduction. Counselors also bring a set of expectations about how counseling should occur and about clients' orientation to HIV/AIDS prevention. These expectations often are deeply rooted in counselors' socialization and training, but through the strategies incorporated within the integrated framework counselors can reshape their approach to be more individualized and focused on harm reduction for clients and others in their community.

Similarly, clients' and counselors' expectations and behavior shape the return for results session in which clients are told whether their test was positive for HIV. To facilitate an effective follow-up session, clients should be given a harm reduction assessment survey as they are waiting for their follow-up counseling session. This survey would ask what the client remembers from the HIV prevention strategies discussed at the first session and their safer-sex and other HIV prevention behaviors since the previous session. After perusing the survey prior to the session, counselors could pinpoint issues for individually focused discussion during the follow-up session. Instead of emphasizing the results of the HIV blood test (i.e., regardless of result), the counselor should utilize this opportunity for further HIV prevention for the client and others.

As the concentric circles in the model illustrate, an integration of risk reduction and harm reduction can be accomplished during VCT, the notion being that HIV prevention is heightened when harm reduction and risk reduction approaches intersect via the goals (i.e., increasing knowledge, providing access to those at risk), principles (i.e., confidentiality, responsive and appropriate counseling and testing), and guidelines (i.e., personalized risk assessment, negotiation about and specific skills to aid accomplishment) of VCT. Infusing the current risk reduction–oriented objectives and activities of VCT with the tenets of HRT would further centralize the concerns of clients by emphasizing respect and focusing on their immediate goals and choices given the realistic barriers to healthier and less harmful behavior that they are facing. In this way, both risk minimization and harm reduction become mindful to the counselor and permeate the discussion with the client.

To further explain the model, we bring our integrated approach to the level of practice by reframing a portion of the two excerpts introduced previously. Note that the counselor's reframed language is less paternalistic, and more pragmatic and responsive to the client's unique concerns and needs in the moment while maintaining the spirit of the goals, principles, and guidelines of VCT. In addition, the counselor supports the accurate knowledge, positive choices, and good decision making exhibited by the client.

### Reframed Excerpt 1

HP: OK, looking back now are you comfortable with the choices you made [actual discussion]?

C: Pregnancy is a big deal, it changes your life but AIDS pretty much kills you, so no, I guess I was focusing on the wrong thing.

HP: So, what will happen if this comes up again, you meet someone you are attractive to him and he is attracted to you?

*I understand why you would be focused on just pregnancy but you are also right—if you are having or intend to have unprotected sex, you should also be concerned about AIDS. But what will you do if this situation happens again, where you meet someone you are attracted to?* [reframed discussion in italics]

C: No, I wouldn't sleep with him unless I was in a relationship.

*It's not like I would sleep with him, unless I was in a relationship.*

HP: He offers a relationship and things are going well, so do you have unprotected sex with him?

*That's great but what if he offers you a relationship?*

C: Yeah, well, I don't know. I wouldn't have unprotected sex unless I knew. First of all, I would still be on birth control but that doesn't affect AIDS, hmm. I would want to know if he has been tested.

*I would either make sure that I had protected sex or make sure I know his sexual history and want to make sure he has been tested. I am on birth control but it's not like that's protecting me from AIDS.*

HP: OK, so he shows you a piece of paper and oh he's everything, totally groovy, he shows you the lab result and has been tested negative, he tells you he has only been with a few other women in his life and that you are so beautiful. That's all going great and you know you have been tested negative. Do you have unprotected sex with him?

*That's true; you should make sure he has been tested. But, you should also keep in mind that doesn't mean he is 100% safe either. Because the tests are only valid from six months after the last intercourse, so you also want to make sure he has been tested after his last relationship and/or intercourse.*

C: I mean, I guess I would, I would feel guilty if I didn't.

*That's good to know, otherwise I would have felt guilty not to have unprotected sex, after seeing his papers.*

HP: Are you telling me what you think I want to hear or what you believe?

*You know, you always have a choice and perhaps, if you feel uncomfortable or guilty, you should consider asking him to wait until both of you are tested.*

C: Obviously, unless I didn't trust him.

*Well, I wouldn't have unprotected sex if I didn't trust him.*

HP: You trust him; from the short amount of time he seems very trustworthy and very honest.

*Yes, that might be the case. But, what if it is just someone you have recently met? In this case, for you to trust him you might need for him to be tested first and using protection until then. Of course, if you have been with the same partner for a longer time then you might be able to trust him since you already know his history.*

C: Yes, I would do the same.


## Reframed Excerpt 2

HP: OK, so when you guys are off and on and you are off and he normally does things and sees other people and when it's on hmm, you

guys go six months no sex or safe sex and then he takes a test
and after the test you go back to not using protection.

*During this on-and-off time, do you know if your boyfriend
has had any other sexual partners?*

C: (interrupting) Oh now, it's not like we have a set pattern or this calendar
here. No, it's not like that, OK?

*We were monogamous for two and a half years and then we
didn't see each other for two years and he had a girlfriend in that
period of time and was monogamous with her and we just got
back together since like January.*

HP: OK, and after the breakup with his girlfriend he waited six months and
took the HIV test.

*Since you have been back together, have either of you or both
of you been tested?*

C: No, he's taken them in between.

*Yes, he has been tested since we were back together.*

HP: So he waited less than six months and so it's been less than six months
since the last time he has been with his ex-girlfriend, right?

*OK, to make sure we have the right time frame, are you saying
that he took his test in less than six months since the last time he
was with his ex-girlfriend?*

C: Just about.

HP: Yeah, so just about but not totally.

*OK, looking at this time frame, he might not have been covered
from his last intercourse. Which means that he might have to be
retested again to cover those last six months.*

C: Well, in December.

*(probably won't need this)*

HP: Which means the test he took is totally inaccurate.

*(probably won't need this)*

C: But if he has been with the same girl.

*Does that matter even if he has been with the same girl?*

HP: It doesn't matter. And if she never got tested. Do you know if she
got tested?

*It wouldn't matter as much, if she has also been tested. Do you
know if she has been tested?*

C: I believe so, but I wouldn't say I am positive on that.

HP: Well, if she never got tested and she did things you know during the
time of the breakup, it doesn't mean a thing.

*In that case, for now let's assume she hasn't been tested. If you
find out later that she was tested then that's good, but for now let's
see what we can do to ensure you are safe.*

C: But they weren't together after the breakup.

> *OK. So if she was tested and they haven't been together after the breakup, I'm OK? And if she wasn't tested and they were together after the breakup, then I'm not?*

HP: Even before they got together and if she didn't get tested before that and she did and it was less than six months, then it's an inaccurate test. You have to remember that what the person does six months before the test or after does not make that test accurate. So, even though you might feel that you are safe, think about it, you may not be.

> *Yes, but remember, even if she was tested but the test occurred less than six months before her last intercourse then the test wouldn't have been accurate. From the information we have now, it seems there are too many ifs—so let's just see what we can do to keep you safe under these circumstances.*

Although the integrated harm reduction model of HIV test counseling incorporates many aspects of the current CDC protocol and further emphasizes client-centered care, we do not suspect this approach will take more than the current average appointment block of approximately 20 minutes per session.[3] Because the client is filling out the risk assessment prior to the start of the session, the time with the counselor can be optimally utilized to address the client's specific risk behaviors from a more personalized harm reduction approach without adding costly minutes to the average per-session time frame.

Now that our integrated harm reduction model of HIV test counseling has been introduced and illustrated using reframed dialogue, we recognize the limitations of this approach and offer ideas for future research and praxis.

## Limitations and Future Directions

Although proposing a revised framework for HIV test counseling is an exciting, albeit idealistic, project, we acknowledge the limitations of this exercise and, in turn, offer viable future directions for research and practice. One obvious limitation of the proposed approach to HIV test counseling stems from its infancy. Although the model was generated from empirical discourse recorded during actual HIV test counseling sessions, this chapter was not a research report and we have yet to test this model. Future research and practice could address this limitation in three ways. First, it would be interesting to gather reactions about the feasibility of the model from administrators of VCT programs and HIV test counselors. Based on this input, the model could be revised accordingly. We have already begun such a research project in Katmandu, Nepal, where VCT sessions are mandated by funding agencies and are accomplished in collaboration with the government at four testing centers. We chose to start our research on this model abroad because these VCT programs are already expressly based on the principles of harm reduction. In Katmandu, all counselors attend the same VCT program training and every 6 months they are required to attend a refresher course. In addition, we learned that the counselors are forming a coalition to network about their VCT experiences in an effort to support each other and maintain consistent program goals within and across sites. When asked about the feasibility of our integrated model, both the administrators and counselors appreciated how it incorporated the tenets of harm reduction and the CDC protocol because this is how they practice VCT, especially given that most of their clients are drug users and commercial sex workers. Our next step in this research project is to revise the model based on the suggestions we received. For example, a few of the HIV test counselors recommended that our model reflect the flexibility required to respond to clients' needs for the timing of their pretest and posttest. Some clients are ready to take the HIV test and receive results on the same day (via rapid testing) with the time between testing and result available to discuss unique concerns about HIV/AIDS identified by the client. Other clients want to receive information about the VCT process with the option to return another day for testing and counseling. An HRT approach would better incorporate both of these (and other) possibilities.

Second, an HIV test counselor training program could be developed based on the revised model. The training program could feature a modular curriculum including the integrated harm reduction model for HIV test counseling, testing and lab procedures, performance standards, role plays with participants at different knowledge levels and with different reasons for being tested, sources of counselor support (e.g., take-home materials to reinforce key learning points, buddy counselor support system), and a visit to a VCT site for a realistic job preview. This program could then be used to train VCT trainers and service providers. Third, comparative field studies could be designed and conducted to determine the effectiveness of the proposed model in practice.

Another limitation of this project is that we run the risk of offending those already involved in HIV test counseling work by suggesting that their current approach is not sufficiently individualized or client centered to encourage both risk and harm reduction. On the contrary, we appreciate the challenges faced by practicing VCT counselors and applaud them for their dedication. Many VCT practitioners are seasoned veterans who were probably socialized in one primary approach to counseling and over time were retrained in another more contemporary approach (and in some cases were retrained again and again). In keeping with this progression, our model and the companion training program we allude to would become a recurrent training opportunity, possibly for continuing education credit, for these veteran counselors and their more novice counterparts. Although we recognize the limitations of this modeling project, mere mention does not preclude the need to further address these concerns in future research. Proposing a reconceptualization of current thinking and practice is never easy, but progress, especially in the realm of HIV/AIDS prevention, is always worth the effort.

HIV/AIDS continues to be a pandemic that threatens personal and community safety but many do not realize this because they do not consider themselves susceptible, despite engaging in risky behaviors. Given the precarious situation in the United States and around the world, HIV prevention counselors simply cannot provide information about risk reduction and expect people to stop putting themselves and others at risk. These rather conservative and standardized messages are likely to be rejected, producing no change in behavior. Instead, we propose infusing HIV test counseling with the tenets of HRT, which allows room for dialogue that can promote and empower clients to realize the ramifications of their actions for themselves and others with an emphasis on behavior change. This approach also celebrates counselors' respect for clients and willingness to encourage them to own the agenda for the counseling session. This includes allowing clients to change the course of the conversation to meet their individual needs, as illustrated in the reframed HIV test counseling excerpts. Although HRT is controversial and there are limitations to incorporating HRT into a revised VCT framework, integrating this contemporary approach into the already accepted CTR protocol may compound the success rate of

HIV test counseling to promote behavior change, which could be an influence factor in reducing the spread of HIV/AIDS.

## Notes

1. The two excerpts presented here were selected from 45 audiotape recordings of HIV test counseling sessions that were collected for a comprehensive research project by Mattson (1999, 2000; Mattson & Roberts, 2001). After carefully listening to a random sample of the recordings and reading the transcripts, the second author chose the two excerpts we build on in this chapter based on their representativeness across counselors in both content and execution of the protocol.
2. The Harm Reduction Network serves regions throughout the world including Australia (http://www.ihra.net), Asia (http://www.ahrn.net), Canada (http://www.canadianharmreduction.com), and Central and Eastern Europe (http://www.ceehrn.org).
3. Although a random sample of testing sites revealed that the average appointment block for an HIV test is 20 minutes, the actual HIV test counseling session is often shorter. When asked why these sessions are generally short in duration, a number of organizational constraints were listed with the most often being limited staff and financial resources.

## References

Aidala, A. A., Lee, G, Garbers, S., & Chiasson, M. A. (2006). Sexual behaviors and sexual risk in a prospective cohort of HIV-positive men and women in New York City, 1994–2002: Implications for prevention. *AIDS Education and Prevention, 18,* 12–32.

Amaro, H., Morrill, A. C., Dai, J., Cabral, H., & Raj, A. (2005). Heterosexual behavioral maintenance and change following HIV counseling and testing. *Journal of Health Psychology, 10*(2), 287–300.

American Medical Association. (2002). *Universal, routine screening of pregnant women for HIV infection.* Chicago: Author.

Bradley-Springer, L. (1996). Patient education for behavior change: Help from the transtheoretical and harm reduction models. *The Journal of the Association of Nurses in AIDS Care, 7*(1), 23–33.

Centers for Disease Control and Prevention. (2001a). *HIV prevention strategic plan through 2005.* Atlanta, GA: Author.

Centers for Disease Control and Prevention. (2001b). *Revised guidelines for HIV counseling, testing, and referral.* Atlanta, GA: Author.

Centers for Disease Control and Prevention. (2001c). Revised guidelines for HIV counseling, testing, and referral: Technical expert panel review of CDC HIV counseling, testing, and referral guidelines. *Morbidity and Mortality Weekly Report, 50*(RR19), 1–58.

Centers for Disease Control and Prevention. (2003a). Advancing HIV prevention: New strategies for a changing epidemic—United States, 2003. *Morbidity and Mortality Weekly Report, 52*(15), 329–332.

Centers for Disease Control and Prevention. (2003b). HIV testing—United States, 2001. *Morbidity and Mortality Weekly Report, 52*(23), 540–545.

Centers for Disease Control and Prevention. (2005a). *HIV/AIDS surveillance report: Cases of HIV infection and AIDS in the United States, 2004* (Vol. 16). Atlanta, GA: Author.

Centers for Disease Control and Prevention. (2005b, June). National HIV Prevention Conference, Atlanta, GA. Retrieved August 4, 2005, from http://www.kaisernetwork.com.

Conley, P., Hewitt, D., Mitic, W., Polin, C., Riley, D., Room, R., et al. (1998). Harm reduction: Concepts and practices. Retrieved March 3, 2006, from http://www.ccsa.ca/wgharm.htm.

Des Jarlais, D. (1995). Harm reduction: A framework for incorporating science into drug policy (Editorial). *American Journal of Public Health, 85*(1), 10–11.

Fylkesnes, K., & Siziya, S. (2004). A randomized trial on acceptability of voluntary HIV counseling and testing. *Tropical Medicine and International Health, 9*(5), 566–572.

Hilton, A., Thompson, R., Moore-Dempser, L., & Janzen, R. (2001). Harm reduction theories and strategies for the control of human immunodeficiency virus: A review of the literature. *Journal of Advanced Nursing, 33,* 357–370.

Hollander, D. (2001). Personalized HIV counseling and testing show promise in reducing risk behaviors. *International Family Planning Perspectives, 27*(1), 49–50.

Hopkins, S. G., Gelfand, S. E., Buskin, S. E., Kent, J. B., Kahle, E. M., & Barkan, S. E. (2005). HIV testing behaviors and attitudes after adoption of name-to-code HIV case surveillance in Washington state. *Journal of Public Health Management Practice, 11*(1), 25–28.

Ickovics, J. R., Morrill, A. C., Beren, S. E., Walsh, U., & Rodin, J. (1994). Limited effects of HIV counseling and testing for women: A prospective study of behavior and psychological consequences. *Journal of the American Medical Association, 272,* 443–448.

Institute of Medicine. (2000). *No time to lose: Getting more from HIV prevention.* Washington, DC: National Academy Press.

Janssen, R., Holtgrave, D., Valdiserri, R., Shepherd, M., Gayle, H., & De Cock, K. M. (2001). The serostatus approach to fighting the HIV epidemic: Prevention strategies for infected individuals. *American Journal of Public Health, 91,* 1019–1024.

Judson, F. N., & Vernon, T. M., Jr. (1988). The impact of AIDS on state and local health departments: Issues and a few answers. *American Journal of Public Health, 78*(4), 387–393.

Kalichman, S. C. (2000). HIV transmission risk behaviors of men and women living with HIV-AIDS: Prevalence, predictors, and emerging clinical interventions. *Clinical Psychology: Science and Practice, 7,* 32–47.

Kalichman, S. C. (Ed.). (2005). *Positive prevention: Reducing HIV transmission among people living with HIV/AIDS.* New York: Springer.

Kalichman, S. C., Rompa, D., & Cage, M. (2000). Sexually transmitted infections among HIV seropositive men and women. *Sexually Transmitted Infections, 76,* 350–354.

Kalichman, S. C., Rompa, D., DiFonzo, K., Simpson, D., Kyomugisha, F., Austin, J., et al. (2001). Initial development of scales to assess self-efficacy for disclosing HIV status and negotiating safer sex in HIV-positive persons. *AIDS and Behavior, 5,* 291–296.

Kamb, M. L., Dillon, B. A., Fishbein, M., & Willis, K. L. (1996). Quality assurance of HIV prevention counseling in a multi-center randomized controlled trial: Project RESPECT study group. *Public Health Reports, 111*(Suppl. 1), 99–107.

Kamb, M. L., Fishbein, M., Douglas, J. M., Jr., Rhodes, F., Rogers, J., Bolan, G., et al. (1998). Efficacy of risk-reduction counseling to prevent human immunodeficiency virus and sexually transmitted diseases: A randomized controlled trial. *Journal of the American Medical Association, 280,* 1161–1167.

Kelly, J. A., Hoffman, R., Rompa, D., & Gray, M. (1998). Protease inhibitor combination therapies and perceptions of gay men regarding AIDS severity and the need to maintain safer sex. *AIDS, 12,* F91–F95.

Luginaah, I. N., Yiridoe, E. K., & Taabazuing, M. M. (2005). From mandatory to voluntary testing: Balancing human rights, religious and cultural values, and HIV/AIDS prevention in Ghana. *Social Science & Medicine, 61,* 1689–1700.

MacCoun, R. (1998). Toward a psychology of harm reduction. *American Psychologist, 53,* 1199–1208.

Mattson, M. (1999). Reconceptualizing communication cues to action in the health belief model: HIV test counseling. *Communication Monographs, 66,* 240–265.

Mattson, M. (2000). Empowerment through agency-promoting dialogue: An explicit application of harm reduction theory to reframe HIV test counseling. *Journal of Communication, 5,* 333–347.

Mattson, M., & Roberts, F. (2001). Overcoming truth telling as an obstacle to initiating safer sex: Discussing deception in pre-HIV test counseling sessions. *Health Communication, 13,* 343–362.

McHale, A. (1996). Risk reduction strategies in the control of AIDS. *Professional Nursing, 11,* 731–733.

McKee, N., Bertrand, J. T., & Becker-Benton, A. (2004). *Strategic communication in the HIV/AIDS epidemic.* Thousand Oaks, CA: Sage.

Miller, W. R., & Rollnick, S. (1991). *Motivational interviewing: Preparing people to change addictive behavior.* New York: Guilford.

Prochaska, J. O., Redding, C., Harlow, L., Rossi, J., & Velicer, W. (1994). The transtheoretical model of change and HIV prevention: A review. *Health Education Quarterly, 21,* 471–486.

Pronyk, P. M., Kim, J. C., Makhubele, M. B., Hargreaves, J. R., Mohlala, R., & Hausler, H. P. (2002). Introduction of voluntary counselling and rapid testing for HIV in rural South Africa: From theory to practice. *AIDS Care, 14*(6), 859–865.

Reid, R. (2002). Harm reduction and injection drug use: Practical lessons from a public health model. *Health and Social Work, 27,* 223–226.

Riley, D. (1993). *The harm reduction model: Pragmatic approaches to drug use from the area between intolerance and neglect.* Retrieved March 6, 2006, from http://www.ccsa.ca/harmred.html.

Roche, A., Evans, K., & Staton, W. (2001). Harm reduction: Road less travelled to the Holy Grail. *Addiction, 92,* 1207–1212.

Rosenberg, J. (2003). Not all Ohio physicians offer HIV testing during standard prenatal care. *Perspectives on Sexual and Reproductive Health, 35*(4), 194–195.

Schiltz, M. A., & Sandfort, T. M. (2000). HIV-positive people, risk and sexual behaviour. *Social Science and Medicine, 50,* 1571–1588.

Strathdee, S. A., & Patterson, T. L. (2005). HIV-positive and HCV-positive drug users. In S. C. Kalichman (Ed.), *Positive prevention: Reducing HIV transmission among people living with HIV/AIDS* (pp. 135–162). New York: Springer.

Sweat, M., Gregorich, S., Sangiwa, G., Furlonge, C., Balmer, D., Kamenga, C., et al. (2000). Cost-effectiveness of voluntary HIV-1 counseling and testing in reducing sexual transmission of HIV-1 in Kenya and Tanzania. *Lancet, 356*(9224), 113–121.

van de Perre, P. (2000). HIV voluntary counselling and testing in community health services. *Lancet, 356,* 86–87.

Voluntary HIV-1 Counseling and Testing Efficacy Study Group. (2000). Efficacy of voluntary HIV-1 counseling and testing in individuals and couples in Kenya, Tanzania, and Trinidad: A randomised trial. *Lancet, 356*(9224), 103–112.

Weinhardt, L. S., Carey, M. P., Johnson, B. T., & Bickham, N. L. (1999). Effects of HIV counseling and testing on sexual risk behavior: A meta-analytic review of published research, 1985–1997. *American Journal of Public Health, 89,* 139–1405.

# 6

# Talking About HIV and AIDS
## *A Focus on Parent–Child Discussions*

*Colleen K. DiIorio*

*Frances McCarty*

*Erika Pluhar*
Emory University

Mary, the mother of Derrick, a 6-year-old boy, was surprised when her son asked her what "AIDS" meant. Mary recalled reading that the best first step to take when a child asks an unexpected question is to ask what the child thinks the word or phrase means. "That's a good question, and I'm glad you asked me. What do you know about what 'AIDS' is, Derrick?" Mary asked, carefully monitoring the tone of her voice and her body language. Derrick replied that he did not know; he thought it was something bad because his classmates were kidding his friend, who was mad about being told by other kids that he had AIDS. Mary used the opportunity to talk with Derrick about AIDS, noting it was a disease that affected adults, but not many children.

Mary was not always comfortable talking to her children about AIDS. She recalled that when her older son, Liam, was 9, and her daughter Renee was 6, Renee asked her what "AIDS" was. Mary attempted to find a way to answer. Liam laughed and declared that he knew. Mary didn't want Liam to give Renee the information (whether it was accurate or not) but she felt too embarrassed to answer herself. She finally mumbled that it was a bad disease that Renee didn't need to know about, and she instructed Liam not to talk to Renee about it. Mary quickly changed the subject and asked the kids about their homework. Later Mary thought about the incident, and though she felt relief that she had averted the conversation, she also wondered if she had missed an opportunity to give her children accurate information. This conversion motivated Mary to learn how she could provide age-appropriate HIV and AIDS information to her children.

The questions and concerns, successes and missed opportunities that Mary faces talking to her children about HIV and AIDS are not unlike those of most parents. Parents often admit to not always knowing what to say, when to say it, and how best to explain these complex issues. One reason for the confusion and discomfort in discussing HIV/AIDS is the fact that the predominant mode of HIV transmission is through sexual intercourse. Thus, frank parent–child discussions about HIV prevention often involve messages about sexual intercourse and disease prevention strategies including abstinence and condom use. The pervasiveness of sexual messages in the media and sexually explicit advertising adds to the challenge of effectively imparting age-appropriate and accurate information while communicating family values about sexuality.

Parents' interest in being informed and developing communication skills about sexuality, in general, and HIV/AIDS, in particular, is reflected in the number of books and magazine articles devoted to the topic. For example, more than 50 books were located on Amazon.com with titles such as *Lynda Madaras Talks to Teens About AIDS: An Essential Guide for Parents, Teachers, and Young People; Ten Talks Parents Must Have with Their Children About Sex and Character; Talking to Your Children About Sex: A Go Parents! Guide;* and *How to Talk with Teens About Love, Relationships, & S-E-X: A Guide for Parents.* Numerous Web sites are also available for parents to learn the facts about HIV and AIDS and gather ideas about how to discuss HIV prevention with their children and adolescents.

Researchers too have been drawn to the topic. Within the past 25 years, since the beginning of the AIDS era, more than 100 research studies have been conducted to assess the prevalence, content, factors, and outcomes associated with parent–child sex-based communication (DiIorio, Pluhar, & Belcher, 2003), and the motivation for much of this research has been to understand how to best promote HIV/AIDS discussions between parents and children.

The increased interest in studying parent–child HIV/AIDS communication corresponds to the rise in the number of AIDS cases among young adults and adolescents, and parental concerns about HIV/AIDS prevention for their children. The latest statistics show that 38,490 adolescents and adults between 13 and 24 years of age have been diagnosed with AIDS (Centers for Disease Control and Prevention [CDC], 2003). An alarming trend among this group is that the proportion of AIDS cases attributed to young people is increasing. In 1999, adolescents and young adults comprised 3.9% of all persons diagnosed with AIDS, and by 2003 the proportion had increased to 4.7%. To be successful in reducing and ultimately eliminating HIV transmission, public health initiatives must use a variety of approaches. Currently, HIV prevention for adolescents and young adults is focused within school systems and is generally included within the sex education curricula. Although this is one avenue for teaching youth about HIV and prevention strategies, other approaches to prevention are needed to reinforce learning and prevention messages. Because of their unique relationship to their children, parents can serve an important role to deliver and reinforce HIV prevention messages as their children progress from pre-adolescence through young adulthood.

Researchers have recognized the unique role that parents can play in HIV prevention and have studied content, process, and factors associated with parent–child discussions about HIV/AIDS. In this chapter, we present an overview of parent–child HIV/AIDS communication. The following review focuses on three areas: (a) HIV/AIDS communication prevalence, content, and process, (b) predictors of HIV/AIDS communication, and (c) influence of parent–child HIV/AIDS communication on adolescent sexual health outcomes. We end the chapter with a brief discussion of the limitations of parent–child sex-based communication research.

## Communication Prevalence, Content, and Process

Most studies assessing parent–child HIV/AIDS communication have been embedded within larger studies assessing sex-based communication between parents and children (DiIorio et al., 2003) and most have focused on prevalence and content of discussions. Overall, the studies show that when queried, most parents (72% to 98%) state that they had "talked to their child about sex." In a nationally representative survey among 880 parents, children, and adolescents, 70% to 78% of parents reported talking with kids about sex-based topics including AIDS, basic facts of sexual reproduction, relationships, becoming sexually active, and how to prevent pregnancy and sexually transmitted diseases (STDs; Kaiser Family Foundation, 1999). Percentages were less for parents of children ages 10 to 12 years. Children as young as 10 years, however, reported wanting more information on how to deal with such issues as personal readiness for sex, protection against HIV/AIDS, and handling peer pressure to have sex.

In one study of predominantly Black and Hispanic parents and adolescents, 92% of mothers and 71% of adolescents reported discussing HIV and AIDS, and 85% of mothers and 70% of adolescents reported discussing STDs (Miller, Kotchick, Dorsey, Forehand, & Ham, 1998). In contrast, parents living in rural settings and those with younger children reported fewer discussions about HIV/AIDS-related issues (Jordan, Price, & Fitzgerald, 2000; Sly et al., 1995). Jordan et al. found that only 40% of parents living in a rural area said they had talked about STDs, and only 36% had talked about abstinence with their children. However, 92% of these parents believed education should include prevention information including condoms and birth control. In a study of first- through fifth-grade students, only 70% of mothers talked to their children about AIDS, and only 41% noted that their children had asked questions about AIDS (Sly et al., 1995).

When asked about specific topics, parents often rated HIV/AIDS as one of the more frequently discussed topics (DiIorio, Hockenberry-Eaton, Maibach, Rivero, & Miller, 1996; DiIorio, Kelley, & Hockenberry-Eaton, 1999; Miller, Kotchick et al., 1998). Other frequently discussed topics include condom use, homosexuality, abstinence, menstruation, reproduction, pregnancy, birth, and sexual values (DiIorio et al., 2003). Parents are less likely to discuss wet dreams/erections, masturbation, and abortion/abortion alternatives. Children, on the other hand, show more variability in their responses to "talking about sex with their parents." The percentage of children and adolescents reporting communication about "sex," "sexuality," or "sexual issues" with one or both of their parents ranges from 13% to 83% (DiIorio et al., 2003). When asked about specific sex-based topics, children reported discussions of STDs, HIV/AIDS, condoms, how to resist sexual pressure, abstinence/postponing sex, sexual intercourse, menstruation, dating relationships, and contraception/birth control (DiIorio, et al., 1999; Fox & Inazu, 1980a, 1980b; Holtzman & Rubinson, 1995; Hutchinson & Cooney, 1998; Kaiser Family Foundation, 1999; Miller, Kotchick et al., 1998; Newcomer

& Udry, 1985; Pistella & Bonati, 1998; Raffaelli, Bogenschneider, & Flood, 1998; Shoop & Davidson, 1994; Tucker, 1989).

Despite the relatively high rates of reported parent–child discussions about HIV/AIDS, some investigators have found that parents are susceptible to common HIV myths and often have misinformation about HIV and AIDS (Crawford, Thomas, & Zoller, 1993; Sly et al., 1995). Crawford et al. found that among a sample of homeless women, mothers with more education had more HIV/AIDS knowledge and communicated more with their children about HIV/AIDS as did mothers who had higher levels of self-esteem. However, mothers often did not perceive themselves at risk of contracting HIV.

Through the use of qualitative methodologies, researchers have identified several distinct components of the sex-based communication process, including openness (Miller, Kotchick et al., 1998), direct versus indirect communication (Hepburn, 1983), interactive versus didactic communication (Lefkowitz, Kahlbaugh, Au, & Sigman, 1998; Lefkowitz, Kahlbaugh, & Sigman, 1996; Lefkowitz, Romo, Corona, Au, & Sigman, 2000; Pluhar, 2001), and nonverbal/behavioral versus verbal communication (Ward & Wyatt, 1994). Lefkowitz and her colleagues conducted a series of studies designed to explore the nature and quality of mother and adolescent communication about sexual issues including HIV and AIDS. In the first study, the investigators filmed mothers and adolescents between the ages of 11 and 14 years discussing two types of conversations: those about sexuality and those that involved a conflict situation (Lefkowitz et al., 1996). They found that sexuality conversations were less interactive with less turn taking between the mother and her adolescent. Mothers tended to dominate sexuality conversations, and children expressed higher levels of shame compared to discussions about a conflict topic. Knowledge of HIV/AIDS was more highly correlated for mother and adolescent dyads whose conversations were interactive.

In subsequent studies exploring dominance in conversations, the investigators found that conversational dominance remained fairly consistent over time (Lefkowitz et al., 1998). That is, mothers who dominated sexuality conversations at the first assessment also tended to dominate conversations when assessed 2 years later. Discrepancies were noted in AIDS knowledge between mothers and their children who were ages 10 to 14 years at the first assessment. Mothers who dominated conversations at the first assessment showed greater differences in their knowledge compared to their children's at the second assessment. Although Latino mothers were more likely to dominate AIDS and sexuality conversations compared to Euro-American mothers, there was a tendency for all mothers to dominate sexuality and AIDS conversations when compared to conversations about conflicts (Lefkowitz, Romo et al., 2000).

Lefkowitz, Sigman, and Au (2000) also found that communication style could be altered with training. In an experimental study, they found that mothers who received training to promote a more conversational style of discussing sexuality and AIDS with their children were able to reduce their amount of speaking time, asked more open-ended questions, acted less judgmental, and discussed dating and sexuality more than were mothers who did not receive the training. Adolescents of mothers who received training showed some increase in AIDS knowledge, but there was no change in AIDS-related beliefs. This series of studies indicates that an interactive style of communication about sexuality and HIV/AIDS is a more effective way of transmitting information from parent to child. Pluhar (2001) supported these findings about an interactive communication process. In a qualitative study of communication about dating, teen sexual behavior, and birth control/safer-sex practices among African-American mothers and adolescent daughters, mother–daughter pairs who communicated interactively also had more close and connected relationships.

The style of conversations about AIDS has also been examined by gender of both the parent and the adolescent. In a study of children in Grades 6 to 8 and their parents, Whalen, Henker, Hollingshead, and Burgess (1996) found that AIDS conversations for both parents tended to be directive for sons and mutual for daughters. When examined by gender of the adolescent, boys tended to be withdrawn and girls more expressive. Father and daughter conversations tended to be mutual and included humor, whereas father and son conversations were more reserved and less interactive. Mothers also tended to be more directive with sons than daughters. O'Sullivan, Meyer-Bahlburg, and Watkins (2001) found that when urban Latina and African-American mothers talked to their daughters, they tended to focus on the dire consequences associated with sexual behavior, the daughter's responsibility in avoiding or controlling sexual encounters, and the daughter's reassurance of her intentions to avoid sex and pursue educational goals. Mothers rarely acknowledged positive aspects of sexuality outside the context of harm.

Investigators also have identified strategies parents use both to communicate with children about sexuality issues and to avoid such discussions. Strategies used to promote communication include using resources such as books and videos, role modeling, using a step-by-step approach, referring to religion and spirituality, being honest or "real," storytelling, and using persuasive arguments (Nwoga, 2000; Pluhar, Jennings, & DiIorio, 2006). Conversational dynamics parents and teens use to *avoid* discussing sexual issues include being flippant, making cut-off remarks, and using verbal platitudes (Aldous, 1983).

## Factors Associated with HIV/AIDS Communication

An enduring finding in the literature is that gender matters when parents talk to their children about sex. The results of numerous studies across race/ethnicity, socioeconomic status, and different age groups of children consistently indicate that mothers are more likely to communicate with children about sex-related topics than are fathers, that mothers are more likely to talk with daughters than with sons, and that fathers are more likely to talk with sons than with daughters (Bennett & Dickinson, 1980; DiIorio et al., 2003; Whalen et al., 1996). Investigators who have studied parental gender differences in communication about HIV/AIDS have also identified the mothers as the primary communicator (CDC, 1991; Miller, Kotchick et al., 1998). For example, Sly et al. (1995) found that although sons and daughters were equally likely to ask mothers questions about AIDS, mothers were more likely to talk to daughters than sons.

In general, fathers have not been included nearly as much as mothers in research on parent–child sexuality communication. The findings of studies that have included fathers as well as mothers consistently show less father–child compared to mother–child communication (Coreil & Parcel, 1983; Downie & Coates, 1999; Geasler, Dannison, & Edlund, 1995; Young & Core-Gebhart, 1993). The findings of some studies also suggest that parents communicate different amounts and about different sexuality topics with sons and daughters (DiIorio et al., 1996; Downie & Coates, 1999; Fisher, 1985; Geasler et al., 1995; Miller, Levin, Whitaker, & Xu, 1998; Nolin & Petersen, 1992; Sly et al., 1995). Nolin and Petersen found that parent–daughter communication was more wide-ranging than parent–son communication, and Downie and Coates concluded that parental messages for girls were more protective and focused on sexual limit setting and physical development than those for boys.

A few studies that focused on father–child communication reveal interesting findings. Lehr, Demi, DiIorio, and Facteau (2005) examined predictors of father–child communication about sexuality among a sample of fathers of adolescent sons. Fathers were more likely to talk with sons who were further along in pubertal development. Fathers who had more permissive sexual values were more likely to share information with their sons but permissive values were not predictive of fathers being more likely to share their values with their sons. Fathers with lower education levels reported more sexuality communication with sons, as well as fathers who had more communication with their own fathers about sexuality, and fathers who had more positive outcome expectations and greater self-efficacy for sexuality communication. Kirkman, Rosenthal, and Feldman (2005) explored the role of fathers as sexuality educator and suggested that fathers' difficulties in sexuality communication stem from two important but conflicting discourses—traditional masculinity and involved fatherhood.

In a group of African-American fathers and stepfathers who participated in an HIV intervention study and who were living with or saw their adolescent sons on a regular basis, communication about HIV and HIV-related topics was found to be relatively high (DiIorio, McCarty, Resnicow, Lehr, & Denzmore, 2007). In the HIV intervention group, approximately 77% of fathers and 80% of sons reported at least some discussion of the following topics: what the act of sexual intercourse is, sexually transmitted diseases, dangers of many sex partners, using a condom during sex, and getting AIDS. The percentage of those reporting some discussion in the study control group was somewhat lower with about 64% of fathers and 69% of sons reporting some discussion. The percentage of fathers indicating they had discussed getting AIDS with their sons was 83% in the HIV intervention group and 68% in the control group. The percentages were slightly higher for sons with 87% of sons in the intervention group and 75% of sons in the control group reporting some discussion. For these particular topics, fathers and sons tended to be in agreement about whether or not the topic had been discussed with the percentage of agreement ranging from about 74% for discussion of sexually transmitted diseases and 66% for discussion of the dangers of many sex partners. About 91% of fathers indicated that they would prob-ably or definitely discuss these topics with their adolescent sons in the future.

According to fathers, the primary reason for discussing a topic was to provide information. Only about 3% indicated talking about one of the aforementioned topics because of a problem. Generally, fathers dominated the discussion with about 66% of fathers indicat-ing that they talked more than the adolescent. Approximately 29% of fathers noted that they and their sons talked equally when discussing the topic. In this sample of fathers and adolescent sons, HIV knowl-edge was relatively high with fathers having a mean score of 85% and sons having a mean score of 75%. In addition, both fathers and sons reported a low perceived risk of ever having HIV. About 56% of fathers indicated that they had no chance at all of having HIV whereas only 9% to 25% indicated "no chance at all" for illnesses like heart attack and kidney disease. The same was true for sons with about 69% stat-ing no chance at all for HIV whereas the percentages ranged from 36% to 52% for illnesses like heart attack and kidney disease.

Several researchers have also examined age and race as potential predictors of sex-based communication. The findings related to age of the child and frequency or amount of discussions are few and inconsistent. Some researchers have found that discussions increase with age of the child (DiIorio et al., 2000; Hepburn, 1983; Rothen-berg, 1980; White, Wright, & Barnes, 1995) whereas others noted the opposite finding (Leland & Barth, 1993) or no difference with age (Pistella & Bonati, 1998). There is evidence, however, to suggest that most parents have discussed HIV/AIDS with their younger children (Sigelman, Derenowski, Mullaney, & Siders, 1993; Sigelman, Mukai, Woods, & Alfeld, 1994; White et al., 1995). As with studies of ado-lescents, parents of younger children are more likely to talk to their daughters than sons (Sly et al., 1995).

Pluhar, McCarty, and DiIorio (2007) assessed a broader set of sexu-ality related communication topics between a sample of urban, Afri-can-American mothers and 6- to 12-year-old children. Their results suggested that a wide range of sexuality topics is being addressed. Mothers of 6- to 10-year-old children reported communicating the most about physical sex differences, gender role differences, self-esteem, friendship, and physical appearance. Mothers of 11- to 12-year-old children reported communicating the most about the aforementioned topics in addition to being friends with boys/girls, pubertal changes, peer pressure, and names of sexual body parts. Mothers in both groups also reported talking about HIV and AIDS, although more focused discussions on when to have sex and preventive behaviors were more common among the older children. In this sample, there was an age-related increase in the percentage of mothers indicating they had talked to their child about HIV. About 33% of mothers with a 6-year-old indicated they had talked to their child, whereas 89% of mothers with a 12-year-old noted they had talked about HIV with their child. Although the age-related pattern was the same, the percentage of mothers in each child age group who indicated talking about sexual intercourse was lower—21% of mothers with a 6-year-old and 73% of mothers with a 12-year-old. Overall, older children and mothers of older children reported communicating about more topics than did younger children and mothers of younger children. As noted in other studies, a higher percentage of mothers reported communicating with female children compared to male children. For the topic of sexual intercourse, 47% of mothers of female children indicated talking about the topic compared to 35% of mothers with male children. Interestingly, about 80% of mothers with a female child noted they had talked about HIV with about 73% of mothers with a male child indicating they had talked about HIV.

The results were also mixed in the few studies in which discussions were compared by race or ethnicity (Coreil & Parcel, 1983; Crawford et al., 1993; Fox & Inazu, 1980a, 1980b; Leland & Barth, 1993; Rothenberg, 1980; Sly et al., 1995). Black parents have been found to be more involved in sexuality education than White or Hispanic parents in one study (Coreil & Parcel, 1983), whereas in another study both African-American and White parents reported talking more frequently to their children than did Latino parents (Crawford et al., 1993). In an early study, Fox and Inazu (1980a) found that the content of discussions varied by the race of the mother, with Black mothers more willing to talk about birth control and White mothers more likely to discuss a variety of sex topics. Researchers who focused on HIV and AIDS discussions also found no consistent patterns by race/ethnicity. In one study, non-Hispanic parents were more likely than Hispanics to discuss AIDS with their children (CDC, 1991), whereas in another, African-American young-adult women were more likely to recall communication about sexual risk reduction than were White women (Hutchinson & Cooney, 1998).

In addition to personal characteristics, researchers have examined attitudes, values, and beliefs as predictors of amount or frequency of sex-based discussions. In general, the more comfortable parents feel discussing sexual matters with their children, the more likely they are to report having had such discussions (Russo, 1991). More specifically, several researchers have found that mothers' self-reported confidence and positive outcome expectations for talking with their children about sexual issues were predictive of the frequency or amount of sex communication (DiIorio et al., 2000; Raffaelli et al., 1998). Furthermore, parents who have higher self-esteem, in general, appeared to report more frequent communication with their children about AIDS (Crawford et al., 1993). Brock and Jennings (1993) found that highly involved parents felt more comfortable talking about STDs and that teens of highly involved parents talked more openly about sex, AIDS, and STDs compared to noninvolved parents. Furthermore, uninvolved parents reported more barriers to parent–adolescent communication about sex and had less certain knowledge about AIDS facts. In a CDC (1991) study, parents with more self-reported knowledge about AIDS were more likely to discuss AIDS.

Cultural context and values are critical in understanding the sexual socialization that occurs through parent–child communication. For example, qualitative research with African-American families has shown that mothers have a tendency to use religious and spiritual messages to teach adolescents about sexual values (Pluhar, 2001). The use of religion as a vehicle for sexual socialization makes sense given the important role the church plays in the African-American community (Billingsley & Morrison-Rodriguez, 1998). In the study by Pluhar, McCarty, and DiIorio (2007) of urban, African-American mothers and 6- to 12-year-old children, there appears to be some association between importance of religious beliefs and discussion of HIV. The percentage of mothers who indicated talking about HIV was higher for those noting that their religious beliefs were quite or very important compared to those who indicated a moderate importance of religious beliefs. Other studies have identified storytelling as an important method for African-American mothers to accomplish socialization and discourage daughters from repeating maternal patterns such as early sexual activity and adolescent pregnancy (Nwoga, 2000; Pluhar, 2001). Pluhar and Kuriloff (2004) observed that affect and style were critical components of determining the perceived effectiveness of sexuality communication between

African-American mothers and adolescent daughters. Wilson and Donenberg (2004) found less mutuality in sex-based conversations between African-American parents and adolescents compared to Whites, which was protective against adolescent sexual risk taking.

Various aspects of family interactions and relationships form the context of parent–child communication about sexuality. Researchers have identified associations between several family-level factors and sexuality communication. The process of communication in general, especially when it is open and problem-free, has been found to be related to a higher likelihood of sexuality discussions between parents and children (Fisher, 1990; White et al., 1995). Similarly, Coreil and Parcel (1983) found that parents who described relationships with their children as very close reported greater involvement in sexual communication and instruction compared to parents who said they were average in closeness, whereas parents who were more strict were less likely to communicate about sex with children. Raffaelli et al. (1998) found that teens who reported one good talk with their mother about personal issues in the past year were more likely also to report discussing sexual topics. A retrospective study with Latino college students examined several family structure variables (Raffaelli & Green, 2003). The authors found that sexual communication between mothers and daughters was negatively associated with having older brothers. The absence of older brothers also predicted sexual communication between fathers and both daughters and sons.

## Communication About HIV/AIDS and Sexual Health Outcomes

One of the areas of most interest to researchers has been the predictive power of sex-based discussions in fostering risk reduction practices among adolescents. These behaviors include abstinence and delayed sexual behavior, and condom use. Some researchers have found that the frequency or amount of discussion is associated with abstinence, delay of sexual intercourse (DiIorio et al., 1999; Furstenberg, Moore, & Peterson, 1985; Karofsky, Zeng, & Kosorok, 2001; Lehr, DiIorio, Dudley, & Lipana, 2000; Leland & Barth, 1993; Pick & Palos, 1995; Romer et al., 1999), and prevention practices (Fisher, 1987; Fox & Inazu, 1980a; Hutchinson, Jemmott, Jemmott, Braverman, & Fong, 2003; Pick & Palos, 1995). Yet others have found no association (Casper, 1990; Cvetkovich & Grote, 1983; Fisher, 1988, 1993; Furstenberg, Herceg-Baron, Shea, & Webb,

1984; Hovell et al., 1994; Kotva & Schneider, 1990; Liebowitz, Castellano, & Cuellar, 1999) or mixed findings (Fisher, 1989; Jaccard, Dittus, & Gordon, 1996).

Both Miller, Kotchick et al. (1998) and Whitaker and Miller (2000) found that parent–adolescent discussions about condoms were strongly associated with greater use of condoms among adolescents. Sexual-risk communication with mothers has also been found to be associated with greater condom use self-efficacy and sexual communication with partners (Hutchinson & Cooney, 1998). Similarly, Leland et al. (1993) found that students who had used safer-sex behaviors to avoid AIDS were more likely to have discussed a number of sexuality topics with parents. In this study, students who communicated with parents were more likely to have not had sexual intercourse, to have had fewer pregnancies, to have tried to avoid AIDS by using condoms and by having fewer sexual partners, and to show greater intentions for not engaging in high-risk sexual behaviors (Leland et al., 1993).

Clawson and Reese-Weber (2003) found that fathers played an equally important role as mothers in predicting later onset of sexual activity. Specifically, fathers who initiated discussions with their children before their children's first sexual-intercourse experience resulted in older age at first sexual intercourse. At the same time, discussions that occurred after first sexual intercourse, along with more frequent sexual communication, resulted in earlier age of first sexual intercourse. The differential effects of communication based on the gender of the child, the quality of communication, and parental values help clarify some results. For example, Moore, Peterson, and Furstenberg (1986) found that sexual communication with parents was related to a *reduced* probability of daughters having had intercourse, though related to an *increased* probability of intercourse among teenage sons. Darling and Hicks (1982) found that the frequency of sexual discussions between parents and teens was not related to the subsequent sexual behavior of daughters, whereas the frequency of communication of both positive and negative messages about sex were related to increased sexual activity of the son. In regard to quality of communication, some studies suggest that parent–child communication is a significant predictor of sexual-risk reduction *only* if teens felt their parents were open, skilled, and comfortable in their discussions (Whitaker, Miller, May, & Levin, 1999), and perceived their parents as having friendly and attentive styles of communication (Mueller &

Powers, 1990). However, in another study of African-American and Latino families, high levels of mutuality were associated with greater sexual risk taking, which led the authors to suggest that less mutuality in conversations about sexuality may be protective for urban, minority adolescents (Wilson & Donenberg, 2004).

In a nationally representative sample, Holtzman and Rubinson (1995) found that students who discussed HIV with their parents were less likely than those who did not to have multiple sex partners and unprotected intercourse, and to have ever injected drugs. Young women were more influenced by parental discussions of HIV, whereas young men were more influenced by peers. Students who had received HIV instruction in school were more likely to have talked about HIV with both parents and peers.

Timing of parental discussion may also be important as it appears that discussions about condom use that occurred prior to sexual debut may have a greater protective effect than discussions occurring after sexual debut (Miller, Levin et al., 1998). In other studies, parental values were important in the expression of the association. Jaccard and Dittus (1991) found that the influence of parent–child communication about sex was moderated by the values of the parent concerning teen sex behavior. In this study, conservative mothers who communicated with their children about sex were more effective in influencing the future sex behavior of their adolescents than were more permissive mothers. Similarly, Moore et al. (1986) found that sexual communication with conservative parents was related to a reduced probability of daughters having had intercourse. Satisfaction with the maternal relationship, maternal beliefs about sex, and the number of topics discussed between adolescent and mother have also been found to be predictive of adolescent sexual behavior and consistent condom use (DiIorio et al., 2000; Jaccard, Dittus, & Gordon, 2000; Romer et al., 1999).

## Limitations

The study of parent–child HIV/AIDS communication has increased our understanding of who talks, how they talk, and the effects of talking. Most of what we know about parent–child HIV/AIDS and sex-based communication is based on studies of conversations between mothers and their adolescents, most of whom are girls. As we continue to explore this area and use information to develop parent-based HIV prevention programs for children and adolescents, we need to identify gaps in our knowledge and limitations of the present group of studies. With this in mind, we present areas of focus for future research.

## Populations

Because sexuality education in the home begins at birth, it is important for parents to communicate with children about sexuality throughout childhood. However, most studies and programs have focused on parental communication about sexuality with *adolescents*. We lack sufficient information on sexuality communication and in particular HIV/AIDS communication between parents and their younger children. Existing data suggest that the topic of HIV/AIDS comes up for parents throughout their children's development. Despite the salience of sexuality, many parents experience considerable challenges in dealing effectively with sexuality communication with their younger children. Like Mary, the mother at the beginning of the chapter, many parents are unsure of when to begin talking to their children about sexual issues and how to answer questions of a sexual nature.

More research is needed to understand parent–child HIV/AIDS communication within African-American and Hispanic families. African-American youth are more likely than youth in other racial and ethnic groups to engage in early sexual behavior, to become pregnant or be involved in a pregnancy as adolescents, and to acquire a sexually transmitted infection (STI) (CDC, 2004). Young African Americans account for 56% of all HIV infections among 13- to 24-year-old individuals (CDC, 2003). Moreover, previous research suggests that cultural context and values are important in understanding the association between parent–child communication and outcomes such as abstinence and condom use. Understanding differences will be important in the development of effective interventions. For these reasons, researchers have begun to focus increased attention on sexual socialization among African-American and Hispanic families. Nevertheless, still only 13 of the 95 studies reviewed by DiIorio et al. (2003) specifically focused on African-American families and fewer on Hispanic families.

Finally, fathers have not been included as much as mothers in research on parent–child sexuality communication. Studies consistently show less father involvement in sexuality discussions compared to mothers. Fathers also tend to talk more to sons than daughters. More research is needed to understand how fathers view their role as sexuality educators and the barriers to fully participating in the sexual education of their children.

## Methods

Well over 100 research studies have been conducted focusing on parent–child communication about sex-based discussions and many of these have included HIV/AIDS and prevention as aspects of these discussions. As we consider future research, it is important to note some of the limitations of the studies and suggest ways to improve the methodology. One of the most important limitations is the fact that researchers who study parent–child HIV/AIDS communication have not always defined what is meant by communication. However, the meaning can be gleaned from measures used to assess the variable. Some researchers use a global question such as "Have you ever talked to your child about HIV/AIDS?" to obtain some idea of the extent to which parents talk to their children about the topic. In these cases, the participants are permitted to define "HIV/AIDS discussions" as whatever that meant to them at the time. More specific measures include a list of topics to which participants respond *yes* or *no* that they talked about the topic. With more refined versions, participants are asked to rate on a scale the amount or frequency of discussions of a particular topic. HIV/AIDS topics generally assessed include general facts about HIV (e.g., incurable), routes of HIV transmission, and types of protective behaviors including abstinence and condom use. Some researchers also include items on their questionnaires that assess affective aspects of HIV/AIDS, such as what it would be like living with AIDS. A few researchers who have conducted qualitative studies have examined nonverbal and indirect aspects of parent–child communication such as how information is presented to the child. Though researchers have measured many aspects of the definition proposed earlier, they have not always explicitly stated their definition of HIV/AIDS discussions, and there does not seem to be a consensus about the meaning of the terms or tools for measuring the variables.

A second limitation of the studies is the use of self-report as the primary means to measure the occurrence of discussions. Self-report of events is influenced by a variety of factors that can add to measurement error. These factors include interpretation, memory, and judgment. As noted previously, general questions such as "Have you ever talked to your child about HIV/AIDS?" can be interpreted in different ways. A mother who has merely asked her child if he or she has heard about AIDS may answer the query in the same manner as a mother who has talked at length to a child about what AIDS is and how it is transmitted. Depending on the time period requested ("have you ever talked to your child" vs. "have you talked to your child in the last month"), parents or children might easily forget that they discussed the topic. Likewise, social desirability may be a factor if parents or children believe that such discussions should occur. Social desirability may result in greater agreement that such discussions took place than actually occurred.

Most of the studies have asked parents and children to remember if a conversation about a particular topic ever took place. Asking participants to recall information even over a short period of time can lead to less than accurate responses. One way to address this deficiency in the studies is to conduct a longitudinal study in which parents and children record discussions. Obviously, this approach has it limitations. However, some questions about the value of parent–child communication and the link to outcomes such as sexual initiation cannot be effectively answered without studies based on longitudinal designs. Similarly, studies are needed to determine when parents choose to talk to their children. Questions raised by the current group of studies include the timing of discussions. Do parents talk to children when they believe that they are becoming more interested in dating and intimate relationships or sexually active? Do parents tend to talk more to give information or when there is a problem? Future research in these areas will help round out our understanding of the context of these conversations.

A final area of consideration is the development of a theoretical framework to guide the development of future research. Most of the parent–child sex-based communication studies have been atheoretical, descriptive studies. However, behavioral theories and theories of communication might be useful in providing a context in which to raise research questions and test hypotheses. A sufficient number of studies have been conducted that could be used as a basis for the development of a theory that can be applied to parent–child communication.

## Summary

The role of the parent as a sexuality educator has received more attention since the beginning of the HIV epidemic. Parents have shown an interest in providing accurate and timely information to their children, and researchers are describing the content and context of parent-child sex-based discussions. The findings of these studies show that gender of both the parent and child matters in terms of what is discussed and who participates in the discussions. Less is known about the context and factors that facilitate these discussions. The volume of work in the area suggests that it is a growing field, which portends a greater understanding of this important parent–child bond.

## Acknowledgments

The data collection described in this chapter was funded by Grant 5 R01 MH59010 from the National Institutes of Mental Health and Grant R01 HD039541 from the National Institute of Child Health and Human Development.

## References

Aldous, J. (1983). Birth control socialization: How to avoid discussing the subject. *Population and Environment, 6*(1), 27–38.
Bennett, S. M., & Dickinson, W. B. (1980). Student–parent rapport and parent involvement in sex, birth control, and venereal disease education. *The Journal of Sex Research, 16*(2), 114–130.
Billingsley, A., & Morrison-Rodriguez, B. (1998). The Black family in the 21st century and the church as an action system: A macro perspective. In L. See (Ed.), *Human behavior in the social environment from an African American perspective* (pp. 31–47). Binghamton, NY: Haworth.

Brock, L. J., & Jennings, G. H. (1993). Sexuality education: What daughters in their 30s wish their mothers had told them. *Family Relations, 42*(1), 61–65.

Casper, L. M. (1990). Does family interaction prevent adolescent pregnancy? *Family Planning Perspectives, 22*(3), 109–114.

Centers for Disease Control and Prevention. (1991). Effectiveness in disease and injury prevention characteristics of parents who discuss AIDS with their children—United States, 1989. *Morbidity and Mortality Weekly Report, 40*(46), 789–791.

Centers for Disease Control and Prevention. (2003). *HIV/AIDS surveillance report, 2003.* Atlanta, GA: Author.

Centers for Disease Control and Prevention. (2004). Youth risk behavior surveillance—United States, 2003. *Morbidity and Mortality Weekly Report, 53*(SS-2), 1–100.

Clawson, C., & Reese-Weber, M. (2003). The amount and timing of parent–adolescent sexual communication as predictors of late adolescent sexual risk-taking behaviors. *Journal of Sex Research, 40*(3), 256–265.

Coreil, J., & Parcel, G. S. (1983). Sociocultural determinants of parental involvement in sex education. *Journal of Sex Education and Therapy, 9*(2), 22–25.

Crawford, I., Thomas, S., & Zoller, D. (1993). Communication and level of AIDS knowledge among homeless African-American mothers and their children. *Journal of Health & Social Policy, 4*(4), 37–53.

Cvetkovich, G., & Grote, B. (1983). Adolescent development and teenage fertility. In D. W. A. F. Byrne (Ed.), *Adolescents, sex, and contraception* (pp. 109–123). Hillsdale, NJ: Lawrence Erlbaum Associates.

Darling, C. A., & Hicks, M. W. (1982). Parental influence on adolescent sexuality: Implications for parents as educators. *Journal of Youth and Adolescence, 11*(3), 231–245.

DiIorio, C., Hockenberry-Eaton, M., Maibach, E., Rivero, T., & Miller, K. (1996). The content of African American mothers' discussions with their adolescents about sex. *Journal of Family Nursing, 2*(4), 365.

DiIorio, C., Kelley, M., & Hockenberry-Eaton, M. (1999). Communication about sexual issues: Mothers, fathers, and friends. *Journal of Adolescent Health, 24*(3), 181–189.

DiIorio, C., McCarty, F., Resnicow, K., Lehr, S., & Denzmore, P. (2007). R.E.A.L. MEN: A group-randomized trial of an HIV prevention intervention for adolescent males. *American Journal of Public Health, 97*(6) 1084–1089.

DiIorio, C., Pluhar, E., & Belcher, L. (2003). Parent–child communication about sexuality: A review of the literature from 1980–2002. *Journal of HIV/AIDS Prevention & Education for Adolescents & Children, 5*(3/4), 7–31.

DiIorio, C., Resnicow, K., Dudley, W. N., Thomas, S., Wang, D. T., van Marter, D. F., et al. (2000). Social cognitive factors associated with mother–adolescent communication about sex. *Journal of Health Communication, 5*(1), 41–51.

Downie, J., & Coates, R. (1999). The impact of gender on parent–child sexuality communication: Has anything changed? *Sexual & Marital Therapy, 14*(2), 109–121.

Fisher, T. D. (1985). An exploratory study of parent–child communication about sex and the sexual attitudes of early, middle, and late adolescents. *Journal of Genetic Psychology, 147*(4), 543–557.

Fisher, T. D. (1987). Family communication and the sexual behavior and attitudes of college students. *Journal of Youth & Adolescence, 16*(5), 481–495.

Fisher, T. D. (1988). The relationship between parent–child communication about sexuality and college students' sexual behavior and attitudes as a function of parental proximity. *Journal of Sex Research, 24,* 305–311.

Fisher, T. D. (1989). An extension of the findings of Moore, Peterson, and Furstenberg (1986) regarding family sexual communication and adolescent sexual behavior. *Journal of Marriage & the Family, 51*(3), 637–639.

Fisher, T. D. (1990). Characteristics of mothers and fathers who talk to their adolescent children about sexuality. *Journal of Psychology & Human Sexuality, 3*(2), 53–70.

Fisher, T. D. (1993). A comparison of various measures of family sexual communication: Psychometric properties, validity, and behavioral correlates. *The Journal of Sex Research, 30*(3), 229–238.

Fox, G. L., & Inazu, J. K. (1980a). Mother–daughter communication about sex. *Family Relations, 29*(3), 347–352.

Fox, G. L., & Inazu, J. K. (1980b). Patterns and outcomes of mother–daughter communication about sexuality. *Journal of Social Issues, 36*(1), 7–29.

Furstenberg, F. F., Jr., Herceg-Baron, R., Shea, J., & Webb, D. (1984). Family communication and teenagers' contraceptive use. *Family Planning Perspectives, 16*(4), 163–170.

Furstenberg, F. F., Jr., Moore, K. A., & Peterson, J. L. (1985). Sex education and sexual experience among adolescents. *American Journal of Public Health, 75*(11), 1331–1332.

Geasler, M. J., Dannison, L. L., & Edlund, C. J. (1995). Sexuality education of young children: Parental concerns. *Family Relations: Journal of Applied Family & Child Studies, 44*(2), 184–188.

Hepburn, E. E. (1983). A three-level model of parent–daughter communication about sexual topics. *Adolescence, 18*(71), 523–534.

Holtzman, D., & Rubinson, R. (1995). Parent and peer communication effects on AIDS-related behavior among U.S. high school students. *Family Planning Perspectives, 27*(6), 235–240.

Hovell, M., Sipan, C., Blumberg, E., Atkins, C., Hofstetter, C. R., & Kreitner, S. (1994). Family influences on Latino and Anglo adolescents' sexual behavior. *Journal of Marriage and the Family, 56*(4), 973–986.

Hutchinson, M. K., & Cooney, T. M. (1998). Patterns of parent–teen sexual risk communication: Implications for intervention. *Family Relations, 47(2)*, 185–194.

Hutchinson, M. K., Jemmott, J., Jemmott, L. S., Braverman, P., & Fong, G. T. (2003). The role of mother–daughter sexual risk communication in reducing sexual risk behaviors among urban adolescent females: A prospective study. *Journal of Adolescent Health, 33*, 98–107.

Jaccard, J., & Dittus, P. J. (1991). *Parent–teen communication: Toward the prevention of unintended pregnancies.* New York: Springer-Verlag.

Jaccard, J., Dittus, P. J., & Gordon, V. (1996). Maternal correlates of adolescent sexual and contraceptive behavior. *Family Planning Perspectives, 28*(4), 159–165.

Jaccard, J., Dittus, P. J., & Gordon, V. V. (2000). Parent–teen communication about premarital sex: Factors associated with the extent of communication. *Journal of Adolescent Research, 15*(2), 187–208.

Jordan, T. R., Price, J. H., & Fitzgerald, S. (2000). Rural parents' communication with their teen-agers about sexual issues. *Journal of School Health, 70*(8), 338–344.

Kaiser Family Foundation. (1999). *Talking with kids about tough issues: A national survey of parents and kids.* Menlo Park, CA: Author.

Karofsky, P. S., Zeng, L., & Kosorok, M. R. (2001). Relationship between adolescent–parental communication and initiation of first intercourse by adolescents. *Journal of Adolescent Health, 28*(1), 41–45.

Kirkman, M., Rosenthal, D., & Feldman, S. (2005). Being open with your mouth shut: The meaning of "openness" in family communication about sexuality. *Sex Education, 5*(1), 49–66.

Kotva, H. J., & Schneider, H. G. (1990). Those "talks" —General and sexual communication between mothers and daughters. *Journal of Social Behavior and Personality, 5*(6), 603–613.

Lefkowitz, E. S., Kahlbaugh, P., Au, T. K., & Sigman, M. (1998). A longitudinal study of AIDS conversations between mothers and adolescents. *AIDS Education & Prevention, 10*(4), 351–365.

Lefkowitz, E. S., Kahlbaugh, P. E., & Sigman, M. D. (1996). Turn-taking in mother–adolescent conversations about sexuality and conflict. *Journal of Youth and Adolescence, 25*(3), 307–321.

Lefkowitz, E. S., Romo, L., Corona, R., Au, T., & Sigman, M. (2000). How Latino American and European American adolescents discuss conflicts, sexuality, and AIDS with their mothers. *Developmental Psychology, 36*(3), 315–325.

Lefkowitz, E., Sigman, M., & Au, T.K. (2000). Helping mothers discuss sexuality and AIDS with adolescents. *Child Development, 17,* 1383–1394.

Lehr, S., Demi, A., DiIorio, C., & Facteau, J. (2005). Predictors of father–son communication about sexuality. *Journal of Sex Research, 42*(2), 119–129.

Lehr, S. T., DiIorio, C., Dudley, W. N., & Lipana, J. A. (2000). The relationship between parent–adolescent communication and safer sex behaviors in college students. *Journal of Family Nursing, 6*(2), 180–197.

Leland, N. L., & Barth, R. P. (1993). Characteristics of adolescents who have attempted to avoid HIV and who have communicated with parents about sex. *Journal of Adolescent Research, 8*(1), 58–76.

Liebowitz, S. W., Castellano, D. C., & Cuellar, I. (1999). Factors that predict sexual behaviors among young Mexican American adolescents: An exploratory study. *Hispanic Journal of Behavioral Sciences, 21*(4), 470–479.

Miller, K. S., Kotchick, B. A., Dorsey, S., Forehand, R., & Ham, A. Y. (1998). Family communication about sex: What are parents saying and are their adolescents listening? *Family Planning Perspectives, 30*(5), 218–222.

Miller, K. S., Levin, M. L., Whitaker, D. J., & Xu, X. (1998). Patterns of condom use among adolescents: The impact of mother–adolescent communication. *American Journal of Public Health, 88*(10), 1542–1544.

Moore, K. A., Peterson, J. L., & Furstenberg, F. F. (1986). Parental attitudes and the occurrence of early sexual activity. *Journal of Marriage & the Family, 48*(4), 777–782.

Mueller, K. E., & Powers, W. G. (1990). Parent–child sexual discussion: Perceived communicator style and subsequent behavior. *Adolescence, 25*(98), 469–482.

Newcomer, S. F., & Udry, J. R. (1985). Parent–child communication and adolescent sexual behavior. *Family Planning Perspectives, 17*(4), 169–174.

Nolin, M. J., & Petersen, K. K. (1992). Gender differences in parent–child communication about sexuality: An exploratory study. *Journal of Adolescent Research, 7*(1), 59–79.

Nwoga, I. A. (2000). African American mothers use stories for family sexuality education. *The American Journal of Maternal/Child Nursing, 25*(1), 31–36.

O'Sullivan, L., Meyer-Bahlburg, H., & Watkins, B. (2001). Mother–daughter communication about sex among urban African American and Latino families. *Journal of Adolescent Research, 16*(3), 269–292.

Pick, S., & Palos, P. A. (1995). Impact of the family on the sex lives of adolescents. *Adolescence, 30*(119), 667–675.

Pistella, C. L. Y., & Bonati, F. A. (1998). Communication about sexual behavior among adolescent women, their family, and peers. *Families in Society, 79*(2), 206–211.

Pluhar, E. I. (2001). Sexuality communication in the family: A qualitative study with African American mothers and their adolescent daughters (Doctoral dissertation, University of Pennsylvania, 2001). *Dissertation Abstracts International, 62*(02A), 478.

Pluhar, E. I., Jennings, T., DiIorio, C. (2006). Getting an early start: Communication about sexuality among mothers and children 6–10 years old. *Journal of HIV/AIDS Prevention in Children & Youth, 7*(1), 7–35.

Pluhar, E., & Kuriloff, P. (2004). What really matters in family communication about sexuality? A qualitative analysis of affect and style among African American mothers and adolescent daughters. *Sex Education, 4*(3), 303–322.

Pluhar, E., McCarthy, F., & DiIorio, C. (2007). *Communication about sexuality between African-American mothers and their children ages 12–16.* Unpublished manuscript.

Raffaelli, M., and Green, S. (2003). Parent–adolescent communication about sex: Retrospective reports by Latino college students. *Journal of Marriage and Family, 65*, 474–481.

Raffaelli, M., Bogenschneider, K., & Flood, M. F. (1998). Parent-teen communication about sexual topics. *Journal of Family Issues, 19*(3), 315-333.

Romer, D. P., Stanton, B. M. D., Galbraith, J. M. A., Feigelman, S. M. D., Black, M. M. P., & Li, X. P. (1999). Parental influence on adolescent sexual behavior in high-poverty settings. *Archives of Pediatrics & Adolescent Medicine October, 153*(10), 1055-1062.

Rothenberg, P. B. (1980). Communication about sex and birth control between mothers and their adolescent children. *Population and Environment, 3*(1), 35-50.

Russo, T. S. (1991). *Factors influencing parents to discuss general and specific sexuality with their adolescent children.* Unpublished doctoral dissertation, Kansas State University, Manhattan.

Shoop, D. M., & Davidson, P. M. (1994). AIDS and adolescents: The relation of parent and partner communication to adolescent condom use. *Journal of Adolescence, 17*(2), 137–148.

Sigelman, C. K., Derenowski, E. B., Mullaney, H. A., & Siders, A. T. (1993). Parents' contributions to knowledge and attitudes regarding AIDS. *Journal of Pediatric Psychology, 18*(2), 221–235.

Sigelman, C. K., Mukai, T., Woods, T., & Alfeld, C. (1994). Parents' contributions to children's knowledge and attitudes regarding AIDS: another look. *Journal of Pediatric Psychology, 20*(1), 61–77.

Sly, D. F., Riehman, K., Wu, C., Eberstein, I., Quadagno, D., & Kistner, J. (1995). Early childhood differentials in mother-child AIDS-information interaction. *AIDS Education & Prevention, 7*(4), 337–354.

Tucker, S. K. (1989). Adolescent patterns of communication about sexually related topics. *Adolescence, 24*(94), 269–278.

Ward, L. M., & Wyatt, G. E. (1994). The effects of childhood sexual messages on African-American and White women's adolescent sexual behavior. *Psychology of Women Quarterly, 18,* 183–201.

Whalen, C., Henker, B., Hollingshead, J., & Burgess, S. (1996). Parent–adolescent dialogues about AIDS. *Journal of Family Psychology, 10*(3), 343–357.

Whitaker, D. J., & Miller, K. S. (2000). Parent–adolescent discussions about sex and condoms: Impact on peer influences of sexual risk behavior. *Journal of Adolescent Research, 15,* 251–273.

Whitaker, D. J., Miller, K. S., May, D. C., & Levin, M. L. (1999). Teenage partners' communication about sexual risk and condom use: The importance of parent–teenager discussions. *Family Planning Perspectives, 31*(3), 117–121.

White, C. P., Wright, D. W., & Barnes, H. L. (1995). Correlates of parent–child communication about specific sexual topics: A study of rural parents with school-aged children. *Personal Relationships, 2,* 327–343.

Wilson, H., & Donenberg, G. (2004). Quality of parent communication about sex and its relationship to risky sexual behavior among youth in psychiatric care: A pilot study. *Journal of Child Psychology and Psychiatry, 45*(2), 387–395.

Young, M., & Core-Gebhart, P. (1993). Parental evaluation of the Living Smart sexuality education program. *Psychological Reports, 73*(3, Pt. 2), 1107–1110.

# 7

# Culture and the Development of HIV Prevention and Treatment Programs

*Ken Resnicow*
University of Michigan

*Colleen K. DiIorio*
Emory University

*Rachel Davis*
University of Michigan

## Introduction

This chapter addresses the issue of cultural sensitivity (CS) as it relates to developing HIV prevention and sex education programs for racial/ethnic-minority populations. The chapter begins with a rationale for culturally targeted and tailored behavior change programs and then presents a conceptual framework for developing culturally sensitive HIV and sexual education interventions. Next we discuss examples for how general cultural differences as well as differences directly related to HIV and sexual behaviors can be used to tailor HIV and sexual education programs. We conclude with recommendations for future research priorities. The chapter focuses on the predominant ethnic/racial groups in the United States, although many of the principles discussed apply to populations outside the United States.

### Rationale for Cultural Sensitivity

The rationale for culturally targeted and tailored health promotion programs derives from essentially four observations: (a) changes in the demographic composition of the U.S. population, (b) differences in disease prevalence rates across racial/ethnic groups, (c) differences in the prevalence of behavioral risk factors across racial/ethnic groups, and (d) differences in the determinants of health behavior and behavior change across groups. Whereas the first three factors provide the rationale for *targeted* (i.e., delivery of programs to subpopulations) prevention programs, it is the latter that provides the basis for *tailoring* (adapting programs and messages for subpopulations) programs. As noted in the Institute of Medicine report, *Speaking of Health,* "[Some] groups are so heterogeneous that if they are to be affected by a campaign, [programs and messages have] to be adapted closely to their unique characteristics." When subgroup heterogeneity is sufficient, program developers are encouraged, therefore, to "create largely distinct campaigns ... varying the behavioral focus, the essential message strategies, the channel choices, and the message executions" (Institute of Medicine, 2002, p. 97). In other words, the need for tailored interventions is determined by the degree to which the target audience may be motivated by culturally specific message content, format, or channel of delivery.

Ethnic/Racial Diversity.    The United States is increasingly becoming racially diverse. Non-White residents comprise 30.9% of the total population, up from 24.4% in 1990 (U.S. Census Bureau, 2001). Minority racial and ethnic groups grew at a rate of 43.2% during the past decade, which was more than three times the overall 13.1% population growth rate and more than 10 times faster than the 3.5% increase in Whites (U.S. Census Bureau, 2001). The fastest growth rates are among Hispanic and Asian groups. Individuals who report being multiracial are an emerging ethnic/racial group that numbered about 7 million in the 2000 Census (U.S. Census Bureau, 2001). The proportion of Whites in the United States is projected to continue decreasing, and, as soon as 2050, Whites may no longer represent the "majority" population.

*Differences in HIV and STD Prevalence
and Related Risk Behaviors*

The incidence, prevalence, and risk factors for HIV and sexually transmitted diseases (STDs) differ across ethnic groups. Minorities currently account for a disproportionately large, and increasing, share of

AIDS cases. Of people diagnosed with AIDS in 2003, 50% were non-Hispanic Black, 28% were non-Hispanic White, 20% were Hispanic, 1% were Asian/Pacific Islander, and less than 1% were American Indian/Alaska Native (Centers for Disease Control and Prevention [CDC], 2004a, 2004c). Although African Americans make up only around 13% of the U.S. population, they account for approximately 40% of AIDS cases diagnosed since the epidemic began (CDC, 2004a, 2004c). African-American women represent approximate 60% of all AIDS cases among women, and children represent almost 71% of all pediatric AIDS cases. Similarly, whereas Hispanics comprise approximately 14% of the U.S. population, they account for almost 20% of the total AIDS cases reported (CDC, 2004a, 2004c).

AIDS is the sixth leading cause of death for African-American men, whereas it is not even among the top 10 causes of death for Whites. Among African-American men ages 25 to 44, AIDS is the leading cause of death, yet it ranks sixth for the population overall in this age group (CDC, 2004a, 2004c). African Americans are more likely to be diagnosed later after infection and are less likely to be alive 9 years postdiagnosis compared with other ethnic/racial groups (CDC, 2004c). Although advances in treatment and prevention have led to declines in AIDS incidence and mortality rates in recent years, these declines are not as pronounced for African Americans and may have plateaued. Between 1999 and 2003, AIDS diagnoses among African Americans increased by 7%, compared to a 3% decline among Whites. Deaths among African Americans with AIDS remained fairly stable between 1999 and 2003, but declined by 18% among Whites over this period.

African-American women compared to women of other racial backgrounds are more likely to be infected with HIV as a result of sex with men (CDC, 2004c). They may be less aware of their male partners' HIV infection status and risk behaviors (Hader, Smith, Moore, & Holmberg, 2001). Among African-American men who have sex with men (MSM), approximately 20% reported having had a female sex partner during the preceding 12 months (CDC, 2004b). Approximately half of the cases of HIV among MSM have been minority men. More African-American and Hispanic MSM identify themselves as heterosexual than White MSM (CDC, 2000, 2003). As a result, African-American and Hispanic MSM may not attend or respond to prevention messages tailored for men who identify themselves solely as bisexual or homosexual.

Rates of STDs are also higher among African Americans than among Whites. In 2003, African Americans were 20 times as likely as Whites to have gonorrhea and five times as likely to have syphilis. Having an STD can increase one's chances of contracting HIV, and individuals with STDs also have a greater chance of spreading HIV to others (Fleming & Wasserheit, 1999).

In terms of determinants of HIV and sexual behaviors, numerous differences have been identified. For example, in one study, self-efficacy was significantly associated with condom use in White but not Black college females (Soet, DiIorio, & Dudley, 1998). Other differences such as conspiracy beliefs, cultural values regarding homosexuality, and gender identity and their relationship to HIV and sexual practices are discussed later.

In general, African-American male adolescents tend to initiate sexual intercourse at younger ages than White or Hispanic male adolescents (CDC, 2005b; DiIorio, Dudley, & Soet, 1998) and to report a greater number of sexual partners (CDC, 2005b). However, a larger percentage of both young and older African-American men reports using condoms than among their White and Hispanic counterparts (CDC, 2005b; Soler et al., 2000).

Differences are also apparent in contraception use among women. Among young women, Whites are most likely to use the birth control pill to prevent pregnancy, whereas African-American and Hispanic women are more likely to rely on long-term (3-month injectable) contraceptives. African-American and Hispanic women are also more likely to use abortion as a method of birth control, as are women of other minority groups. African-American and Hispanic women are 3.0 and 2.5 times, respectively, more likely than White women to have had an abortion (Guttmacher Institute, 2005).

Risk behaviors such as injection drug use also vary across cultural groups. Several studies have documented unique patterns of nonrecreational injection drug use among U.S. Latinos. For example, many Latinos use injectable forms of antibiotics, vitamins, birth control, and other medications (Flaskerud & Nyamathi, 1996, 2000). Qualitative data suggest that injectable forms of routine medications may be preferred because they are believed to be more effective, faster acting, higher quality, less expensive, and available without a prescription. One study of 216 low-income Latina women found that 43.5% of respondents had used injectable medications in the preceding 6 months (Flaskerud & Nyamathi, 1996). Among these respondents, almost half reported that needles and syringes had been reused in their households. Though some families injected medications themselves, others paid a small fee to a neighborhood "injection woman" to receive their medications (Flaskerud & Nyamathi, 1996). It is unknown whether these injection women reuse disposable needles and syringes, although some qualitative data suggest that they do. One reason for the prevalence of reuse is that many Latinos obtain injectable medications from Mexico, by either traveling there themselves or ordering supplies from those who make the journey through neighborhood shops, swap meets, or flea markets. Because it has been illegal to bring these medications or disposable needles and syringes across the border, paraphernalia is smuggled into the country. The needles and syringes are difficult to hide, so quantities are limited and users often reuse the disposable needles and syringes that they have. Needles and syringes are often cleaned using soap and water or alcohol instead of bleach (Flaskerud & Nyamathi, 1996, 2000). Some Latinos may believe that bleach is required only for needles and syringes used to inject illegal, recreational drugs.

## Sociodemographic Factors

Socioeconomic status adversely affects HIV prevention efforts. Nearly one in four African Americans lives in poverty, and HIV incidence outside the gay population is inversely associated with income (Diaz, Chu, & Buehler, 1994). Constraints of poverty, such as limited access to health care and HIV prevention education, both directly and indirectly increase HIV risk. Education level has been shown to be a particularly strong predictor of AIDS knowledge among Latinos (Miller, Guarnaccia, & Fasina, 2002), and Latinos with higher educational statuses are less likely to use injectable forms of medications (Flaskerud & Nyamathi, 1996). African-American women with HIV are more likely than noninfected women to be unemployed, receive public assistance, have had 20 or more lifetime sexual partners, have a lifetime history of genital herpes infection, have used crack or cocaine, or have traded sex for drugs, money, or shelter (CDC, 2005a).

An additional sociodemographic factor affecting Latinos and possibly other immigrant groups is acculturation. Several studies have demonstrated that Latinos at lower levels of acculturation are less likely to report accurate knowledge about HIV transmission and

AIDS (Flaskerud & Uman, 1993; Miller et al., 2002). However, lower levels of acculturation may also have a protective influence on HIV practices. In a study of 190 recently immigrated Latino men and women, Mikawa et al. (1992) concluded that less acculturated men were more likely to endorse *machismo* beliefs such as the responsibility of protecting women, which, in turn, was associated with increased condom use.

## Cultural Sensitivity Further Defined

CS can be conceptualized in terms of two primary dimensions (Resnicow, Braithwaite, Ahluwalia, & Baranowski, 1999): *surface structure* and *deep structure*. *Surface structure* involves matching intervention materials and messages to observable social and behavioral characteristics of a target population. For audiovisual materials, surface structure may involve using people, places, language, music, foods, brand names, locations, and clothing that are familiar to and preferred by the target audience. Surface structure includes identifying the sources, channels (e.g., media), and settings (e.g., churches, schools) that are most appropriate for delivery of messages and programs (Kreuter & McClure, 2004). Such *contextualization* entails understanding characteristics of the behavior in question such as the product brands that are used (e.g., condoms), behavioral patterns (e.g., sexual behaviors, birth control practices), and the environmental and social context in which behaviors occur. In sum, surface structure refers to the extent to which interventions correspond to the behavioral preferences of the target population and how well interventions *fit* within the culture and experience of the target audience. In this sense, surface structure is analogous to face validity of psychologic measures: a necessary but insufficient prerequisite for construct validity. Like face validity, surface structure is generally achieved through formative research with the target population (Resnicow, Braithwaite, et al., 1999).

With regard to HIV prevention and sexual education, surface-structure issues include the language used around sexual behavior (e.g., down-low, homo thugz), gender, and beauty (e.g., thick, tight, big) (Airhihenbuwa, DiClemente, Wingood, & Lowe, 1992; Mays, Cochran, & Zamudio, 2004; Wingood & DiClemente, 1992), as well as specific sexual preferences. For example, there is some evidence that African-American and Hispanic youth are less likely to give (though perhaps paradoxically not receive) oral sex than Whites, whereas they are more likely to engage in anal intercourse (CDC, 2005b). Among adults, African Americans are less likely to report engaging in oral sex than Hispanics or Whites, whereas Hispanics are more likely to engage in anal intercourse (Quadagno, Sly, Harrison, Eberstein, & Soler, 1998).

Culture may also affect the channel and mode of delivery. For example, African-American youth may respond more positively to HIV messages presented with rap music or in video format (Airhihenbuwa et al., 1992; Wingood & DiClemente, 1992), whereas some Hispanic youth may respond more favorably to a *novela* or storytelling format.

The second dimension of intervention sensitivity, *deep structure,* reflects how cultural, social, psychologic, environmental, and historical factors may influence health behaviors differently across racial/ethnic populations. This dimension requires understanding how members of the target population perceive the cause, course, and treatment of illnesses, as well as perceptions regarding the determinants of specific health behaviors. Deep structure involves appreciation for how religion, family, society, economics, and the government, both in perception and in fact, influence the target behavior. Whereas surface structure generally increases the receptivity, comprehension, or acceptance of messages (Simons-Morton, Donohew, & Crump, 1997), deep structure conveys *salience.* Surface structure establishes feasibility, whereas deep structure determines program impact.

With regard to HIV programs, potential deeper structure cultural factors may include gender roles, the social meaning and value of sex, attitudes toward homosexuality, religiosity, ethnic identity, culturally specific stressors such as racism, homophobia, or concerns over immigration status and/or deportation (Airhihenbuwa et al., 1992; Weeks, Schensul, Williams, Singer, & Grier, 1995).

In addition to beliefs and values specific to HIV and sexuality, core cultural values may also impact sexual behavior and response to behavior change interventions. Core cultural values for African Americans include: communalism, religion/spiritualism, expressiveness, respect for verbal communication skills, connection to ancestors and history, unity, cooperation, extended family, commitment to family, and intuition and experience versus empiricism (Akbar,

1984; Cochran & Mays, 1993; Harris, 1992; Nobles, Goddard, Cavil, & George, 1993). African culture is also characterized by a unique sense of time, rhythm, and communication style (Butler, 1992; Nobles et al., 1993). The use of oral communication (i.e., interpersonal versus print interventions) as well as stories, religious/spiritual themes, and historical references to convey messages should be considered when developing health promotion programs for African Americans.

Core values among many Hispanic/Latino groups include *familismo,* or a central importance placed on family relationships. On one hand, *familismo* may have a detrimental impact on HIV risk, as many unmarried Latino MSM live with their parents and may seek to hide their sexual activity so as not to bring disrepute upon their families. On the other hand, *familismo* may provide a protective force for MSM and other Latinos, as they may draw important emotional and material support from their families (Zamora-Hernández & Patterson, 1996). Other Latino cultural values include *machismo, marianismo, simpatia, personalismo,* and *respeto.* The impact of these values on HIV behavior is unclear. For example, some researchers have speculated that *simpatia,* the desire for conflict-free social interactions, and *marianismo,* the traditional submissive role of women, may impede women from initiating conversations about condom use with their male partners or rejecting unwanted sexual advances. However, there is evidence that Latino women and men are comfortable discussing condom use, which raises questions about the role of submissiveness in sexual communication (Mikawa et al., 1992).

### The Importance of Heterogeneity

An essential principle of CS and multiculturalism is the recognition of heterogeneity not only between ethnic (and racial) subgroups, but also within. African Americans and other racial groups cannot be considered homogeneous "communities" with single mind-sets (Longshore, 1997; Trimble, 1990–1991). Such ethnic "glossing" has been commonplace in public health (Trimble, 1990–1991). To achieve CS at the level of surface or deep structure, it is essential to understand the heterogeneity of the target population (Pasick, D'Onofrio, & Otero-Sabogal, 1996; Sabogal, Otero-Sabogal, Pasick, Jenkins, & Perez-Stable, 1996).

One important factor by which many racial/ethnic populations differ within groups is ethnic identity (EI). EI involves the extent to which individuals identify with and gravitate to their racial/ethnic group. EI includes elements such as racial/ethnic pride, affinity for in-group culture (e.g., food, media, and language), attitudes toward majority culture, involvement with in-group members, experience with and attitudes regarding racism, attitudes toward intermarriage, and the importance placed on preserving one's culture and aiding others of similar backgrounds.

For some African Americans, for example, African and/or African-American culture and heritage play central roles in their personal identity and daily psychosocial functioning, whereas, for others, ethnicity and race may be only peripheral elements of self (Cross, 1991; Cross, Parham, & Helms, 1991). Some African Americans define themselves in relation to Whites and/or majority culture, whereas others do not view the world through a "race tinted" lens. According to Cross (Cross, 1991; Cross et al., 1991), personality comprises two primary dimensions, personal identity (PI) and racial identity (RI). PI includes traits common to all individuals regardless of race and ethnicity, such as nonculturally bound self-esteem, whereas RI refers to those aspects of personality that are linked to culture and ethnicity. Three aspects of racial identity included by most racial/ethnic identity theorists are: (a) awareness of and pride in African/Black heritage, also referred to as "pro-Black"; (b) recognition of racism and distrust of majority culture, also referred to as "anti-White" or "racial mistrust"; and (c) bicultural orientation (Belgrave et al., 1994; Burlew & Smith, 1991; Cross, 1991; Parham & Helms, 1985). Strong EI has been generally associated with lower rates of substance use and other problem behaviors (Gary & Berry, 1985; Herd & Grube, 1996; Resnicow, Soler, Braithwaite, Selassie, & Smith, 1999), as well as other psychologic characteristics and health behaviors in adults and youth (Baldwin, 1984; Belgrave et al., 1994; Brook, Whiteman, Balka, Win, & Gursen, 1998; Helms, 1990; Herd & Grube, 1996; Oyserman, Gant, & Ager, 1995; Parham & Helms, 1985; Vega, Zimmerman, Warheit, Apospori, & Gil, 1993). Deep-structure concepts such as EI have been applied to the development of HIV prevention programs, and the impact of these programs has generally been positive (Baldwin et al., 1996; Damond, Breuer, & Pharr, 1993; DiClemente et al., 2004; Jemmott, Jemmott, Braverman, & Fong, 2005; Jemmott, Jemmott, & Fong, 1998; Kalichman, Kelly,

Hunter, Murphy, & Tyler, 1993; Quimby, 1993; Weeks et al., 1995; Wingood, Hunter-Gamble, & DiClemente, 1993).

## Developing CS Interventions

The process of developing CS health promotion programs should begin with an analysis of disease and behavioral risk factors and, more important, the unique behavioral predictors in the target population. Whereas much of this information can be culled from the scientific literature, this process will likely require collection of new data, particularly to elucidate the predictors of use. Data for this analysis can be obtained through both quantitative and qualitative techniques. Qualitative data collection can include exploratory or formative focus groups as well as pretesting strategies based on principles of social marketing and health communications (Andreasen, 1995; Resnicow, Braithwaite et al., 1999). Quantitative methods may include the administration of surveys and secondary analyses of existing datasets or archival information.

Focus groups (FGs) are a potentially valuable means for developing CS intervention messages. At the formative level, members of the target population are convened to explore thoughts, feelings, experiences, associations, language, assumptions, and environmental enabling and constraining factors regarding HIV and sexual behaviors. Specific guidelines for conducting FGs can be found elsewhere (Basch, 1987; Krueger, 1988).

Exploratory FGs also provide an opportunity to examine the possible role of culturally based messages. Although potentially costly, they can also be valuable when developing interventions for minority groups to conduct a few groups with Euro-Americans. Though some might view this as ethnocentric (by establishing White values and practices as the norm) or simply a waste of resources, contrasting responses from racial/ethnic populations with those of the majority culture can help crystallize the extent of tailoring required. Such groups can also elucidate the language used around a particular topic. For example, FGs conducted by the first author with African-American smokers in Harlem revealed the term "loosies" as a reference to single cigarettes purchased generally for 25¢ at newspaper stands. Incorporating such terminology can increase the surface-structure sensitivity of an intervention.

It can also be useful to explore how the target population perceives that the prevalence, expression, and determinants of the target health behavior may differ in their community relative to Euro-Americans. For instance, when conducting exploratory groups for a smoking cessation program for low-income African Americans, participants reported that for many African Americans smoking served as a stress reduction technique, whereas "White folk," they felt, "can just take a vacation" (Resnicow, Vaughan, Futterman, Weston, & the Harlem Health Conection Study Group, 1997).

When conducting exploratory FGs, another strategy that can be used to delineate cultural differences is what we have called "ethnic mapping" (Resnicow, Braithwaite et al., 1999). This procedure entails asking participants to rate aspects of the target behavior along a continuum similar to the following:

Mostly a Black Thing---Equally Black and White Thing---Mostly a White Thing

When using this continuum, the process begins by first presenting several "anchors" for which responses have been generally consistent across African-American populations. Examples include rap music and Kwanzaa (generally rated mostly Black things), skiing and caviar (generally rated mostly White things), and Christmas and television (generally rated equally Black and White things). Once participants become comfortable with the classification schema, elements of the target behavior are introduced and classified using the same categories. This process provides information that is generally not available through quantitative data sources. The ethnic-mapping technique may be useful for examining HIV and sexual behaviors such as perceived prevalence and acceptability of particular sexual behaviors, birth control practices, brands of condoms, and so forth.

FGs can also be used for pretesting, during which members of the target audience are exposed to materials and messages to obtain feedback regarding format and content and both surface and deep structure. Pretesting should be distinguished from pilot testing. The former typically involves exposing potential participants, under controlled conditions, to subelements of an intervention, such as specific messages, artwork, or intervention themes, to determine appropriateness and potential salience. Pilot testing usually entails delivering the actual intervention under "real world" circumstances to a small number of participants to determine feasibility of the intervention delivery process. During pretesting, participants are typically asked to rate materials using dimensions such as comprehension, interest, and attractiveness. It can also be useful to specifically inquire about the sensitivity of the materials and messages. This is often done with questions such as "how appropriate are these materials for people like yourself, or people with your background?"

Occasionally, racial/ethnic populations may prefer audiovisual materials that represent or are designed for multiple racial/ethnic groups, as opposed to materials featuring only their race and ethnicity. In some cases, audiences may perceive targeted interventions as singling out or casting an unfavorable light on their community. This reaction may be more likely to surface when addressing behaviors or illnesses associated with social stigma such as HIV and substance use, or issues for which there is a belief that the government contributes to the problem (e.g., guns, drugs, HIV). Additionally, among low-income groups, there may be a preference for images that portray individuals from their same racial/ethnic group but from a higher socioeconomic bracket. Similarly, it cannot always be assumed that racial/ethnic groups prefer, or are more responsive to, in-group practitioners (Parham & Helms, 1981).

Can existing models be adapted to various ethnic populations or do we need to delineate entirely new approaches to working with these groups? Some scholars contend that conceptual models developed from a Eurocentric perspective fail to adequately incorporate the social, psychologic, cultural, historical, and genetic characteristics of African Americans and other groups (Airhihenbuwa et al., 1992; Akbar, 1984; Asante, 1988; Resnicow, Braithwaite, & Kuo, 1997). For example, the theory of reasoned action and social cognitive theory both emphasize individual psychologic and behavioral determinants such as self-efficacy, personal goals, self-management, and assertiveness (Bandura, 1997), which are rooted in what have been considered the Eurocentric, predominantly male values of competitiveness, materialism, personal achievement, impulse control, and self-determinism (Cochran & Mays, 1993; Nobles et al., 1993). Such individual-centered models, it has been argued, fail to adequately account for environmental determinants such as stress, racism, and poverty or the importance of community empowerment that, for many African Americans, may be more influential than individual motivation (Cochran & Mays, 1993; Mays et al., 2004). Moreover, many Eurocentric models situate "Whites" as the norm for what constitutes "normative" and "appropriate," if not acceptable and desired. Furthermore, such ethnocentric contrasts often impose a deficit model on nonmajority groups, whose performance may not "measure up" to White standards or whose cultures may operate by different principles. For instance, the Afrocentric view asserts, to some degree, that individual and social learning principles may operate differently in African Americans. For example, assumptions regarding the centrality of individual-level motivation may not be appropriate for African or other non-Western cultures. Instead, greater emphasis could be placed on communal benefits, inter- rather than intrapersonal motivation, and collective rather than individual goals. Hispanic culture has also been characterized as having a strong sense of collectivism (*colectivismo*), which includes high levels of personal interdependence, conformity, and sacrifice for the communal good (Bagley, Angel, Dilworth-Anderson, Liu, & Schinke, 1995; Schinke, Botvin, Orlandi, Schilling, & Gordon, 1990). Emphasis on communal versus individual-centered motivation for behavior may also be appropriate for this population.

A contrasting approach assumes that the fundamental determinants of behavior operate similarly in all populations, and psychologic and behavioral models, can, despite their Eurocentric origins, be successfully adapted for a range of sociodemographic, racial, and ethnic populations. For example, many cultural values could be absorbed in social cognitive theory as variations in outcome expectancies or social norms. Similar to designing interventions according to factors such as age and gender, culture simply represents another construct through which these models can be applied. Adaptation, however, requires an integrative understanding of the unique personal and environmental characteristics of the target population and the surface- and deep-structure determinants of behavior that can be translated into culturally sensitive messages and behavior change strategies (Resnicow, Braithwaite et al., 1997).

## Ethnic Differences That May Impact HIV and Sexual Behaviors

### Gender Identity and Sex Roles

Culture can have a significant influence on gender identity and sex roles. For example, there is evidence that the sexual identity of

Mexican-American MSM is determined by the sex roles they generally assume in these interactions (Magaña & Carrier, 1991). Latino MSM are more apt to engage in anal intercourse than oral sex, and, over the course of many sexual engagements, individual men tend to primarily adopt either an anal-insertive role or an anal-receptive role. Men who play the insertive role are called *activos* and tend to assume the more desired, traditional, dominant masculine role. In contrast to Anglo culture, sexual activity between men does not necessarily affect the sexual identities of the men involved. As long as *activos* maintain their *activo* status and continue to have sexual relations with women, they tend to be both self- and publicly identified as heterosexual (Magaña & Carrier, 1991). In fact, sexual activity with men may even be viewed as enhancing the masculinity of *activos*. Men who predominantly assume the anal-receptive role are labeled *pasivos* and are characterized as playing a more feminine, passive, and receptive sex role. *Pasivos* are more likely than *activos* to identify as homosexual, particularly if they have sex exclusively with men. One study of HIV-positive blood donors found that 34% of Latino MSM identified themselves as heterosexual (Zamora-Hernández & Patterson, 1996). At least one additional study suggests that more Latino men report bisexual activity than do men from any other racial and ethnic group in the United States. Bisexual activity was particularly frequent among Latino men who were born outside the United States or recently immigrated. Approximately 22% of Latino men engaged in bisexual relations were married, in contrast to an average marital rate of 7% for men from other racial and ethnic groups (Zamora-Hernández & Patterson, 1996). However, regardless of sex role, many Latino MSM identify more with their ethnic group than with the gay community. Thus, many Latino MSM disregard health communication initiatives tailored for bisexual, "gay," or homosexual men.

Whitehead (1997) explored the meaning of masculinity and attributes associated with masculinity among African-American males. One theme, *male strength*, is reflected in the masculine attributes of *respectability* and *reputation*. *Respectability* includes conventional masculine attributes such as higher education, marriage, family, and income. *Reputation* attributes include "sexual prowess, toughness, fathering numerous children, defying authority, outwitting others, and sweet talking women" (Aronson, Whitehead, & Baber, pp. 735–736). The roots of the respectability–reputation dialectic can be traced to oppression during and after the era of slavery. Historically,

African-American men, who faced obstacles in higher education and the job market, were less able to display male strength through respectability attributes, and as a result, reputation attributes emerged to counter the inability to express masculine self-identity in a more conventional manner. The reputation attributes are most evident among young, low-income African-American men. Wolfe (2003) refers to this phenomenon as *hypermasculinity* and notes that the sexual expression of hypermasculinity is reflected in behaviors such as having multiple current partners, fathering children with multiple mothers, unprotected sexual intercourse, and "manipulative and exploitative" attitudes toward African-American women. These high-risk and coercive sexual behaviors have been implicated in the higher rates of sexually transmitted infections among African-American men and the transmission of HIV to African-American women (Wolfe, 2003).

The fragmentation of masculine self-identify (Whitehead, 1997) has also been implicated in the pervasive homophobia found within the African-American community. Research has shown that African Americans have more negative attitudes toward homosexuals than do Whites and that African-American men report more negative attitudes than do African-American women (Waldner, Sikks, & Baig, 1999). Thus, like Latinos, many African-American MSM identify themselves as heterosexual (CDC, 2000, 2003). These findings underscore the importance of understanding sex roles within cultural groups as a foundation for effective health communication efforts.

Because sexual behaviors of adults tend to be enduring and difficult to change, messages about risky sexual behaviors may be delivered best prior to sexual debut before these behaviors become firmly established (Wolfe, 2003). For young men in particular, prevention efforts might also include discussions about sexual identity and what it means to be a man in their respective cultures. Providing opportunities for young men to develop life skills can allow them to develop a masculine self-identity through work and education and counter the need to adopt risky sexual behaviors as a mark of manhood (Wolfe, 2003).

A related issue is perceived power regarding sexual negotiations. There is evidence that Hispanic couples are more likely than White and Black couples to engage in joint decision making about when sex occurs, what sexual acts will be performed, and method of birth control (Quadagno et al., 1998; Soler et al., 2000). On the other hand, African-American women may be more likely than Hispanic and

White women to make such decisions unilaterally (Quadagno et al., 1998). Black women may feel a greater sense of control over their relationships than do White women (Soet, Dudley, & DiIorio, 1999). Establishing which, if any, of these gender patterns exist within a particular population is important in program design.

## Religiosity

Several studies of adults and adolescents have found higher levels of religiosity among Blacks than Whites (Headen, Bauman, Deane, & Koch, 1991; Taylor & Chatters, 1991). Blacks are more likely to attend church, place a higher value on religion, and use religion as a coping strategy. The salience of religion in African-American life is supported by the finding that religiosity is a stronger predictor of life satisfaction for Blacks than Whites, whereas among Black adolescents, religion appears more protective of substance use than for Whites (Thomas, Bethlehem, & Holmes, 1992). Additionally, the church serves different functions in Black and White communities. Beyond spiritual sustenance, Black churches also provide a forum for social discourse and political activism; the Black church was a major contributor to the civil rights movement. Many Black churches also provide social and medical services such as health screenings, voter registration campaigns, and feeding programs for the disadvantaged (Thomas, Quinn, Billingsley, & Caldwell, 1994; Thomas et al., 1992).

Religiosity may be used to motivate HIV-preventive health behaviors. For example, health messages can be linked to religious or spiritual themes such as those contained within the biblical commandments. Health educators can also seek partnerships with religious leaders, who may be willing to serve as respected and trustworthy message sources or role models for their parishioners. The norms of a particular faith community may also provide a source of positive or negative sanctions. Additionally, self-evaluative expectations, for example, emphasizing personal feelings of spiritual/religious pride, can be used to encourage positive health behaviors.

Increased involvement in religion may also be associated with an increased responsiveness to fear messages among African Americans. Preaching in Black religious institutions is often evangelical and replete with passionate messages of salvation and damnation, virtue and sin. African Americans, as a result, may be more receptive to fear messages regarding sexual behavior when tied to religious themes. Whether the use of fear messages in the church reflects a motivational predisposition that operates outside of this context, however, has not been adequately examined. Research is needed to determine the effectiveness of fear messages in African Americans and the degree to which responsiveness to such messages is related to religiosity.

Despite the positive influence of the church in the lives of many African Americans, the Black church may also promote beliefs and values that can have a detrimental impact on HIV risk behaviors. One example is anti-gay values. Lemelle and Battle (2004) found that religious attendance among African-American men was an important predictor of negative attitudes toward gay men. Ward (2005) noted that the roots of homophobia within the Black church may be explained by a literal interpretation of the Bible, fear of sexuality emanating from White exploitation during slavery, and racial consciousness. Racial consciousness as presented by Crichlow (2004) holds that the construction of Black masculinity in response to White racism has resulted in the perception that homosexuality reflects weakness. Thus, fear of being labeled homosexual and anti-gay messages by ministers may exacerbate hypersexuality behaviors as men attempt to prove their heterosexuality to themselves and their peers. Likewise, outwardly heterosexual MSM may resist any gay or bisexual identity to avoid the social stigma it carries in the Black community. Black churches may encourage men to keep their homosexuality secret or "down low" (Woodyard, Peterson, & Stokes, 2000). Another related potential problem is that individuals who may contract HIV through same-sex contact may be reluctant to disclose their HIV status or acknowledge homosexual activity. This, in turn, may increase the likelihood of transmitting the disease and decrease the likelihood of seeking care. Inhibition to disclose HIV status among religious individuals may increase their stress response, as well as eliminate potentially valuable sources of instrumental and emotional support.

This paradoxical impact of religion on sexual health is reflected in a recent longitudinal study of adolescents who reported taking a pledge of sexual abstinence (Bruckner & Bearman, 2005). Although pledgers over time tend to initiate sex later than nonpledgers, to have fewer sexual partners, and to get married earlier than nonpledgers, most pledgers do not wait to get married before having first sex.

Moreover, STD infection rates did not differ from nonpledgers. One reason for the lack of protection against STDs among pledgers is that they are less likely than others to use condoms at sexual debut and less likely to be tested for STDs. Most notably, nonpledging females were almost twice as likely as pledging females to be tested for STDs, and pledgers were significantly less likely to report seeing a doctor because they are worried about an STD.

Religious individuals, perhaps due to shame or guilt, may be less able to take responsibility for their sexual behavior and may partly dissociate themselves from their actions. As a result, they may be less able to implement harm reduction strategies such as condom use.

Application to Other Racial/Ethnic Groups    Hispanic youth may also have higher levels of religiosity than majority youth, and culturally sensitive interventions for this population should also consider religion as a possible motivational factor in health behavior decisions (Neff & Hoppe, 1992). However, it is important to investigate how religiosity may play a role in specific health behaviors. For example, contrary to earlier hypotheses, studies indicate that stronger religious ties to the Catholic Church are not associated with lower rates of condom use (Mikawa et al., 1992; Organista, Organista, García de Alba, Castillo-Morán, & Carrillo, 1996). Another aspect of spirituality that is often cited as a Latino trait is the tendency to be fate oriented, or to put one's fate in the hands of God. Though less acculturated Latinos have been shown to endorse a fate orientation, data suggest that fate orientation is not related to condom use (Organista et al., 1996).

## Mistrust of the Medical System

Mistrust of the medical system poses a great challenge for the prevention and treatment of HIV among African Americans and other minority groups. Inequities in the quality and availability of care have generated legitimate concerns among African Americans about bias in the health care system. In a study of attitudes about care, African-American patients were more likely than Whites to perceive racism and express lower levels of trust and less satisfaction with their care (LaVeist, Nickerson, & Bowie, 2000). Moreover, both perception of racism and mistrust of the medical care system were associated with less satisfaction with care.

Feelings of mistrust fueled by social inequities have contributed to the endorsement of a variety of conspiracy theories related to the origins of HIV, the treatment of HIV-infected African Americans, and the intentions of health professions promoting safer-sex behaviors. Several studies have documented that many African Americans believe that the U.S. government may have intentionally brought HIV into the Black community or that it covertly encourages the spread of HIV (as well as guns and drugs) (Airhihenbuwa et al., 1992; Bogart & Bird, 2003; Bogart & Thorburn, 2005; Cochran & Mays, 1993; Gasch, Poulson, Fullilove, & Fullilove, 1991). In one study of conspiracy beliefs about HIV and AIDS, Bogart and Thorburn (2005) found that 58% of Black adults sampled believed that information about AIDS is being withheld from the public, 53% felt that a cure for AIDS is being withheld from poor people, and 61% disagreed that HIV medications are saving lives in the Black community. Nearly as many respondents (48%) believed that "HIV is a man-made virus" and that the government is telling the truth (37%). Conversely, 75% of the sample agreed that "medical and public health institutions are trying to stop the spread of HIV in the Black community." For most of the items, men demonstrated more negative attitudes than did women. Such beliefs may impact sexual practices. Bogart (Bogart & Bird, 2003; Bogart & Thorburn, 2005) found that among Black men, stronger conspiracy beliefs were significantly associated with more negative condom attitudes and less consistent condom use. Some minorities perceive programs that promote condom use and birth control as "eugenics," that is, attempts to reduce reproduction among minorities in order to help Whites maintain majority status and retain political and economic power.

Distrust of the medical care system can be attributed in part to the U.S. Public Health Service Syphilis Study, which is more commonly known as the Tuskegee Study. To elucidate its impact on participation in research studies, Freimuth et al. (2001) assessed knowledge and attitude about medical research and the Tuskegee Study among African Americans. Using focus group interviews, they found that participants had strong beliefs about interactions with the government and medical agencies, noting that African Americans must be "very cautious." They also expressed distrust of researchers, citing racism as a motivation for mistreatment. Many participants endorsed beliefs that placed the researchers' legal and financial interests above those of the participants. Many also confused research with standard treatment, noting that they probably "unknowingly" participated in research at some time. Although most of the participants were aware of the Tuskegee Study, most were not able to provide specific details about the study, the participants, or the reasons for termination. One participant noted that lack of information about the study seemed to breed conspiracy theories such as those associated with the prevention and treatment of AIDS. Many believed that AIDS was made in a laboratory to harm people of African descent.

Culturally sensitive interventions may include messages that acknowledge though not necessarily dismantle or refute these beliefs. Additionally, for new community-based programs, extra effort may be needed on the front end to build trust with potential clients.

## Conclusion

Differences in the prevalence and determinants of HIV and related risk factors provide a compelling rationale for tailoring HIV education programs for ethnic and racial subgroups. Numerous cultural differences, both global and specific to HIV-related behavior, provide program developers with opportunities for tailoring HIV and sexual education programs. For example, addressing constructs such as conspiracy beliefs, cultural mistrust, attitudes toward homosexuality, and gender identity can increase the personal relevance and salience of such programs, and, thereby, program impact.

Yet, despite the numerous studies that have reported the results of culturally tailoring HIV and sexual education programs, in most studies the cultural tailoring was not isolated experimentally (Damond et al., 1993; DiClemente & Wingood, 1995; DiClemente et al., 2004; Jemmott et al., 1998, 2005; Quimby, 1993; Wingood et al., 1993). That is, the intervention and comparison group programs differed in ways beyond the cultural tailoring. Therefore, it is difficult to attribute intervention effects solely to cultural variations. To investigate the independent efficacy of culturally tailored HIV and sexual education programs with a high degree of internal validity, it is important to use comparison materials that are similar in as many dimensions as possible to the tailored materials. For example, it may be possible to hold constant key scientific content and health education messages as well as the length, graphics, and production value of audiovisual materials and only vary source, graphics, or text of the communication, that is, the tailored elements of the intervention. A limited number of studies have experimentally manipulated cultural elements of health communications (Ahluwalia, Richter, Mayo, & Resnicow 1999; Herek et al., 1998; Kalichman & Coley, 1995; Kreuter et al., 2004; Sussman et al., 1995), but more research is needed to determine the independent contribution of cultural tailoring on key consumer variables such as perceived relevance and salience, and, ultimately, behavioral impact.

## References

Ahluwalia, J., Richter, K., Mayo, M., & Resnicow, K. (1999, April-May). *Quit for Life: A randomized trial of culturally sensitive materials for smoking cessation in African Americans (Abstract).* Paper presented at the annual meeting of the Society of General Internal Medicine.

Airhihenbuwa, C. O., DiClemente, R. J., Wingood, G. M., & Lowe, A. (1992). HIV/AIDS education and prevention among African-Americans: A focus on culture. *AIDS Education & Prevention, 4*(3), 267–276.

Akbar, N. (1984). Afrocentric social sciences for human liberation. *Journal of Black Studies, 14*(4), 395–414.

Andreasen, A. (1995). *Marketing social change: Changing behavior to promote health, social development, and the environment* (1st ed.). San Francisco: Jossey-Bass.

Aronson, R. E., Whitehead, T. L., & Baber, W. L. (2003). Challenges to masculine transformation among urban low-income African American males. *American Journal of Public Health, 93,* 732–741.

Asante, M. (1988). *Afrocentricity.* Trenton, NJ: Africa World Press.

Bagley, S. P., Angel, R., Dilworth-Anderson, P., Liu, W., & Schinke, S. (1995). Adaptive health behaviors among ethnic minorities. *Health Psychology, 14*(7), 632–640.

Baldwin, J. (1984). African self-consciousness and the mental health of African-Americans. *Journal of Black Studies, 15*(2), 177–194.

Baldwin, J. A., Rolf, J. E., Johnson, J., Bowers, J., Benally, C., & Trotter, R. T. (1996). Developing culturally sensitive HIV/AIDS and substance abuse prevention curricula for Native American youth. *Journal of School Health, 66*(9), 322–327.

Bandura, A. (1997). *Self efficacy: The exercise of control.* New York: Freeman.

Basch, C. (1987). Focus group interview: An underutilized research technique for improving theory and practice in health education. *Health Education Quarterly, 14*(4), 411–448.

Belgrave, F. Z., Cherry, V. R., Cunningham, D., Walwyn, S., Letkala-Rennert, K., & Phillips, F. (1994). The influence of Africentric values, self-esteem, and Black identity on drug attitudes among African American fifth graders: A preliminary study. Special Section: Africentric values, racial identity, and acculturation: Measurement, socialization, and consequences. *Journal of Black Psychology, 20*(2), 143–156.

Bogart, L. M., & Bird, S. T. (2003). Exploring the relationship of conspiracy beliefs about HIV/AIDS to sexual behaviors and attitudes among African-American adults. *Journal of the National Medical Association, 95*(11), 1057–1065.

Bogart, L. M., & Thorburn, S. (2005). Are HIV/AIDS conspiracy beliefs a barrier to HIV prevention among African Americans? *Journal of Acquired Immune Deficiency Syndrome, 38*(2), 213–218.

Brook, J. S., Whiteman, M., Balka, E. B., Win, P. T., & Gursen, M. D. (1998). Drug use among Puerto Ricans: Ethnic identity as a protective factor. *Hispanic Journal of Behavioral Sciences, 20*(2), 241–254.

Bruckner, H., & Bearman, P. (2005). After the promise: The STD consequences of adolescent virginity pledges. *Journal of Adolescent Health, 36*(4), 271–278.

Burlew, A. K., & Smith, L. R. (1991). Measures of racial identity: An overview and a proposed framework. Special Issue: Incorporating an African world view into psychology: II. *Journal of Black Psychology, 17*(2), 53–71.

Butler, J. (1992). Of kindred minds: The ties that bind. In M. Orlandi, R. Weston, & L. Epstein (Eds.), *Cultural competence for evaluators: A guide for alcohol and other drug abuse prevention practitioners working with ethnic communities* (pp. 23–54). Washington, DC: USDHHS/OSAP.

Centers for Disease Control and Prevention. (2000). HIV/AIDS among racial/ethnic minority men who have sex with men—United States, 1989–1998. *Morbidity & Mortality Weekly Report, 49,* 4–11.

Centers for Disease Control and Prevention. (2003). HIV/STD risks in young men who have sex with men who do not disclose their sexual orientation—six US cities, 1994–2000. *Morbidity & Mortality Weekly Report, 52,* 81–85.

Centers for Disease Control and Prevention. (2004a). Diagnoses of HIV/AIDS—32 states, 2000–2003. *Morbidity & Mortality Weekly Report, 53,* 1106–1110.

Centers for Disease Control and Prevention. (2004b). HIV transmission among black college student and non-student men who have sex with men—North Carolina, 2003. *Morbidity & Mortality Weekly Report, 53,* 731–734.

Centers for Disease Control and Prevention. (2004c). HIV/AIDS surveillance report, 2003. *HIV/AIDS Surveillance Report, 15,* 1–46.

Centers for Disease Control and Prevention. (2005a). HIV transmission among Black women—North Carolina, 2004. *Morbidity & Mortality Weekly Report, 54,* 89–93.

Centers for Disease Control and Prevention. (2005b). Sexual behavior and selected health measures: Men and women 15–44 years of age, United States, 2002. *Advance Data from National Survey of Family Growth, 362*(September 15).

Cochran, S., & Mays, V. (1993). Applying social psychological models to predicting HIV-related sexual risk behaviors among African Americans. *Journal of Black Psychology, 19,* 142–154.

Crichlow, W. (2004). *Buller men and batty boys: Hidden men in Toronto and Halifax Black communities.* Toronto, Ontario, Canada: University of Toronto Press.

Cross, W. (1991). *Shades of black: Diversity in African American identity.* Philadelphia: Temple University Press.

Cross, W., Parham, T., & Helms, J. (1991). The stages of Black identity development: Nigrescence models. In R. Jones (Ed.), *Black psychology* (3rd ed., pp. 319–338). Berkeley, CA: Cobb & Henry.

Damond, M. E., Breuer, N. L., & Pharr, A. E. (1993). The evaluation of setting and a culturally specific HIV/AIDS curriculum: HIV/AIDS knowledge and behavioral intent of African American adolescents. Special Issue: Psychosocial aspects of AIDS prevention among African Americans. *Journal of Black Psychology, 19*(2), 169–189.

Diaz, T., Chu, S., & Buehler, J. (1994). Socioeconomic differences among people with AIDS: Results from a multi-state surveillance project. *American Journal of Preventive Medicine, 10,* 217–222.

DiClemente, R. J., & Wingood, G. M. (1995). A randomized controlled trial of an HIV sexual risk-reduction intervention for young African-American women. *Journal of the American Medical Association, 274*(16), 1271–1276.

DiClemente, R. J., Wingood, G. M., Harrington, K. F., Lang, D. L., Davies, S. L., Hook, E. W., III, et al. (2004). Efficacy of an HIV prevention intervention for African American adolescent girls: A randomized controlled trial. *Journal of the American Medical Association, 292*(2), 171–179.

DiIorio, C., Dudley, W. N., & Soet, J. (1998). Predictors of HIV risk among college students: A CHAID analysis. *Journal of Applied Biobehavioral Research, 3*(2), 119–134.

Flaskerud, J. H., & Nyamathi, A. M. (1996). Home medication injection among Latina women in Los Angeles: Implications for health education and prevention. *AIDS Care, 8*(1), 95–102.

Flaskerud, J. H., & Nyamathi, A. M. (2000). Collaborative inquiry with low-income Latina women. *Journal of Health Care for the Poor and Underserved, 11*(3), 326–342.

Flaskerud, J. H., & Uman, G. (1993). Directions for AIDS education for Hispanic women based on analyses of survey findings. *Public Health Reports, 108*(3), 298–304.

Fleming, D., & Wasserheit, J. (1999). From epidemiological synergy to public health policy and practice: the contribution of other sexually transmitted diseases to sexual transmission of HIV infection. *Sexually Transmitted Infections, 75,* 3–17.

Freimuth, V. S., Quinn, S. C., Thomas, S. B., Cole, G., Zook, E., & Duncan, T. (2001). African Americans' views on research and the Tuskegee Syphilis Study. *Social Science & Medicine, 52*(5), 797–808.

Gary, L., & Berry, G. (1985). Predicting attitudes toward substance use in a Black community: Implications for prevention. *Community Mental Health Journal, 21*(1), 42–51.

Gasch, H., Poulson, D. M., Fullilove, R. E., & Fullilove, M. T. (1991). Shaping AIDS education and prevention programs for African Americans amidst community decline. *Journal of Negro Education, 60*(1), 85–96.

Guttmacher Institute. (2005). *Induced abortion in the United States.* Retrieved November 11, 2005, from http://www.Guttmacher.org/pubs/ib_induced_abortion.html.

Hader, S., Smith, D., Moore, J., & Holmberg, S. (2001). HIV infection in women in the United States: status at the millennium. *Journal of the American Medical Association, 285,* 1186–1192.

Harris, N. (1992). A philosophical basis for an Afrocentric orientation. *The Western Journal of Black Studies, 6*(3), 154–159.

Headen, S., Bauman, K., Deane, G., & Koch, G. (1991). Are the correlates of cigarette smoking initiation different for Black and White adolescents? *American Journal of Public Health, 81*(7), 854–858.

Helms, J. E. (1990). *Black and White racial identity: Theory, research, and practice.* New York: Greenwood.

Herd, D., & Grube, J. (1996). Black identity and drinking in the US: A national study. *Addiction, 91*(6), 845–857.

Herek, G., Gillis, J., Glunt, E., Lewis, J., Welton, D., & Capitanio, J. (1998). Culturally sensitive AIDS education videos for Africa American audiences: Effects of source, message, receiver, and context. *American Journal of Community Psychology, 26,* 705–743.

Institute of Medicine. (2002). *Speaking of health: Assessing health communication strategies for diverse populations.* Washington, DC: National Academy of Science Press.

Jemmott, J. B., III, Jemmott, L. S., Braverman, P. K., & Fong, G. T. (2005). HIV/STD risk reduction interventions for African American and Latino adolescent girls at an adolescent medicine clinic: A randomized controlled trial. *Archives of Pediatrics & Adolescent Medicine, 159*(5), 440–449.

Jemmott, J. B., III, Jemmott, L. S., & Fong, G. T. (1998). Abstinence and safer sex HIV risk-reduction interventions for African American adolescents: A randomized controlled trial. *Journal of the American Medical Association, 279*(19), 1529–1536.

Kalichman, S., & Coley, B. (1995). Context framing to enhance HIV-antibody testing messages targeted to African American women. *Health Psychology, 14,* 247–254.

Kalichman, S. C., Kelly, J. A., Hunter, T. L., Murphy, D. A., & Tyler, R. (1993). Culturally tailored HIV-AIDS risk-reduction messages targeted to African-American urban women: Impact on risk sensitization and risk reduction. *Journal of Consulting & Clinical Psychology, 61*(2), 291–295.

Kreuter, M. W., & McClure, S. M. (2004). The role of culture in health communication. *Annual Review of Public Health, 25,* 439–455.

Kreuter, M. W., Skinner, C. S., Steger-May, K., Holt, C. L., Bucholtz, D. C., Clark, E. M., et al. (2004). Responses to behaviorally vs culturally tailored cancer communication among African American women. *American Journal of Health Behavior, 28*(3), 195–207.

Krueger, R. A. (1988). *Focus groups: A practical guide for applied research* (Vol. 197). Newbury Park, CA: Sage.

LaVeist, T. A., Nickerson, K. J., & Bowie, J. V. (2000). Attitudes about racism, medical mistrust and satisfaction with care among African American and White cardiac patients. *Medical Care Research and Review, 57*(Suppl. 1), 146–161.

Lemelle, A. J., Jr., & Battle, J. (2004). Black masculinity matters in attitudes toward gay males. *Journal of Homosexuality, 47*(1), 39–51.

Longshore, D. (1997). Treatment motivation among Mexican American drug-using arrestees. *Hispanic Journal of Behavioral Sciences, 19*(2), 214–229.

Magaña, J. R., & Carrier, J. M. (1991). Mexican and Mexican American male sexual behavior and spread of AIDS in California. *The Journal of Sex Research, 28*(3), 425–441.

Mays, V. M., Cochran, S. D., & Zamudio, A. (2004). HIV prevention research: Are we meeting the needs of African American men who have sex with men? *Journal of Black Psychology, 30*(1), 78–105.

Mikawa, J. K., Morones, P. A., Gomez, A., Case, H. L., Olsen, D., & Gonzales-Huss, M. (1992). Cultural practices of Hispanics: Implications for the prevention of AIDS. *Hispanic Journal of Behavioral Sciences, 14*(4), 421–433.

Miller, J. E., Guarnaccia, P. J., & Fasina, A. (2002). AIDS knowledge among Latinos: The roles of language, culture, and socioeconomic status. *Journal of Immigrant Health, 4*(2), 63–72.

Neff, J., & Hoppe, S. (1992). Acculturation and drinking patterns among U.S. Anglos, Blacks, and Mexican Americans. *Alcohol & Alcoholism, 27*(3), 293–308.

Nobles, W., Goddard, L., Cavil, W., & George, P. (1993). *An African-centered model of prevention for African-American youth at high risk* (No. SMA 93-2015). Rockville, MD: USDHHS/CSAP.

Organista, K. C., Organista, P. B., García de Alba, J. E., Castillo Morán, M. A., & Carrillo, H. (1996). AIDS and condom-related knowledge, beliefs, and behaviors in Mexican migrant laborers. *Hispanic Journal of Behavioral Sciences, 18*(3), 392–406.

Oyserman, D., Gant, L., & Ager, J. (1995). A socially contextualized model of African American identity: Possible selves and school persistence. *Journal of Personality & Social Psychology, 69*(6), 1216–1232.

Parham, T., & Helms, J. (1981). The influence of Black students' racial identity attitudes on preferences for counselor's race. *Journal of Counseling Psychology, 28*(3), 250–257.

Parham, T., & Helms, J. (1985). Attitudes of racial identity and self-esteem of Black students: An exploratory investigation. *Journal of College Student Personnel, 26,* 143–147.

Pasick, R., D'Onofrio, C., & Otero-Sabogal, R. (1996). Similarities and differences across cultures: Questions to inform a third generation for health promotion research. *Health Education Quarterly, 23*(Suppl.), S142–S161.

Quadagno, D., Sly, D. F., Harrison, D. F., Eberstein, I. W., & Soler, H. R. (1998). Ethnic differences in sexual decisions and sexual behavior. *Archives of Sexual Behavior, 27*(1), 57–75.

Quimby, E. (1993). Obstacles to reducing AIDS among African Americans. Special Issue: Psychosocial aspects of AIDS prevention among African Americans. *Journal of Black Psychology, 19*(2), 215–222.

Resnicow, K., Braithwaite, R., Ahluwalia, J., & Baranowski, T. (1999). Cultural sensitivity in public health: Defined and demystified. *Ethnicity and Disease, 9,* 10–21.

Resnicow, K., Braithwaite, R., & Kuo, J. (1997). Interpersonal intervention for African American adolescents. In D. Wilson, J. Rodrigue, & W. Taylor (Eds.), *Adolescent health promotion in minority populations* (pp. 201–228). Washington, DC: American Psychological Association.

Resnicow, K., Soler, R., Braithwaite, R., Selassie, M., & Smith, M. (1999). Development and validation of a racial identity scale for African American adolescents: The Survey of Black Life. *Journal of Black Psychology, 25*(2), 171–188.

Resnicow, K., Vaughan, R., Futterman, R., Weston, R., & the Harlem Health Connection Study Group. (1997). A self-help smoking cessation program for inner-city African Americans: Results from the Harlem Health Connection Project. *Health Education & Behavior, 24*(2), 201–217.

Sabogal, F., Otero-Sabogal, R., Pasick, R., Jenkins, C., & Perez-Stable, E. (1996). Printed health education materials for diverse communities: Suggestions learned from the field. *Health Education Quarterly, 23*(Suppl.), S123–S141.

Schinke, S., Botvin, G., Orlandi, M., Schilling, R., & Gordon, A. (1990). African-American and Hispanic-American adolescents, HIV infection, and preventive intervention. *AIDS Education & Prevention, 2*(4), 305–312.

Simons-Morton, B. G., Donohew, L., & Crump, A. D. (1997). Health communication in the prevention of alcohol, tobacco, and drug use. *Health Education & Behavior, 24*(5), 544–554.

Soet, J. E., DiIorio, C., & Dudley, W. N. (1998). Women's self-reported condom use: Intra and interpersonal factors. *Women & Health, 27*(4), 19–32.

Soet, J. E., Dudley, W. N., & DiIorio, C. (1999). The effects of ethnicity and perceived power on women's sexual behavior. *Psychology of Women Quarterly, 23*(4), 707–723.

Soler, H., Quadagno, D., Sly, D. F., Riehman, K. S., Eberstein, I. W., & Harrison, D. F. (2000). Relationship dynamics, ethnicity and condom use among low-income women. *Family Planning Perspectives, 32*(2), 82–88.

Sussman, S., Parker, V. C., Lopes, C., Crippens, D. L., Elder, P., & Scholl, D. (1995). Empirical development of brief smoking prevention videotapes which target African-American adolescents. *International Journal of the Addictions, 30*(9), 1141–1164.

Taylor, L., & Chatters, R. (1991). Religious life. In J. Jackson (Ed.), *Life in Black America* (pp. 105–123). Newbury Park, CA: Sage.

Thomas, M., Bethlehem, L., & Holmes, B. (1992). Determinants of satisfaction for Blacks and Whites. *Sociological Quarterly, 33*(3), 459–472.

Thomas, S., Quinn, S., Billingsley, A., & Caldwell, C. (1994). The characteristics of northern Black churches with community health outreach programs. *American Journal of Public Health, 84,* 575–580.

Trimble, J. (1990–1991). Ethnic specification, validation prospects, and the future of drug use research. *The International Journal of the Addictions, 25*(2A), 149–170.

U.S. Census Bureau. (2001). *National population projections.* Retrieved May 3, 2007, from http://www.census.gov/population/www/pop-profile/natproj.html.

Vega, W., Zimmerman, R., Warheit, G., Apospori, E., & Gil, A. (1993). Risk factors for early adolescent drug use in four ethnic and racial groups. *American Journal of Public Health, 83*(2), 185–189.

Waldner, L. K., Sikks, A., & Baig, S. (1999). Ethnicity and sex differences in university student's knowledge of AIDS, fear of AIDS, and attitudes toward gay men. *Journal of Homosexuality, 37*(3), 117–133.

Ward, E. G. (2005). Homophobia, hypermasculinity and the US Black church. *Culture, Health & Sexuality, 7*(5), 493–504.

Weeks, M. R., Schensul, J. J., Williams, S. S., Singer, M., & Grier, M. (1995). AIDS prevention for African-American and Latina women: Building culturally and gender-appropriate intervention. *AIDS Education & Prevention, 7*(3), 251–264.

Whitehead, T. L. (1997). Urban low-income African American men, HIV/AIDS, and gender identity. *Medical Anthropology Quarterly, 11*(4), 411–447.

Wingood, G. M., & DiClemente, R. J. (1992). Cultural, gender, and psychosocial influences on HIV-related behavior of African-American female adolescents: Implications for the development of tailored prevention programs. *Ethnicity & Disease, 2*(4), 381–388.

Wingood, G. M., Hunter-Gamble, D., & DiClemente, R. J. (1993). A pilot study of sexual communication and negotiation among young African American women: Implications for HIV prevention. Special Issue: Psychosocial aspects of AIDS prevention among African Americans. *Journal of Black Psychology, 19*(2), 190–203.

Wolfe, W. A. (2003). Overlooked role of African-American males' hypermasculinity in the epidemic of unintended pregnancies and HIV/AIDS cases with young African-American women. *Journal of the National Medical Association, 95*(9), 846–852.

Woodyard, J. L., Peterson, J. L., & Stokes, J. P. (2000). "Let us go into the house of the Lord": Participation in the African American churches among young African American men who have sex with men. *The Journal of Pastoral Care, 54,* 451–460.

Zamora-Hernández, C., & Patterson, D. (1996). Homosexually active Latino men: Issues for social work practice. *Journal of Gay & Lesbian Social Services, 5*(2/3), 69–91.

# 8

# Mass Media Campaigns as a Tool for HIV Prevention

*Philip Palmgreen*

*Seth M. Noar*

*Rick S. Zimmerman*
University of Kentucky

The mass media have been employed with great frequency around the world in interventions to help prevent the spread of HIV/AIDS and other sexually transmitted diseases (STDs) (DeJong, Wolf, & Austin, 2001; Holtgrave, 1997; Myhre & Flora, 2000; Ratzan, Payne, & Massett, 1994; Singhal & Rogers, 2003). These mass communication campaigns have employed single or multiple media at the national, regional, and local levels, either as stand-alone efforts or as part of multicomponent programs involving strategies such as needle-sharing programs, community coalitions, counseling, support groups, and peer education. Mass media campaigns, because of their ability to reach huge and diverse audiences in a cost-effective manner, have tremendous potential as a tool in fighting the spread of the HIV/AIDS pandemic and other STDs. Cohen, Wu, and Farley (2005) estimated through mathematical modeling that media campaigns were the sixth most cost-effective strategy (out of 24 tested) for preventing HIV infection in the United States. This estimate did not take into account that three of the five strategies rated above media campaigns in cost-effectiveness (community mobilization, STD screening, and needle exchange) have often utilized the media to facilitate the strategy.

Unfortunately, more is assumed than is actually known about the effectiveness of HIV/STD media campaigns for a variety of reasons, including a scarcity of well-funded and sophisticated evaluation efforts and the difficulty of isolating media effects in multicomponent interventions (Noar, 2006). In addition, whereas HIV prevention interventions in the United States have traditionally been focused at the individual level in counseling, small-group, and school-based programs (e.g., Centers for Disease Control and Prevention [CDC], 2001; Peterson & DiClemente, 2000), although recent years have witnessed increasing calls for more interventions that incorporate the mass media and other community-wide elements (DiClemente, 2000; Frieden, Das-Douglas, Kellerman, & Henning, 2005; Keller & Brown, 2002; Kelly, 1999; Ross & Williams, 2002).

## Purpose of the Chapter

The goal of the current chapter is to explore the very real potential of HIV prevention mass media campaigns and to provide guidelines to researchers and practitioners for their effective execution. This is accomplished by: (a) a brief review of the literature on health mass communication campaigns where solid evidence now exists of campaign effectiveness; (b) a discussion of well-accepted principles of effective media campaigns derived from this literature, with illustrative examples of how these principles either have or have not been successfully applied to media-based HIV/STD prevention efforts; (c) a discussion of recent quantitative reviews that suggest that HIV/ AIDS media campaigns can be successful in changing behavior; and (d) for illustrative purposes, a relatively detailed examination of one recent successful mass media campaign to promote safer sexual practices that employed several principles of successful health communication campaigns coupled with a rigorous evaluation design. The current chapter is *not* intended to be a new systematic review of HIV prevention media campaigns, as such reviews already exist in the literature (e.g., Holtgrave, 1997; Johnson, Flora, & Rimal, 1997; Myhre & Flora, 2000; Vidanapathirana, Abramson, Forbes, & Fairley, 2005). However, the combination of existing review articles and an updated (but not exhaustive) search conducted in preparation for this chapter give us a strong sense of where this literature stands. Thus, where possible, generalizations about the state of the HIV prevention campaign literature are made.

Furthermore, in the current chapter we confine ourselves to conventional mass media HIV/STD campaigns that involve the purposive and organized use of "traditional media" such as television, radio, and print to disseminate relatively short messages to both mass and more differentiated audiences, although some of the campaigns discussed also utilized "small" media such as leaflets, brochures, billboards, and newsletters. We do not concern ourselves with other uses of the media in HIV/STD prevention, involving much more extensive messages such as television or radio programs in "entertainment-education," or in press coverage of issues, which has been very effective in "setting the agenda" for efforts to combat the epidemic. Nor do we treat the growing use of the Internet to reach both large and targeted audiences with prevention-related information. These are all examined in detail in separate chapters in this volume (see chaps. 9 and 10, this volume).

## Health Communication Campaigns: Evidence of Effectiveness

As noted in a recent review by Randolph and Viswanath (2004):

> Mass media campaigns to promote healthy behavior and discourage unhealthy behaviors have become a major tool of public health practitioners in their efforts to improve the health of the public. Large amounts of money, time, and effort are poured into mass media campaigns, both local and national in scope, each year in various attempts to get the public to eat healthy, get moving, stop smoking, and practice safer sex. (p. 419)

Although most early health communication media campaigns (and even many recent ones) were failures, more sophisticated efforts incorporating many or all of the design elements discussed herein, including more powerful evaluation methodologies, have led to a body of evidence that media health campaigns can produce a variety of important effects (Backer, 1990; Hornik, 2002; Noar, 2006; Perloff, 2003; Rice & Atkin, 2001; Rogers & Storey, 1987). Research generally has shown that mass media used in conjunction with other kinds of interventions are more successful than media campaigns alone (Flora, Maibach, & Maccoby, 1989; Rogers & Storey, 1987). Evidence is accumulating, however, that properly designed media campaigns alone can have significant impacts on health-related knowledge, attitudes, and beliefs. Hornik (2002) has compiled an impressive edited volume of studies that demonstrates important effects of media campaigns on a wide variety of health *behaviors* across a number of contexts and cultures. Moreover, recent meta-analyses of media health campaigns have documented effects on behaviors equivalent to those of in-school smoking and drug abuse prevention programs and family-planning programs around the world, with larger effects on attitudes and knowledge (Derzon & Lipsey, 2002; Snyder & Hamilton, 2002). The success of these campaigns, however, appears to depend on their utilization of a number of principles widely recognized in the campaign literature (e.g., Noar, 2006).

### Principles of Effective Campaign Design

The mass media campaign literature is rich with descriptions of factors associated with more effective and successful campaigns (e.g., Atkin; 2001; Perloff, 2003; Randolph & Viswanath, 2004; Rogers & Storey, 1987; Salmon & Atkin, 2003; Valente, 2001), many of which were derived from the social marketing and advertising literature (e.g., Grier & Bryant, 2005). Though reviewing and discussing all such factors is beyond the scope of this chapter, we focus instead on a core set of principles that can in many ways be viewed as a "recipe book" of how to conduct and evaluate an effective campaign (Noar, 2006). These include (a) conducting *formative research* with the target audience, (b) *using theory* as a conceptual foundation, (c) *segmenting one's audience* into meaningful subgroups, (d) using a *message design approach* that is *targeted* to the audience segment(s), (e) placing messages in *channels* widely viewed by the target audience, (f) conducting *process evaluation* and ensuring *high message exposure*, and (g) using a sensitive *outcome evaluation design* that reduces threats to internal validity. Each principle is discussed next with accompanying examples from the HIV/AIDS campaign literature.

Formative Research.    Conducting formative research is a key to the success of any mass media campaign. Without it, campaign planners will lack a sophisticated understanding of the audience, the targeted behavior(s), as well as knowing how individuals might react to campaign messages. Atkin and Freimuth (2001) discuss two phases of formative research: (a) *preproduction research,* where information regarding audience characteristics, the behavior at issue, and message channels are gathered; and (b) production test-ing, or *pretesting*, where initial messages are tested with target audi-ence members in order to gain feedback on the appropriateness and persuasive impact of those messages.

Recent systematic reviews of HIV/AIDS media campaign stud-ies have *not* examined whether such studies conducted formative research to inform campaign efforts. Thus, generalizations regarding this principle are difficult to make. However, in our updated review of 25 HIV/AIDS media campaign studies published between 1998 and 2005, some excellent examples of formative research were found. For example, Alstead et al. (1999) made extensive use of formative research in the development of an HIV prevention print-media cam-paign targeted toward sexually active teenagers in urban communi-ties in Washington State. They conducted numerous focus groups with the target audience in order to understand issues surrounding condom use for teens, especially why condoms are often used incon-sistently. The focus groups also helped identify the best media chan-nels for reaching sexually active teens. Additional focus groups with youth and other key decision makers examined message concepts developed by a professional advertising agency, and provided valu-able feedback subsequently used to modify the campaign messages.

In addition, Bull, Cohen, Ortiz, and Evans (2002) provide one of the most comprehensive discussions of the application of forma-tive research in developing a media campaign to promote use of both male and female condoms by teen and young-adult women in Denver, Colorado. They conducted 12 focus groups with the target audience regarding knowledge levels, attitudes, and behaviors with respect to condoms. In addition, campaign messages were developed through an iterative process involving focus groups at each stage of message development, including soliciting message concepts and gaining specific feedback on near-final campaign materials.

Use of Theory.    Many theories can and have served as conceptual foundations for mass media campaigns (e.g., Cappella, Fishbein, Hornik, Ahern, & Sayeed, 2001; Murray-Johnson & Witte, 2003; Noar, 2007; Slater, 1999). Theories can serve a number of important roles, including suggesting: (a) important theoretical determinants upon which campaign messages might focus, (b) variables for audience segmentation, and (c) variables to be used in evaluating campaigns. In addition, Murray-Johnson and Witte suggest that when using theory for campaigns, it is useful to think in terms of which variables in one's theory might stimulate thought on the behavior of interest, which might motivate individuals to change, which might promote an individual's appraisal of their environment and resources, and which might suggest important outcomes to measure.

Myhre and Flora (2000) found, in their systematic review of 41 HIV/AIDS media campaigns conducted in 17 countries, that very few campaigns (less than 20%) were theory based. More recent studies appear to be using theories with greater frequency, and this is a promising development. Campaign studies are utilizing such theoretical perspectives as the health belief model (Agha, 2003; Meekers, Agha, & Klein, 2005), theories of reasoned action and planned behavior (Bull et al., 2002; Oh et al., 2002; Yzer, Siero, & Buunk, 2000), social cognitive theory (Bull et al., 2002; Meekers et al., 2005; Ross, Chatterjee, & Leonard, 2004), diffusion of innovations (Geary, Mahler, Finger, & Shears, 2005; Valente & Saba, 1998), the stages of change model (CDC, 1999), and the extended parallel process model (Witte, Cameron, Lapinski, & Nzyuko, 1998). Many recent studies rely on a single theory to inform their campaign, whereas others use multiple theories to form a conceptual basis for their campaign (i.e., Bull et al., 2002). However, other recent studies have either not used theories (Devos-Comby & Salovey, 2002) or not reported what theory guided the campaign, although in some cases campaigns have employed important theoretical concepts without specifying their origin (e.g., attitude change, modeling).

Audience Segmentation.    Grunig (1989) has stated: "The basic idea of segmentation is simple: divide a population, market, or audience into groups whose members are more like each other than members of other segments" (p. 202). Audience segmentation is employed to create homogenous groups that can then be targeted with messages designed specifically for that audience (Atkin, 2001; Slater, 1996), and a failure to segment is often cited as a major contributing factor to failed campaign efforts (Flay & Sobel, 1983; Rogers & Storey, 1987). Numerous HIV nonmedia interventions have segmented audiences into very specific kinds of groups (e.g., Peterson & DiClemente, 2000), but have HIV/AIDS media campaigns followed suit? Johnson et al. (1997) and Myhre and Flora (2000) found that despite the fact that early AIDS cases in the United States occurred in very specific high-risk groups (e.g., homosexual men, injection drug users), the majority of early campaigns were directed toward a broad, undefined audience. Johnson et al. (1997) found that most of 317 televised HIV/AIDS public service announcements (PSAs) from 33 countries (from 1987 to 1993) were directed at heterosexual viewers or to generalized audiences, whereas Myhre and Flora (2000) reported that 24 of 41 (59%) campaigns in 17 countries were directed at general audiences. One example is "America Responds to AIDS" (ARTA), the major U.S. campaign launched in the 1980s by the CDC. ARTA employed a large number of media messages disseminated through numerous channels. ARTA messages usually were quite generic in an attempt to reach virtually the entire U.S. population, although some were directed at specific audiences such as adults with multiple sexual partners (Ratzan et al., 1994). Unfortunately, political pressure led the federal government to abandon concepts that had been developed for ARTA and targeted to specific high-risk audience segments such as men who have sex with men and injection drug users (DeJong et al., 2001).

A minority of campaigns *have* utilized audience segmentation, primarily segmenting on demographic and sexual risk variables, with campaigns directed at youth, families, men, women, college students, commercial sex workers, heterosexuals, injection drug users, and other "high-risk" groups (Myhre & Flora, 2000). More recently published studies appear to be following this template of segmenting audiences on these types of variables (e.g., Agha, 2003; CDC, 1999; Chen, Kodagoda, Lawrence, & Kerndt, 2002; Kaiser Family Foundation, 2004; Ross et al., 2004). This may be related to the fact that newer campaigns are much more focused on influencing behaviors related to HIV/AIDS prevention (e.g., condom use, HIV testing) than on the earlier goal of raising general awareness of the threat posed by HIV/AIDS. A focus on behavioral influence almost mandates concentrating campaign efforts on those groups who are at risk for or currently performing a behavior.

A word of caution, however, is necessary in segmenting audiences for HIV/AIDS campaigns. On the one hand, messages targeted to specific audiences are likely to be the most effective. On the other, messages crafted for these specific audiences (i.e., African Americans, gay men, injection drug users) run the risk of stereotyping certain audience segments as especially prone to HIV/AIDS, and could give the impression that other groups (i.e., heterosexuals) are *not* at risk for AIDS. In fact, some spots early in the ARTA campaign were targeted toward African-Americans, but were pulled off the air because of protests from African-American leaders who thought that they might lead to stereotyping and stigmatization. As already discussed, one method of dealing with this challenging issue is to pretest messages with the target audience, including group leaders, to discover possible adverse reactions in advance. Another method is to "narrowcast" highly targeted messages through channels and media likely to reach only those groups especially at risk. This would avoid dissemination to general audiences and greatly reduce the chances of widespread stereotyping.

Message Design and Targeting.     Once a meaningful audience segment has been created, messages effective with that segment can be developed. This is referred to as message targeting (Kreuter, Strecher, & Glassman, 1999). Reviews of HIV/AIDS campaigns from the 1980s to the mid-1990s (e.g., DeJong et al., 2001; Holtgrave, 1997; Myhre & Flora, 2000) provide little evidence of the use of sophisticated message design and targeting frameworks. For instance, DeJong et al. examined 56 televised PSAs primarily produced by the CDC and found that: (a) The majority provided general information only; (b) few provided prevention messages specific to sexual behavior or condom use; (c) nearly half were fear based; and (d) theories of behavioral change were rarely utilized in the design of the messages. Johnson et al. (1997) also found that the majority of the 317 PSAs they reviewed were "heavy on information but light on recommendations" (p. 231). Furthermore, these findings must be put into context. Early AIDS campaigns in the United States transmitted general messages because their primary aim was to change the perception of AIDS from a "gay" disease to a mainstream threat about which all Americans should be concerned. In addition, the campaigns that took place in the 1980s often used general messages because of political pressure from conservative groups to avoid sexual content in government-sponsored ads. In fact, the first televised PSA to mention the word *condom* did not air until 1994 under the Clinton administration, and this delay in promoting condom use had to do with political rather than public health reasoning (DeJong et al., 2001).

However, the trend toward greater use of both theory and audience segmentation in media campaigns has meant that many of the theories mentioned previously have been applied to message design in more recent safer-sex campaign efforts. These theories have been useful in suggesting message content that addresses important determinants of sexual behaviors (e.g., behavioral beliefs, subjective norms, self-efficacy), and messages can clearly be developed based on these determinants (see Murray-Johnson & Witte, 2003). Despite this, few theoretical approaches help specify themes, content, and formal features of messages that resonate with particular audience segments. One of the few such approaches to do so is sensation-seeking targeting (SENTAR; Noar, Palmgreen, Zimmerman, Lustria, & Lu, 2006; Palmgreen & Donohew, 2003), whose application is illustrated later in this chapter. Other approaches that can inform many of these aspects of message design include the fear appeal approach, social cognitive theory (particularly modeling) and consideration of source credibility, message framing, and cultural targeting approaches (for reviews, see Devos-Comby & Salovey, 2002; Salmon & Atkin, 2003; Witte & Allen, 2000). Moreover, though formative research is often used to pretest campaigns themes and messages, and is very useful for this purpose, message design and targeting should be theoretically based.

Channel Selection.    Channel selection refers to the choice of medium through which one's mass media messages are to be disseminated. Traditional campaigns often use one or a combination of media channels such as television, radio, and print media such as newspapers and magazines, although many traditional mass media campaigns have also utilized nonmedia channels including community mobilization, public relations events, and school-based components (Perloff, 2001). In addition, some campaigns utilize so-called "small" media such as leaflets, brochures, billboards, and newsletters. The choice of channel(s) is important, as channels differ on numerous factors including cost, reach, credibility, ease of use, intrusiveness, depth of content, personalization and interactivity, and stimulation of senses (Salmon & Atkin, 2003). Selected channels should be well-suited to disseminating campaign messages in a way that is consistent with the tendencies of the target audience, and messages should be carefully placed within those channels (e.g., Palmgreen & Donohew, 2003).

In addition to choosing the types of channels for a campaign, campaign planners must also choose the number of different channels to be used in any given campaign. With multiple-channel campaigns, understanding which channels were responsible for campaign impact can be difficult, although a well-designed *scientific* study could allow for inferences about the effects of individual channels as well as any synergistic effects of using multiple channels. From a practitioner perspective, however, using multiple channels is often desirable, as local, state, and federal agencies that conduct campaigns typically want to use all of the resources at their disposal in an attempt to have maximum public health impact. Where funding and research expertise allow, the effects of individual and combined channels might be examined even in these kinds of campaigns, although post hoc separating of channel effects can often be difficult.

HIV/AIDS media campaigns to date have utilized numerous media and nonmedia channels including television, film, radio, and print media such as posters, leaflets, brochures, newspapers, and role model stories, as well as community educators and peer outreach approaches. Though approximately one fourth of campaigns have used just one channel, most campaigns have used multiple channels to disseminate campaign messages (Myhre & Flora, 2000). However, Myhre and Flora noted that only some campaign articles explicitly discussed channel selection. In addition, they noted that campaigns in developing countries have often used a mix of low-cost media such as radio and print materials, whereas campaigns in developed countries have tended to make heavy use of television, often resulting in higher message exposure. More recent campaigns have continued to use a variety of traditional and small media, and several have incorporated the Internet as practitioners have begun to recognize the great potential of this medium to target and tailor a variety of HIV/AIDS messages to specific audiences and individuals (Andersen, Ostergaard, Moller, & Olesen, 2001; Chen et al., 2002; Geary et al., 2005; Kaiser Family Foundation, 2003, 2004; see also chap. 13, this volume).

Process Evaluation and Message Exposure.    Process evaluation, a key component of overall campaign evaluation, is concerned with the monitoring and collection of data on fidelity and implementation of campaign activities (e.g., Valente, 2001). Although campaigns are often *planned* to be executed in a very specific way, without process evaluation it will be unclear *whether* and how the plan "worked." For instance, did the messages *reach* the target audience? If so, with what *frequency*? If not, *what went wrong*? Understanding the target audience's exposure levels to campaign messages is a key component of process evaluation. Traditionally, health mass media campaigns have suffered from poor message exposure, with many achieving less than 20% exposure and with an average of only 36% to 42% reach (Snyder & Hamilton, 2002). Even many large campaign efforts in the "classic" media campaign literature suffered from low exposure, which may explain some of the modest or even nonsignificant results of these trials (Hornik, 2002).

Though Myhre and Flora (2000) did not examine process evaluation generally in their review of campaigns through 1998, they did examine message exposure (reach), finding that 38% of campaigns gave no estimate of campaign exposure. However, of those that did report on message exposure, 68% reported at least one campaign exposure measure of greater than 50% of the target audience, with several reporting maximum reach percentages of 69% to 93%. In addition, message exposure was related to resources available as well as channel selection—televised campaigns appear to have the greatest exposure, whereas print media campaigns have had much poorer exposure (Myhre & Flora, 2000).

By comparison, in our updated review of 25 studies published between 1998 and 2005, only 16% (4 studies) gave no estimate of campaign exposure. Of the 21 studies that did report on exposure, 18 (72%) reported that at least one exposure measure was greater than 50%. In addition, 14 studies (67%) reported maximum reach percentages in an even higher range, (69% to 98%). Again, reach varied by channel and audience subgroup. Thus, it appears that the reach of most HIV/AIDS media campaigns is adequate and improving with time, although very few data are available on exposure *frequency* or on other types of process evaluation. Also, in a number of the studies both reviewed by Myhre and Flora (2000) and examined in our updated review, exposure was treated as an outcome variable rather than a process measure. Process evaluation is most useful when the data produced are used to modify and improve an ongoing campaign.

Outcome Evaluation.    Outcome evaluation is concerned with assessing whether a campaign had its intended impact. For instance, media campaigns are often focused on increasing knowledge, changing perceptions, attitudes or beliefs, and/or changing behaviors. Because campaigns are often community-level efforts that occur in real-world contexts, true experimental designs are often not feasible (Hornik,

2002). However, a number of rigorous quasi-experimental designs are available and well-suited for this context (Valente, 2001).

What outcomes have HIV/AIDS media campaigns focused on, and how have such campaigns typically been evaluated? Myhre and Flora (2000) found that knowledge and attitudes were the most common variables assessed. However, a majority of campaigns (approximately 60%) did assess behaviors such as sexual activity and condom use. Few campaigns examined theoretical variables such as perceived risk or social norms, and just three campaigns looked at STD/HIV incidence or prevalence. However, most campaigns examined in their review used outcome evaluation designs that are best described as *preexperimental*, lacking control/comparison groups or other rigorous design aspects (e.g., time series). In fact, only 7 of 41 campaigns, or 17%, used quasi-experimental designs that included comparison groups, and 5 of these articles were written about differing phases of the same campaign—the CDC Community Demonstration Projects (CDC, 1999). In fact, because of the lack of controlled research designs and the great variability in outcome measures employed, Myhre and Flora were not able to address the question of average effects of HIV/AIDS media campaigns. A similar review by Holtgrave (1997) mirrors these conclusions, as does the newer literature that we reviewed. For instance, we found that 9 of the 22 studies reporting evaluation methods used a posttest-only design, 9 utilized a pretest–posttest independent-samples design (i.e., were not panel studies), and one study used the number of calls to a hotline as the only outcome measure (Oh et al., 2002). Only three studies used a control group, one of which also employed a panel design (Yzer et al., 2000). This lack of strong outcome evaluation designs makes assessments of average campaign effects difficult to estimate.

### Evidence for Effectiveness of HIV/AIDS Media Campaigns

Despite the fact that many HIV/AIDS media campaigns use weak outcome evaluation designs, two recent quantitative reviews were able to synthesize the effects of such campaigns among studies with stronger designs. Vidanapathirana et al. (2005) examined campaigns that promoted voluntary HIV counseling and testing. Of 35 studies identified in their review, the authors judged 14 to have strong evaluation designs, including two randomized controlled trials, three nonrandomized controlled studies, and nine interrupted time-series investigations. Their reanalysis of these studies using sophisticated regression-based interrupted time-series techniques and meta-analytic procedures revealed that all 14 studies documented short-term changes in HIV testing produced by the campaigns. No support was found for long-term effects. In addition, Snyder and Hamilton (2002) examined average behavior change effect sizes of health mass media campaigns conducted in the United States. They found that safer-sex campaigns changed the behavior, on average, of 6% of the target audience (or $r = .04$), comparable to media campaigns targeting other health behaviors such as heart disease, smoking, and mammography screening.

Overall, both of these reviews provide evidence that HIV/AIDS media campaigns have had effects on behavioral change. Although these effects have been relatively small and short term, as noted earlier the wide reach of media campaigns can render them highly cost-effective and capable of having real public health impact (Cohen et al., 2005). In addition, campaigns that closely adhere to principles of effective design may outperform the average effects reported in these quantitative reviews (Noar, 2006).

## Summary

The design, implementation, and evaluation of any HIV/AIDS mass media campaign is a major undertaking. Unfortunately, the literature to date provides more examples of studies with modest or inconclusive outcomes than it does studies with stellar outcomes. However, campaign designers who follow the principles described in this chapter, which are based on decades of research on mass media campaigns, should greatly increase their chances of conducting an effective campaign (Noar, 2006; Randolph & Viswanath, 2004; Salmon & Atkin, 2003).

In the next section, we describe a safer-sex mass media campaign effort funded by the National Institute of Mental Health (NIMH) that was undertaken with the goal of applying all of the major principles described in this chapter. The purpose was to rigorously and empirically test the idea that a televised HIV/AIDS media-only campaign embodying these principles could impact not only safer-sex beliefs but safer sexual behavior as well (i.e., condom use).

## Illustrative Example: Safer Sex Campaign Study

The Safer Sex Campaign (SSC) study was a rigorous evaluation of a televised PSA campaign aimed at increasing condom use and related variables in at-risk young adults (Zimmerman et al., in press). The study employed formative research, theory, audience segmentation, message design and targeting techniques, and channel selection procedures tied to the *sensation-seeking targeting approach* (SENTAR—see Palmgreen & Donohew, 2003). Campaign messages (TV PSAs) were selected/developed to be persuasive with high-sensation seekers and impulsive decision makers, two groups at particular risk for unsafe sexual practices. The PSAs were placed in programming popular with the target audience, and an interrupted time series design with a control community was used to rigorously evaluate the campaign. The next two sections describe the theoretical background for the segmentation of audiences.

## Sensation Seeking

Zuckerman (1994) defines sensation seeking as "the seeking of varied, novel, complex, and intense sensations and experiences, and the willingness to take physical, social, legal, and financial risks for the sake of such experience" (p. 27). Sensation seeking is a moderate to strong predictor of a variety of risky behaviors including drug use, unsafe sex, crime, deviance, drinking and driving, and speeding according to scores of studies spanning four decades across different cultures (e.g., Barnea, Rahav, & Teichman, 1992; Donohew et al., 2000; Zuckerman, 1994; Zuckerman & Neeb, 1980). Hoyle, Fejfar, and Miller (2000) found sensation seeking to be the personality trait with the strongest and most consistent relationships with risky sexual behaviors including numbers of sexual partners, unprotected intercourse, and various "high risk" sexual encounters. Especially important from a campaign-targeting perspective, however, is that high-sensation seekers (HSSs) also have distinct and consistent preferences for particular kinds of messages based on their needs for the novel, the unusual, and the intense (Donohew, Lorch, & Palmgreen, 1991; Zuckerman, 1979, 1990, 1994). HSSs prefer messages that are high in *sensation value* (HSV messages), that is, messages whose content and formal features elicit strong sensory, affective, and arousal responses (Palmgreen et al., 1991). Low-sensation seekers (LSSs) generally prefer lower levels of message sensation value (i.e., LSV messages). In practical terms, this means that HSSs prefer messages that are novel, complex, emotionally powerful, physically arousing, graphic, socially unconventional, fast-paced, or suspenseful. A variety of experimental studies have demonstrated that HSV messages are more effective than LSV messages with HSSs in eliciting changes in drug use attitudes and intentions, as well as greater liking for, attention to, and processing of prevention messages (Lorch et al., 1994; Palmgreen et al., 1991; Palmgreen, Stephenson, Everett, Baseheart, & Francies, 2002; Stephenson, 2003). A campaign study, employing a SENTAR-based controlled time-series design similar to that used in the SSC study described here, showed that all three televised PSA campaigns resulted in large reductions in marijuana use among HSS teens (Palmgreen, Donohew, Lorch, Hoyle, & Stephenson, 2001, 2002).

## Impulsive Decision Making

Decision making can range from a highly rational style involving careful consideration of cognitive cues to a very impulsive "act without thinking" process that relies primarily on affective and physiological cues. Donohew et al. (2000) showed that impulsive decision makers (IDMs) were significantly more likely than rational decision makers (RDMs) to have had sex, to have ever used alcohol or marijuana, and to have had unwanted sex under pressure while drunk. The same study showed an additive relationship of sensation seeking and impulsive decision making (which are moderately correlated), such that those high on both variables took greater sexual risks than those high on only one or none of the variables. Noar, Zimmerman, Palmgreen, Lustria, and Horosewski (2006) found through structural equation modeling that sensation seeking and impulsive decision making were related to more negative condom attitudes and social norms, and lower condom self-efficacy, which were in turn related to condom use. In addition, formative research from the SSC study yielded preliminary indications that IDMs prefer many of the same message characteristics effective with HSSs.

## Study Design

The SSC study involved a 21-month controlled time series design (Cook & Campbell, 1979). Safer-sex PSAs were aired from January through March 2003 in Lexington, Kentucky, whereas no campaign took place in the comparison city, Knoxville, Tennessee. These two moderate-size southeastern cities had similar demographics and nonoverlapping media systems. Data were collected from May 2002 to January 2004, which includes 8 months prior to the onset of the Lexington campaign, 3 months during the campaign (January–March, 2003), and 10 months postcampaign.

### Formative Research and Public Service Announcement Development

The PSAs developed for the campaign were the product of formative research consisting of three waves of focus groups drawn from the target audience. More than 40 focus groups (divided by sensation seeking, impulsive decision making, and gender) were aimed at: (a) gaining a better understanding of sexual risk taking, (b) pretesting existing safer-sex TV PSAs with the target audience, and (c) testing scripts developed by the research team according to SENTAR principles. This led to the production (by a professional producer) of five original 30-second televised PSAs targeted at HSS-IDM young adults. All five PSAs were highly novel, with dramatic narrative frameworks—features with special appeal for HSSs. The PSAs varied in their use of different combinations of other characteristics known to increase the sensation value of messages (e.g, fast pace, unexpected visual and audio formats, loud music, unusual sound effects, strong emotion). Each ad ended with the message (superimposed on the screen) "Use a condom. Every partner. Every time." Permission from the Kaiser Family Foundation was also secured to use five of their safer-sex PSAs in the campaign. All had been rated highly by HSS and IDM focus group participants (Noar et al., 2006).

### Theoretical Frameworks

In addition to the SENTAR approach, several concepts common to behavioral theories in the health arena were used to guide message content and campaign evaluation. Messages encouraged positive attitudes toward condom use, promoted positive safer-sex norms, emphasized increased condom use self-efficacy, encouraged discussion of and negotiation of safer-sex practices, and emphasized and modeled commitment to and planning ahead for safe sex (Noar, Anderman, Zimmerman, & Cupp, 2004; Noar & Zimmerman, 2005; Noar et al., 2006). In addition, campaign messages sought to increase perceived HIV/STD susceptibility, personalize risk, and dispel the myth that intimate relationships protect against STDs (Noar, Zimmerman, & Atwood, 2004). Theoretical factors thought to be strong mediators of condom use, such as self-efficacy and intentions to use condoms, were also used in the evaluation of the campaign. Finally, campaign messages were aired in a manner consistent with stage theories of health behavior (e.g., Prochaska, DiClemente, & Norcross, 1992). Specifically, across the 12-week campaign, messages were "staged" to focus on (a) perceived threat of HIV and other STDs (Weeks 1–3), (b) personalization of HIV/STD risk (Weeks 4–6), (c) benefits of condom use and negative consequences of nonuse (Weeks 7–9), and (d) skills necessary to enact condom use (Weeks 10–12).

## The Televised Campaign

The campaign used television as its only channel for three reasons. First, television was chosen in order to test the idea that a single-channel media-only campaign could be effective with a medium that is easily disseminated and replicated in future campaigns (i.e., TV). Second, television was selected because members of this target audience watch a significant amount of television each day, increasing the chances that exposure to campaign messages might be high. Finally, television was selected for its multimedia characteristics—spots that are developed for TV can include various sound and music features, intense images, and other features that allow the *sensation value* of campaign messages to be maximized.

The campaign was shown (using a 50/50 combination of paid and donated time) from January to March 2003, in Lexington, Kentucky, using the 10 PSAs described. A professional media buyer placed the paid PSAs in programming (especially in narrowly targeted cable programs) popular with the target audience (channel selection), as determined by precampaign survey data. Most pro-bono PSAs were placed in the same programs. Standard industry formulas estimated that 80% of the target audience would be exposed to an average of 33 campaign messages, considered to be high exposure for a 3-month TV ad campaign.

## Sampling, Participants, and Interviewing Methods

Beginning 8 months before the campaign, interviews were conducted with *independent* cross-sectional samples of 100 randomly selected young adults each month in each community. The population cohort followed in each community was initially ages 18 years, 0 months to 23 years, 11 months, and aged 20 months as the cohort was followed to the end of the study. This was accomplished by continuously adjusting the minimum and maximum ages for eligibility upward 1 month at the start of each month. Two sampling methods were used to recruit participants monthly: random-digit dialing and the calling of random samples of undergraduate and graduate students at the University of Kentucky (Lexington) and the University of Tennessee (Knoxville). Of those contacted, 60% agreed to complete a brief screener over the phone. To be eligible, participants had to be: (a) in the appropriate age span for the particular study month, (b) heterosexually active (had sex with an opposite-sex partner) in the past 3 months, and (c) a U.S. citizen (because of logistical factors related to paying participants the incentive). Of those screened and determined to be eligible ($N = 4,989$), 82% completed interviews for the project ($N = 4,032$ individuals across the two cities).

The majority (including all sensitive items) of the private 40- to 45-minute interview was self-administered via a laptop computer, which increased confidentiality and anonymity and improved assessment of message exposure, as participants actually viewed the PSAs on the laptop. Most interviews took place in the respondent's home. Interviewees were paid $30 (this amount increased by $5 every 6 months).

## Measures

A number of valid and reliable measures were used in the study, including questions on demographics, sexual characteristics, condom self-efficacy, condom use intentions, and condom use. All multiple-item scales used 5-point Likert response formats (for more on measures used, see Zimmerman et al., in press). Two particularly important measures are described next.

Sensation Seeking/Impulsive Decision Making. A composite risk variable called sensation seeking/impulsive decision making (SSIDM) was created as the product of two scales: sensation seeking and impulsive decision making. *Sensation seeking* was assessed using Hoyle, Stephenson, Palmgreen, Lorch, and Donohew's (2002) eight-item Brief Sensation Seeking Scale (BSSS). Participants were asked how much they agreed or disagreed with items such as "I like to do frightening things." Coefficient alpha in this study was .74. *Impulsive decision making* was measured with the 12-item decision-making style scale (Donohew et al., 2000). Items included "I do the first thing that comes into my mind." Coefficient alpha was .84. Individuals above the median on the composite scale, within race/gender categories, were classified as high sensation seekers/impulsive decision makers (HSSIDMs), with those below the median classified as low sensation seekers/rational decision makers (LSSRDMs).

Cued PSA Exposure Measure. Respondents in both cities were shown (via the laptop) the five original PSAs developed for the campaign. Time and respondent fatigue prohibited showing the five Kaiser PSAs. Respondents indicated how often they had seen each PSA using five categories (first category = "have not seen"; last category = "more than 10 times"). Responses were conservatively recoded to reflect the category median, or in the case of the highest category, a low estimate (i.e., "more than 10 times" was recoded to 11).

## Results

Both Lexington and Knoxville samples matched closely on most demographic variables, which generally paralleled Census and university figures for each city. With the first number in parentheses indicating the Lexington sample and the second number indicating the Knoxville sample, the samples were (57.4%; 55.7%) female, (80.7%; 86.9%) White, (69.3%; 68.9%) some college to graduate degree, and (21.9; 21.7) years old. The samples matched closely on sensation seeking ($M$ = 3.40; 3.43) and impulsive decision making ($M$ = 2.59; 2.64), and on all variables related to sexual behavior: for example, currently in a relationship (72.0%; 73.3%); age at first intercourse (16.4; 16.7), condom use in past 3 months—sometimes/everytime (68.9%; 69.2%); frequency of intercourse in past 30 days—males (11.6 times; 11.6 times); frequency of intercourse past 30 days—females (10.4 times; 10.9 times); median number of sexual partners in past year—males (2; 2); median number of sexual partners in past year—females (1; 1).

*Process Evaluation and Campaign Exposure (Recall)*

Process evaluation included a major focus on implementation of the televised campaign, with continuous reports provided by the television stations to our media buyer and the research team to monitor implementation. All indications were that the PSA spots actually aired as planned, including targeted placements made in programs specific to gender (e.g., airing male-focused PSAs within sports programming) and HSS/IDM preferences. Figure 8.1 plots campaign message recall (derived from the interviews) as reported by Lexington HSSIDMs from January (the start of the campaign) through the end of the study. This figure examines percentages who recalled seeing any one of the five *original* campaign PSAs (which received the greatest airtime). As expected, recall was lower in the first month of the campaign (67%), and greatly increased to between 93% and 100% recall through August (indicating high memorability). During the peak period of the campaign (February, March), we estimate that 96% of the target audience recalled seeing at least one of the original PSAs, 88% at least 2, 75% at least 3, and 58% recalled four or more such PSAs. Regarding frequency of exposure, it was estimated conservatively (because the category "10 or more times" was coded as "11") that the target audience recalled seeing the five original PSAs 22 times on average during the campaign. Of course, mean recall frequency for all 10 PSAs employed (including the Kaiser PSAs) undoubtedly would have been higher.

*Lexington Time-Series Regression Analyses*

Monthly means for all dependent variables were calculated separately by city for HSSIDMs and LSSRDMs and the means for each category

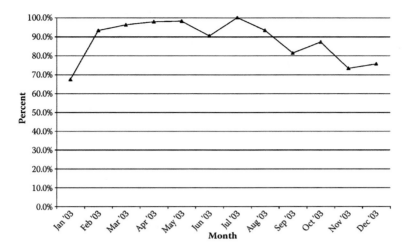

**FIGURE 8.1.** Percentage of Lexington HSSIDM respondents reporting exposure to at least one campaign PSA.

of respondents were analyzed separately with a regression-based interrupted time-series procedure appropriate for datasets with fewer than 50 data points (Lewis-Beck, 1986). The procedure employs dummy variables to model slopes, as well as intercept and slope changes due to the intervention. A series of different analyses using various models were run to clarify a complex pattern of results due to an apparent wearing off of campaign effects a few months after the campaign ended.

## Results for HSSIDMs

For those high on the composite risk variable (HSSIDMs), initial analyses of regression data for all dependent variables were run using five dummy variables: one for the slope prior to the Lexington campaign, slope and intercept change variables for the Lexington campaign "interruption," and slope and intercept change variables for a downward change observed for each dependent variable 2 to 3 months after the campaign, apparently caused by campaign effects eventually wearing off (as ordinarily observed in ad campaigns). Intercept changes had very high $p$ levels in these initial analyses, whereas slope changes, also nonsignificant, nonetheless had $p$ values much closer to conventional significance levels. Therefore, following Lewis-Beck

(1986), the two intercept change terms in each of the models were dropped. This also increased degrees of freedom for estimation in these "reduced" models.

A Lexington reduced-model analysis indicated that the campaign produced a significant immediate upward slope change ($p < .05$) for *condom use* in HSSIDMs that lasted for 3 months after the campaign ended, after which the Lexington sample resumed its precampaign downward trend in condom use ($p < .05$ for slope change—see Fig. 8.2). Autocorrelation was acceptable ($\rho = -0.22$). Comparison of the postcampaign trend line with projected condom use levels (light gray line) in the absence of a campaign indicates that despite the campaign wear-out, participants had higher condom use as measured by the 5-point scale (regression estimate = 2.60) at the end of data collection than the level projected in the absence of a campaign (regression estimate = 2.32). Analyses with *condom self-efficacy* and *condom use intentions* as dependent variables produced almost identical results, and thus are not presented. The conclusion that the effects observed were due to the campaign and not to history factors is strengthened by monthly online content analyses conducted for the major newspapers in each community, which revealed no programs or events during the data gathering that could plausibly have

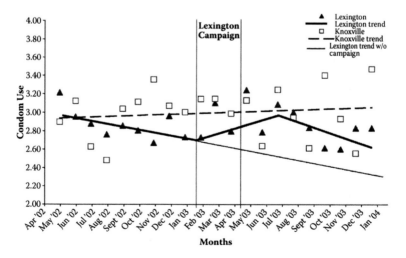

**FIGURE 8.2.**    Lexington and Knoxville 3-month condom use time series regression plots for HSSIDM young adults. (Condom use measured on a 5-point scale.)

affected the dependent variables. National safer-sex campaigns like the Kaiser Family Foundation's campaign were common to both cities, and could not have produced the differential patterns observed.

## Results for LSSRDMs

As expected, LSSRDMs were considerably and significantly lower than HSSIDMs on sexual-risk variables across both cities prior to the campaign in Lexington. Also as expected (because LSSRDMs were not targeted), various Lewis-Beck analyses (including both full and reduced models) involving LSSRDMs showed no campaign effects in Lexington on condom use, condom self-efficacy, or condom use intentions.

## Knoxville Time-Series Regression Analyses

In order to test whether the respondents in the comparison no-campaign city exhibited any patterns similar to those in Lexington on the dependent variables, a series of Knoxville time-series analyses were run with full and reduced models and employing the same "interruption" points as Lexington. As expected, these analyses showed no significant patterns for either HSSIDMs or LSSRDMs.

## Campaign Impact

An effect size for the Lexington campaign was calculated using Cohen's $d$, comparing condom use precampaign with postcampaign means and standard deviations, and taking into account the secular trend in Knoxville. In this case, $d = .26$, or slightly greater than a "small" effect size as defined by Cohen (1988). However, the campaign was considerably more effective than other safer-sex campaigns. Snyder and Hamilton (2002) reported the following effect sizes for safer-sex campaigns: AIDS Community Demonstration Projects ($r = .03$), AIDS Prevention for Pediatric Life ($r = .05$), and America Responds to AIDS ($r = .01$). By comparison, the Cohen's $d$ of .26 converts to $r = .13$.

Furthermore, using number of occasions of *unprotected* intercourse in the past 30 days as a second indicator of campaign impact, estimates derived from regression lines (similar to those in Fig. 8.2) computed both with and without the impact of the Lexington campaign were compared. On average, HSSIDMs engaged in a total of 10.49 fewer occasions of unprotected intercourse during the 12 months after the campaign began than would have been expected if the precampaign pattern of use had simply continued. The 2000 Census estimate of the number of 18- to 26-year-olds in Lexington was divided by 2 to yield an estimated number of HSSIDMs ($N = 20{,}649$). Multiplying by those estimated in the SSC data to be sexually active in a 30-day period (84.4%) yielded 17,276 individuals. Multiplying this figure by the mean number of unprotected intercourse occasions averted as a result of the campaign (10.49) yields an estimate of 181,224 fewer such occasions among HSSIDMs between January and December 2003.

## Discussion

Although the campaign appears to have been quite effective, as expected its impact was relatively short-term. This suggests that a continuing campaign presence is necessary to reinforce and sustain a behavior such as condom use, utilizing a constant supply of novel messages to maintain attention. In fact, reinforcement messages that might come in the form of booster campaigns are likely needed, especially as new cohorts of young adults matriculate and increasingly adopt hormonal birth control methods over condom use (e.g., Noar, Zimmerman et al., 2004). Alternatively, it may be unrealistic to expect that media campaigns alone will have the kind of impact needed to sustain behavioral changes over the long term. Thus, combining media campaigns with other behavioral interventions such as school-based programs may be a manner in which to increase the efficacy and ultimate impact and sustainability of intervention efforts. Although some health campaigns have done this effectively (e.g., Worden & Flynn, 2002, with cigarette use), additional research on synergistic links between health media campaigns and other behavioral interventions is needed. Indeed, many HIV prevention researchers have recently called for mass media campaigns as a complement to individual-level approaches such as counseling and small-group interventions (e.g., DiClemente, 2000; Ross & Williams, 2002).

Overall, the SSC study suggests that mass media campaigns alone can be effective in changing sexual-risk behavior and related variables *if* well-documented principles of campaign design are followed. In this study, these principles included careful audience segmentation and targeting, as well as extensive formative research to design, test, and select campaign messages. Multiple theoretical perspectives, particularly SENTAR, were employed to inform these tasks. High sensation seekers and impulsive decision makers are particularly relevant groups to target because of their proclivity for engaging in risky sexual behaviors. Evaluation of target audience program preferences immediately prior to the campaign allowed more precise placement of the campaign messages, and helped in achieving the high reported exposure levels. Finally, a rigorous independent sample interrupted time-series design with a control community greatly strengthened causal inferences about campaign effects.

## Implications

The overriding implication of this review and discussion of safer-sex campaigns as well as of the illustrative SSC example is the following: Mass media campaigns *can* be an effective tool in the ongoing battle to reduce the incidence of STDs including HIV/AIDS provided that principles of effective campaign design are carefully followed. However, what should campaign planners do in cases where they have limited or even scarce resources? Rigorous evaluation and high exposure to campaign messages often come at a high cost in dollars. If a campaign is limited due to scarce resources, campaign planners will have to make difficult decisions that allow them to maximize the use of these principles for minimal cost. For instance, one focus group of members of the target audience giving their feedback on campaign messages is better than none. Similarly, using an outcome evaluation design with a limited ability to permit causal conclusions is better than not conducting *any* evaluation. Thus, rather than ignoring certain principles when resources are scarce, campaign planners might still consider each principle and do the best they can with the available resources.

In terms of the scientific literature on HIV/AIDS campaigns, what kinds of studies might still be undertaken? The current review suggests that what is urgently needed are additional efforts that utilize numerous campaign design principles and that are rigorously evaluated so that campaign effects can be documented. The literature thus far has provided examples of campaigns that use *some* principles of campaign design. However, there is a lack of studies that use numerous effective principles together in the design, implementation, and evaluation of safer-sex media campaigns. Unfortunately, lack of attention to just one crucial principle, such as careful placement of messages, can easily lead to a failed campaign (i.e., due to inadequate message exposure). In addition, lack of attention to certain principles (i.e., audience segmentation) can affect the ability of campaign designers to effectively use other principles (i.e., message design and targeting). Until additional carefully designed and evaluated media campaigns are undertaken in this area, the potential of such efforts to effectively reach numerous populations at risk for HIV/AIDS and other STDs will remain just that—potential that is yet to be fully realized.

## Acknowledgments

Preparation of this chapter was funded in part by Grant R01-MH63705 from the National Institute of Mental Health (Principal Investigator: Rick S. Zimmerman).

## References

Agha, S. (2003). The impact of a mass media campaign on personal risk perception, perceived self-efficacy and on other behavioral predictors. *AIDS Care, 15*(6), 749–762.

Alstead, M., Campsmith, M., Halley, C.S., Hartfield, K., Goldbaum, G., & Wood, R. W. (1999). Developing, implementing, and evaluating a condom promotion program targeting sexually active adolescents. *AIDS Education and Prevention, 11*(6), 497–512.

Andersen, B., Ostergaard, L., Moller, J.K., & Olesen, F. (2001). Effectiveness of a mass media campaign to recruit young adults for testing of Chlamydia trachomatis by use of home obtained and mailed samples. *Sexually Transmitted Infections, 77*(6), 416–418.

Atkin, C. K. (2001). Theory and principles of media health campaigns. In R. E. Rice & C. K. Atkin, (Eds.), *Public communication campaigns* (3rd ed., pp. 49–68). Thousand Oaks, CA: Sage.

Atkin, C. K., & Freimuth, V. S. (2001). Formative evaluation research in campaign design. In R. E. Rice & C. K. Atkin (Eds.), *Public communication campaigns* (3rd ed., pp. 125–145). Thousand Oaks, CA: Sage.

Backer, T. E. (1990). Comparative synthesis of mass media health behavior campaigns. *Knowledge: Creation, Diffusion, Utilization, 11,* 315–329.

Barnea, Z., Rahav, G., & Teichman, M. (1992). Alcohol consumption among Israeli youth-1989: epidemiology and demographics. *British Journal of Addictions, 87,* 295–302.

Bull, S. S., Cohen, J., Ortiz, C., & Evans, T. (2002). The POWER Campaign for promotion of female and male condoms: Audience research and campaign development. *Health Communication, 14*(4), 475–491.

Cappella, J. N., Fishbein, M., Hornik, R., Ahern, R. K., & Sayeed, S. (2001). Using theory to select messages in antidrug media campaigns: Reasoned action and media priming. In R. E. Rice & C. K. Atkin (Eds.), *Public communication campaigns* (3rd ed., pp. 214–230). Thousand Oaks, CA: Sage.

Centers for Disease Control and Prevention. (1999). Community-level HIV intervention in 5 cities: Final outcome data from the CDC AIDS community demonstration projects. *American Journal of Public Health, 89*(3), 336–345.

Centers for Disease Control and Prevention. (2001). *Compendium of HIV prevention interventions with evidence of effectiveness.* Atlanta, GA: Department of Health and Human Services. Division of HIV/AIDS Prevention.

Chen, J. L., Kodagoda, D., Lawrence, A. M., & Kerndt, P. R. (2002). Rapid public health interventions in response to an outbreak of syphilis in Los Angeles. *Sexually Transmitted Diseases, 29*(5), 277–284.

Cohen, D. A., Wu, S., & Farley, T. A. (2005). Cost-effective allocation of government funds to prevent HIV infection. *Health Affairs, 24*(4), 915–926.

Cohen, J. (1988). *Statistical power analysis for the behavioral sciences* (2nd ed.). Hillsdale, NJ: Lawrence Erlbaum Associates.

Cook, T., & Campbell, D. (1979). *Quasi-experimentation: Design & analysis issues for field settings.* Boston: Houghton Mifflin.

DeJong, W., Wolf, R., & Austin, S. B. (2001). U.S. federally funded television public service announcements (PSAs) to prevent HIV/AIDS: A content analysis. *Journal of Health Communication, 6*(3), 249–263.

Derzon, J. H., & Lipsey, M. W. (2002). A meta-analysis of the effectiveness of mass-communication for changing substance-use knowledge, attitudes, and behavior. In W. D. Crano, & M. Burgoon (Eds.), *Mass media and drug prevention: Classic and contemporary theories and research* (pp. 231–258). Mahwah, NJ: Lawrence Erlbaum Associates.

Devos-Comby, L., & Salovey, P. (2002). Applying persuasion strategies to alter HIV-relevant thoughts and behavior. *Review of General Psychology, 6*(3), 287–304.

DiClemente, R. J. (2000). Looking forward: Future directions for HIV prevention reearch. In J. L. Peterson, & R. J. DiClemente (Eds.), *Handbook of HIV prevention* (pp. 311–324). New York: Kluwer Academic/Plenum.

Donohew, L., Lorch, E. P., & Palmgreen, P. (1991). Sensation seeking and targeting of televised anti-drug PSAs. In L. Donohew, H. E. Sypher, & W. J. Bukoski (Eds.), *Persuasive communication and drug abuse prevention* (pp. 209–226). Hillsdale, NJ: Lawrence Erlbaum Associates.

Donohew, L., Zimmerman, R., Cupp, P. K., Novak, S., Colon, S., & Abell, R. (2000). Sensation seeking, impulsive-decision making, and risky sex: Implications for risk-taking and design of interventions. *Personality and Individual Differences, 28,* 1079–1091.

Flay, B. R., & Sobel, J. L. (1983). The role of mass media in preventing adolescent substance abuse. In T. J. Glynn, C. G. Leukefeld, & J. P. Lundford (Eds.), *Preventing adolescent drug abuse: Intervention strategies* (NIDA Research Monograph Series 47). Rockville, MD: National Institute on Drug Abuse.

Flora, J. A., Maibach, E. W., & Maccoby, N. (1989). The role of media across four levels of health promotion intervention. *Annual Review of Public Health, 10,* 181–201.

Frieden, T. R., Das-Douglas, M., Kellerman, S. E., & Henning, K. J. (2005). Applying public health principles to the HIV epidemic. *The New England Journal of Medicine, 353*(22), 2397–2402.

Geary, C.W., Mahler, H., Finger, W., & Shears, K.H. (2005). *Using global media to reach youth: The 2002 MTV staying alive campaign.* Arlington, VA: Family Health International.

Grier, S., & Bryant, C. A. (2005). Social marketing in public health. *Annual Review of Public Health, 26,* 319–339.

Grunig, J. (1989). Publics, audiences, and market segments: Segmentation principles for campaigns. In C. Salmon (Ed.), *Information campaigns: Balancing social values and social change* (pp. 199–228). Newbury Park, CA: Sage.

Holtgrave, D. R. (1997). Public health communication strategies for HIV prevention: Past and emerging roles. *AIDS, 11*(Suppl. A), S183–S190.

Hornik, R. C. (Ed.). (2002). *Public health communication: Evidence for behavior change.* Mahwah, NJ: Lawrence Erlbaum Associates.

Hoyle, R. H., Fejfar, M. C., & Miller, J. D. (2000). Personality and sexual risk taking: A quantitative review. *Journal of Personality, 68*(6), 1203–1231.

Hoyle, R. H., Stephenson, M. T., Palmgreen, P. P., Lorch, E. P., & Donohew, R. L. (2002). Reliability and validity of a brief measure of sensation seeking. *Personality and Individual Differences, 32,* 401–414.

Johnson, D., Flora, J. A., & Rimal, R. N. (1997). HIV/AIDS public service announcements around the world: A descriptive analysis. *Journal of Health Communication, 2,* 223–235.

Kaiser Family Foundation. (2003). *National survey of teens and young adults on sexual health public education campaigns.* Menlo Park, CA: Author.

Kaiser Family Foundation. (2004). *Assessing public education programming on HIV/AIDS: A national survey of African Americans.* Menlo Park, CA: Author.

Keller, S. N., & Brown, J. D. (2002). Media interventions to promote responsible sexual behavior. *The Journal of Sex Research, 39*(1), 67–72.

Kelly, J. A. (1999). Community-level interventions are needed to prevent new HIV infections. *American Journal of Public Health, 89*(3), 299–300.

Kreuter, M. K., Strecher, V. J., & Glassman, B. (1999). One size does not fit all: The case for tailoring print materials. *Annals of Behavioral Medicine, 21*(4), 276–283.

Lewis-Beck, M. S. (1986). Interrupted time series. In W. D. Berry & M. S. Lewis-Beck (Eds.), *New tools for social scientists: Advances and application in research methods* (pp. 209–240). Beverly Hills, CA: Sage.

Lorch, E. P., Palmgreen, P., Donohew, L., Helm, D., Baer, S. A., & D'Silva, M. U. (1994). Program context, sensation seeking, and attention to televised anti-drug public service announcements. *Human Communication Research, 20*(3), 390–412.

Meekers, D., Agha, S., & Klein, M. (2005). The impact on condom use of the "100% Jeune" social marketing program in Cameroon. *Journal of Adolescent Health, 36,* 530e1–530e12.

Murray-Johnson, L., & Witte, K. (2003). Looking toward the future: Health message design strategies. In T. L. Thompson, A. M. Dorsey, K. I. Miller, & R. Parrott (Eds.), *Handbook of health communication* (pp. 473–496). Mahwah, NJ: Lawrence Erlbaum Associates.

Myhre, S. L., & Flora, J. A. (2000). HIV/AIDS communication campaigns: Progress and prospects. *Journal of Health Communication, 5*(Suppl.), 29–45.

Noar, S. M. (2006). A 10-year retrospective of health mass media campaigns: Where do we go from here? *Journal of Health Communication, 11*(1), 21–42.

Noar, S. M. (2007). An interventionists' guide to AIDS behavioral theories. *AIDS Care, 19,* 392–402.

Noar, S. M., Anderman, E. M., Zimmerman, R. S., & Cupp, P. K. (2004). Fostering achievement motivation in health education: Are we applying relevant theory to school-based HIV prevention programs? *Journal of Psychology & Human Sexuality, 16*(4), 59–76.

Noar, S. M., Palmgreen, P., Zimmerman, R. S., Lustria, M., & Lu, H. Y. (2007). *Perceived message sensation value as a predictor of perceived message impact: Application to safer sex PSAs.* Manuscript submitted for publication.

Noar, S. M., & Zimmerman, R. S. (2005). Health behavior theory and cumulative knowledge regarding health behaviors: Are we moving in the right direction? *Health Education Research: Theory & Practice, 20,* 275–290.

Noar, S. M., Zimmerman, R. S., & Atwood, K. A. (2004). Safer sex and sexually transmitted infections from a relationship perspective. In J. H. Harvey, A. Wenzel, & S. Sprecher (Eds.), *Handbook of sexuality in close relationships* (pp. 519–544). Mahwah, NJ: Lawrence Erlbaum Associates.

Noar, S. M., Zimmerman, R. S., Palmgreen, P., Lustria, M. L. A., & Horosewski, M. L. (2006). Integrating personality and psychosocial theoretical approaches to understanding safer sexual behavior: Implications for message design. *Health Communication, 19*(2), 165–174.

Oh, M. K., Grimley, D. M., Merchant, J. S., Brown, P. R., Cecil, H., & Hook, E. W. (2002). Mass media as a population-level intervention tool for Chlamydia trachomatis screening: Report of a pilot study. *Journal of Adolescent Health, 31,* 40–47.

Palmgreen, P., & Donohew, L. (2003). Effective mass media strategies for drug abuse prevention campaigns. In Z. Slobada & W. J. Bukoski (Eds.), *Handbook of drug abuse prevention: Theory, science, and practice* (pp. 27–43). New York: Kluwer Academic/Plenum.

Palmgreen, P., Donohew, L., Lorch, E. P., Hoyle, R. H., & Stephenson, M. T. (2001). Television campaigns and adolescent marijuana use: Tests of sensation seeking targeting. *American Journal of Public Health, 91,* 292–296.

Palmgreen, P., Donohew, L., Lorch, E. P., Hoyle, R.H., & Stephenson, M.T. (2002). Television campaigns and sensation seeking targeting of adolescent marijuana use: A controlled time series approach. In R. C. Hornik (Ed.), *Public health communication: Evidence for behavior change* (pp. 35–56). Mahwah, NJ: Lawrence Erlbaum Associates.

Palmgreen, P., Donohew, L., Lorch, E., Rogus, M., Helm, D., & Grant, N. (1991). Sensation seeking, message sensation value, and drug use as mediators of PSA effectiveness. *Health Communication, 3,* 217–234.

Palmgreen, P., Stephenson, M. T., Everett, M. W., Baseheart, J. R., & Francies, R. (2002). Perceived message sensation value (PMSV) and the dimensions and validation of a PMSV scale. *Health Communication, 14*(4), 403–428.

Perloff, R. M. (2001). *Persuading people to have safer sex: Applications of social science to the AIDS crisis.* Mahwah, NJ: Lawrance Erlbaum Associates.

Perloff, R. M. (2003). *The dynamics of persuasion: Communication and attitudes in the 21st century* (2nd ed.). Mahwah, NJ: Lawrence Erlbaum Associates.

Peterson, J. L., & DiClemente, R. J. (Eds.). (2000). *Handbook of HIV prevention*. New York: Kluwer Academic/Plenum.

Prochaska, J. O., DiClemente, C. C., & Norcross, J. C. (1992). In search of how people change: Applications to addictive behaviors. *American Psychologist, 47*(9), 1102–1114.

Randolph, W., & Viswanath, K. (2004). Lessons learned from public health mass media campaigns: Marketing health in a crowded media world. *Annual Review of Public Health, 25,* 419–437.

Ratzan, S. C., Payne, J. G., & Massett, H. A. (1994). Effective health message design: The "America responds to AIDS" campaign. *American Behavioral Scientist, 38*(2), 294–309.

Rice, R. E., & Atkin, C. K. (Eds.) (2001). *Public communication campaigns* (3rd ed.). Thousand Oaks, CA: Sage.

Rogers, E. M., & Storey, J. D. (1987). Communication campaigns. In C. R. Berger & S. H. Chafee (Eds.), *Handbook of communication science* (pp. 817–846). London: Sage.

Ross, M. W., Chatterjee, N.S., & Leonard, L. (2004). A community level syphilis prevention programme: outcome data from a controlled trial. *Sexually Trasmitted Infections, 80,* 100–104.

Ross, M. W., & Williams, M. L. (2002). Effective targeted and community HIV/STD prevention programs. *The Journal of Sex Research, 39*(1), 58–62.

Salmon, C. T., & Atkin, C. (2003). Using media campaigns for health promotion. In T. L. Thompson, A. M. Dorsey, K. I. Miller, & R. Parrott (Eds.), *Handbook of health communication* (pp. 285–313). Mahwah, NJ: Lawrence Erlbaum Associates.

Singhal, A., & Rogers, E. M. (2003). *Combating AIDS: Communication strategies in action.* Thousand Oaks, CA: Sage.

Slater, M. D. (1996). Theory and method in health audience segmentation. *Journal of Health Communication, 1*(3), 267–285.

Slater, M. D. (1999). Integrating application of media effects, persuasion, and behavior change theories to communication campaigns: A stages-of-change framework. *Health Communication, 11*(4), 335–354.

Snyder, L. B., & Hamilton, M. A. (2002). A meta-analysis of U.S. health campaign effects on behavior: Emphasize enforcement, exposure, and new information, and beware the secular trend. In R. C. Hornik (Ed.), *Public health communications: Evidence for behavior change* (pp. 357–384). Mahwah, NJ: Lawrence Erlbaum Associates.

Stephenson, M. T. (2003). Examining adolescents' responses to antimarijuana PSAs. *Human Communication Research, 29*(3), 343–369.

Valente, T. W. (2001). Evaluating communication campaigns. In R. E. Rice & C. K. Atkin (Eds.), *Public communication campaigns* (3rd ed., pp. 105–124). Thousand Oaks, CA: Sage.

Valente, T. W., & Saba, W. P. (1998). Mass media and interpersonal influence in a reproductive health communication campaign in Bolivia. *Communication Research, 25*(1), 96–124.

Vidanapathirana, J., Abramson, M. J., Forbes, A. & Fairley, C. (2005). Mass media interventions for promoting HIV testing (Review). *The Cochrane Database of Systematic Reviews, 3,* 1–38.

Witte, K., & Allen, M. (2000). A meta-analysis of fear appeals: Implications for effective public health campaigns. *Health Education & Behavior, 27*(5), 591–615.

Witte, K., Cameron, K. A., Lapinski, M., & Nzyuko, S. (1998). A theoretically based evaluation of HIV/AIDS prevention campaigns along the transafrica highway in Kenya. *Journal of Health Communication, 3*(4), 345–367.

Worden, J. K, & Flynn, B.S. (2002). Using mass media to prevent cigarette smoking. In R. C. Hornik (Ed.), *Public health communications: Evidence for behavior change* (pp. 23–34). Mahwah, NJ: Lawrence Erlbaum Associates.

Yzer, M. C., Siero, F. W., & Buunk, B. P. (2000). Can public campaigns effectively change psychological determinants of safer sex? An evaluation of three Dutch campaigns. *Health Education Research, 15*(3), 339–352.

Zimmerman, R. S., Palmgreen, P., Noar, S. M., Lustria, M. L. A., Lu, H. Y., & Horosewski, M. L. (in press). Effects of a televised two-city safer sex mass media campaign targeting high sensation-seeking and impulsive decision-making young adults. *Health Education & Behavior.*

Zuckerman, M. (1979). *Sensation seeking: Beyond the optimal level of arousal.* Hillsdale, NJ: Lawrence Erlbaum Associates.

Zuckerman, M. (1990). The psychophysiology of sensation seeking. *Journal of Personality, 58,* 313–345.

Zuckerman, M. (1994). *Behavioral expressions and biosocial bases of sensation seeking.* Cambridge, England: Cambridge University Press.

Zuckerman, M., & Neeb, M. (1980). Demographic influences in sensation seeking and expression of sensation seeking in religion, smoking and driving habits. *Personality and Individual Differences, 1,* 197–206.

# 9

# Entertainment Education and HIV Prevention

*May G. Kennedy*
Virginia Commonwealth University

*Vicki Beck*
University of Southern California

*Vicki S. Freimuth*
University of Georgia

Like the ancient fables of Aesop, narratives broadcast through modern mass media communication channels can teach as well as entertain (Brodie et al., 2001). Since the 1970s, an approach called *Entertainment Education* (EE) has used formats such as serialized dramas on radio and television in conscious attempts to educate and prompt positive, voluntary behavior change in large audiences (Singhal & Rogers, 1999). There is evidence that even the earliest EE broadcast projects increased the frequency of health behaviors and/or raised levels of their psychosocial determinants (Brown & Singhal, 1999). Many of the positive EE broadcast outcomes documented to date pertain to HIV prevention either directly (e.g., Kennedy, O'Leary, Beck, Pollard, & Simpson, 2004; Vaughan, Rogers, Singhal, & Swalehe, 2000) or indirectly via common risk factors such as unprotected sex (e.g., Whittier, Kennedy, St. Lawrence, Seeley, & Beck, 2005).

Later in this chapter, we argue that it is theoretically plausible that the EE approach is particularly powerful among communication strategies for HIV prevention. Anecdotal data also support this view:

> Recently, when I returned home from work, I noticed my 18-year-old daughter was extremely upset. I asked her what was the matter. She told

me some guy named Stone died from AIDS and that Stone's girlfriend tested HIV positive. My heart sank until I found out that they were characters in the soap opera, *General Hospital*. It led to an excellent conversation with both my daughters. My older daughter said, "Dad, Stone was a heterosexual. Did you know AIDS could strike anyone?" It was music to my ears that she and her sister have finally gotten through their heads the potential of contracting AIDS. My kids have a lot of exposure to the dangers of this deadly disease in school, through AIDS Awareness Week and lectures from both my wife and me, but they really thought this could never happen to them. *General Hospital* accomplished what the schools and other sources could not.[1]

The present chapter begins with a summary of EE theory and history that draws extensively from a recent book on the topic by leaders in the field (Singhal, Cody, Rogers, & Sabido, 2004). After that, it covers current international and domestic EE applications to HIV/AIDS and sexual health, focusing on evidence of effectiveness. We conclude by raising questions that research should address to advance knowledge in this area.

## EE Theory and History

The British Broadcasting Corporation (BBC) set out in the 1920s to inform and educate as well as to entertain (Cody, Fernandez, & Wilkin, 2004). In the 1970s, Miguel Sabido, a Mexican television writer/director/producer, brought formal theory and audience research to bear on the social uses of commercial television. Sabido recognized the centrality of emotion in changing audience behaviors and the importance of using a systematic method; his approach became known as EE (Sabido, 2004).

As a theater student, Sabido theorized about the influence of acting techniques on the tone of a dramatic presentation, and about how the tone of a dramatic presentation mediates its emotional and intellectual impact on audiences. Later, he focused on the *telenovela*, a serialized Latin American television format similar to American "soap operas" but briefer, usually lasting about 6 months. Sabido knew that thousands of viewers had enrolled in literacy classes after they saw the heroine of a wildly successful Peruvian telenovela enjoy upward mobility when she finished her class. He considered telenovelas well suited for social change because (a) their emotional tone fosters identification, (b) their multiple episodes allow a message to be repeated, (c) their limited length provides narrative closure, and (d) episodes can be followed by short epilogues referring viewers to services needed to support new behaviors (Sabido, 2004).

Before long, Sabido noted parallels between his ideas about the tonal flow of the telenovela and social learning theory (SLT) (Bandura, 1977). He began to use SLT terminology and he recommended that scripts include *role models* to promote observational learning (Singhal & Rogers, 1999). Pure entertainment should come first in EE so that audiences are attracted and engaged before health messages appear in a storyline. An admired character should perform the target behavior and experience positive consequences to create positive behavioral *outcome expectancies* in audience members. A negative role model should fail to perform the behavior and experience bad consequences and generally bad luck. A key transitional character should be crafted to elicit audience identification. Observing this role model face and successfully overcome a series of obstacles to performing the behavior should enhance an audience member's sense of *self-efficacy*, the perceived ability to perform the behavior. The appeal and/or salience and credibility of narrative elements such as character profiles and barriers and rewards should be pretested in audience research.

In 1977, Sabido built tone theory and SLT into the first fully fledged EE television series, a telenovela called *Acompañame* that promoted family planning. It was considered a significant causal factor in a national birthrate decline (Poindexter, 2004).

Sabido integrated other theoretical perspectives into his work as time went on, as have others. Existing theories of archetypes, information processing, drama, communication, individual health behavior change, diffusion of innovations, audience involvement/ parasocial interaction, collective efficacy, and political power have been used to inform EE and predict its effects. Some EE researchers have synthesized their own hybrid theoretical models, incorporating individual behavior change and interpersonal or social/political constructs (Sood, Menard, & Witte, 2004).

## EE History and Trends in Developing Countries

Sabido worked with the Population Communication Center to export the EE telenovela methodology to developing countries interested in family planning. Beginning in 1982, the Johns Hopkins University Center for Communication Programs built the sexual health legacy of EE internationally through some 50 television and radio soap opera projects (Piotrow & de Fossard, 2004). Other entities developed the necessary expertise and there have been at least 200 EE radio and TV broadcast series around the world to date (Singhal & Rogers, 2004). Poindexter (2004) provided a firsthand account of factors that allow implementation of the EE process, even when the idea is perceived as alien, the national (and often government-controlled) media infrastructure is limited, and there is turnover in political and media leaders. He linked success to funding from foundations, UN agencies, and other donors; requests for government cooperation from funders and high-status individuals from other countries; national plans or international resolutions that commit a country to work on a health or social problem; data on EE's effectiveness and cost-effectiveness in other countries; and EE practitioner persistence.

Current EE projects in developing countries rely more on indigenous script writers and less on foreign consultants than in the past. When possible, opportunities for face-to-face interaction are added now to reinforce mediated messages through interpersonal channels. Another trend is partnering with local organizations to provide the health services people need to follow health recommendations in storylines.

Evaluators are gathering qualitative and quantitative data not only to document the effects of these programs, but also to investigate mechanisms and mediators of effects. It has been demonstrated overseas repeatedly that the EE approach can effect behavioral changes ranging from using oral-rehydration therapy to sending girls to school (Singhal, Sharma, Papa, & Witte, 2004); a better understanding of the mechanisms involved may strengthen the effects of future programs. Three examples of ambitious international projects that addressed HIV-relevant issues and investigated mechanisms of change are offered next. The book edited by Singhal and colleagues (2004) details other examples (e.g., the prize-winning South African *Soul City* project).

## Tanzania

Between 1993 and 1995, *Twende na Wakati* (Let's Go With the Times), an EE soap opera, was broadcast by seven stations of Radio

Tanzania, a country of 30 million people with an 8.8% HIV prevalence rate among 15- to 49-year-olds (UNAIDS, 2004). The soap opera dealt with family-planning and HIV/AIDS issues. An eighth station aired other programming during that time slot; its listening area served as a "wait list" comparison condition.[2] Annual household and clinic surveys showed that exposure to the soap opera had strong effects on family planning and its predictors (Vaughn & Rogers, 2000). Listeners had progressed though stages of behavioral change, starting with involvement with the media characters and moving through interpersonal communication about the behaviors with spouses and peers to the eventual adoption of the behaviors. In the process, listener self-efficacy regarding family-planning adoption increased (Rogers et al., 1999). Family-planning messages were not incompatible with HIV messages. By 1997, reported exposure to the broadcast in the treatment area was 58%; compared to those in the comparison area, 17% more respondents in the broadcast area reported having fewer sex partners and 3% reported using condoms more frequently. These changes were mediated by increases in perceived risk of contracting HIV, self-efficacy regarding HIV prevention, and interpersonal communication about the disease (Vaughn et al., 2000). After the first 2 years, the soap opera was aired in the "wait-listed" comparison district and similar movement through the stages of change was observed.

## Botswana

In Botswana, where HIV prevalence is 37.3% among those age 15 to 49 years (UNAIDS, 2004), the Centers for Disease Control and Prevention (CDC) funded an EE project called *Modeling and Reinforcement to Combat HIV/AIDS* (MARCH; Galavotti, Pappas-DeLuca, & Lansky, 2001). A theory-based radio HIV-prevention soap opera, *Makgabaneng* ("a rocky place" or "the ups and downs of life"), served as the modeling component. Written and produced jointly with local talent, it targeted individual factors such as self-efficacy. The reinforcement component consisted of listening groups, listening spots, and road shows; they were designed to reduce barriers to performing the behaviors by changing group norms.

The MARCH project had two interesting process goals as well: (a) to develop a user-friendly technique that would ensure that local script writers infused theory and audience research results into scripts, and (b) to explore the exportability of a series produced in one African country to others with the same language and similar cultures. The first process goal was met by a board game for writers; they progress around the board if they build into scripts items such as explicit consequences of actions.

MARCH focused on mother-to-child transmission (MTCT); preliminary survey results showed that, for regular listeners, exposure to the series was associated with MTCT-relevant outcomes such as HIV testing while pregnant (Pappas-DeLuca, 2004). It is too soon to say whether the reinforcement activities will increase these effects, and questions of exportability remain open pending funding for replication in other African countries.

### India

The third international example comes from Hindi-speaking states in India where seroprevalence is still low but risk factors make the rapid spread of HIV a serious threat. In this EE project, a year-long radio soap opera called *Taru* (the heroine's name) was considered one of three necessary "legs" of a three-legged intervention "stool." The second and third legs were (a) opportunities for audiences to reflect on and discuss the messages in the show, and (b) supportive local services (Singhal et al., 2004).

*Taru* tells the story of an upper-caste girl employed by a village reproductive health care facility. She empowers rural women (e.g., by stopping child marriages) and is assisted by an intelligent, respectful, lower-caste boy. At first, the men in Taru's family scorn or undercut her work (and unspoken romantic attachment to the boy), but they experience changes of heart and begin to take part in the social reform efforts.

Singhal and his co-authors (2004) compare this All India Radio show to "air cover," and the reproductive health care services provided by Janani, a nongovernmental organization, to "ground cover" in an assault on the hide-bound traditions that maintain a social context in which women are at high risk of HIV. Before the soap opera was aired, Janini publicized it through posters, wall paintings, and folk performances so that a large audience would be interested in the show at its initial airing. Janani distributed transistor radios at the folk performances and organized the radio recipients into *Taru* listening groups to create opportunities to reflect on and discuss the show's messages. After the launch of the broadcast, rural health practitioners trained by Janani diagnosed and treated sexually transmitted infections, provided other reproductive and child health services, and sold Janani-branded condoms, pills, and pregnancy tests.

Tens of millions of people tuned into *Taru,* and listening groups took collective action to stop child marriages and improve the lives of low-caste persons through education and inclusion in community life. In interviews, high school girls stressed the importance of protecting oneself from HIV and voiced their intentions to encourage partners to use condoms. In unprompted comments, the girls explained that they made these decisions after listening to *Taru* episodes. Several-fold increases in sales of the branded condoms at sentinel sites also testified to the program's effectiveness.

However, Singhal et al. (2004) caution that EE is no magic bullet. They viewed the EE effects on buying behavior as indirect, mediated not only through parasocial relationships between the characters in the narrative and audience members but also through interpersonal interaction. The researchers predicted that, when power relationships are at stake, community dynamics will be complex, there will be resistance to messages, and social change will be nonlinear and episodic. Their qualitative data indicated distortions of the "take home message" in the direction of the status quo, talk that was not followed by action, and mothers who did not feel empowered to change themselves but vowed that things would be different for their daughters. In short, social change remained a struggle.

## Current Practice in Developed Countries

In the United States today, it would be prohibitively expensive to write a narrative series solely intended to change health behavior, to tape the series with the high production values that television viewers in this country have come to expect, and to buy airtime for the series on a major network, especially during prime viewing hours. Here, national television is big business, driven by bottom-line considerations of audience size and commercial sponsorship (Beck, 2004). But health threats heighten drama and drama draws audiences, so health themes are common in television. Project Daytime at the State

University of New York at Buffalo noted depictions of AIDS and HIV in American soap operas like *As the World Turns* and *General Hospital* starting in the mid-1990s (personal communication, Mary Cassata & Barbara Irwin, October 17, 2005). AIDS themes are still being introduced into scripts; one recent example comes from a telenovela that was broadcast by Telemundo and reached a wide audience of Spanish speakers in the United States beginning in May 2004. Titled *Prisonera*, it portrayed a 16-year-old girl who died of AIDS after being abducted, addicted to cocaine by her abductor, and infected with HIV while exchanging sex for money to support her drug habit.

Entertainment groups and organizations such as the Red Cross have encouraged the inclusion of the topics of HIV and AIDS in television shows (e.g., via the Ribbon of Hope award bestowed by the Academy of Television Arts & Sciences for the last 9 years). Many writers and producers who deal with these topics are willing to work with health experts to ensure the accuracy of the topic treatments. Some writers and producers will even listen to suggestions for dramatizing health issues, but they have the final say regarding program content. As a rule, health experts are viewed simply as resources. They are asked to consult as needed and to help with simulations of medical procedures on the set; in rare instances, they may be hired to develop scripts (Beck, 2004).

Historically, several governmental and nongovernmental organizations in the United States have facilitated the delivery of health expertise to script writers and producers and advocated for the dramatization of particular topics. The organizations partner with the entertainment industry on specific campaigns and conduct studies on the impact of media on the issue they espouse. In most cases, they are insufficiently funded to buy ad time for public service announcements (PSAs). Unfortunately, many single-topic efforts have been short-lived, their outreach to writers and producers limited by the scope of the focal topic, the duration of a campaign, or a lack of ongoing funding.

A striking exception is the well-endowed Kaiser Family Foundation (KFF), which concentrates on sexual health issues. KFF has not only survived but also geometrically expanded the impact of its own work on HIV and AIDS through productive partnerships. Its partners include media organizations in the United States (especially Viacom, Inc., the corporate parent for a host of networks and other media companies) and around the world. The partnerships result in multifaceted public HIV/AIDS education campaigns aimed primarily at young people. KFF outreach initiatives include regional and national meetings (e.g., in India, Russia, Thailand, Asia, and Africa) in which media leaders receive substantive briefings. Follow-up trainings are geared toward staff in news and entertainment divisions to stimulate more HIV/AIDS content in programming. As a result, targeted public service messages are combined with longer-form special programming or editorials and other forms of outreach. Resources needed to support behavior change are provided through toll-free hotlines, Web sites, and other means at no charge (see http://www.kff.org/hivaids/gmai. cfm for details).

An organization with a more diversified portfolio of health issues is also conducting robust, sustained outreach on HIV/AIDS in Hollywood. The *Hollywood, Health and Society* (HH&S) program of the Norman Lear Center at the University of Southern California (USC) is a multi-issue entity that links script writers with HIV experts and fosters network support for using storylines to direct audiences to HIV resources. An example of this work is given later in the subsection A Study of HIV/AIDS Information Seeking.

Positioned as an unbiased resource for the entertainment industry, HH&S grew out of a pilot project at the CDC and was launched in its current, independent form in 2002. Its staff has experience in script development and in public health, and its advisory board includes high-level representatives of the entertainment, academic, and health sectors in the United States. HH&S engages television writers and producers through: (a) a Web site with tip sheets on various health topics and user-friendly links to federal health agency sites, (b) expert panel discussions held at the Writers Guild of America, West, in Los Angeles, (c) introductions to health experts who can provide face-to-face or in-depth telephone consultation on particular health topics, (d) partnership brokering (e.g., between CDC's Office of Women's Health and the American Federation of Television and Radio Executives), and (e) recognition of accurate, compelling health storylines via the Sentinel for Health Awards (Beck, 2004). In addition, HH&S conducts research on: (a) the health themes portrayed on television, (b) the degree to which audience members report getting health information from television, (c) the impact of viewing on health behavior and its psychosocial predictors, and (d) the separate and accumulated effects of additional ways to foster information-seeking behavior, for example, PSAs with 800-numbers and Web links for health information. The program encourages such research by means of the USC Annenberg School for Communications' Everett M. Rogers Award for Achievement in EE, introduced in 2005 (see http://www.learcenter.org/html/projects/?&cm=hhs/Ev_Rogers_Award).

HH&S also conducts outreach to Spanish-language networks and telenovelas produced in the United States because Hispanic audiences are at disproportionately high risk for HIV infection (CDC, 2005) and a number of other health problems.[3] The future plans of HH&S include participating in the university training of budding script writers.

Other highly industrialized countries have the opportunity to influence television content but they face barriers to control over television content similar to those in the United States and they lack organizational infrastructure for lobbying or outreach to the entertainment industry. Nonetheless, there have been a few short-term partnerships between health groups and television writers in continental Europe (Bouman, 2004). As in the United States, health experts in Europe have had to accept the established characters, plots, and tones of existing shows instead of designing a series to change behavior according to the EE soap opera formula. There has been no formal evaluation of the impact of their HIV-related EE work, but ratings have not suffered, so there may be additional collaboration between health experts and the script writers in the future (Bouman, 2004).

Meanwhile, the BBC has featured an HIV-positive character named Mark Fowler in the long-running, highly rated BBC soap opera *EastEnders!* When Mark stopped taking his combination therapy because of its side effects, he contracted a life-threatening case of pneumonia. He recovered after several cliff-hanging episodes. Viewers were referred to Internet resources for HIV information.

Despite many similarities between this BBC storyline and classical EE (Cody et al., 2004), *EastEnders!* differs in having a multi-issue social agenda. Consequently, the HIV themes may have been less salient than they would have been in a series designed specifically to change HIV-relevant behavior or social attitudes. There are no data on HIV prevention outcomes of exposure to this storyline.

Studies of U.S. HIV Storylines

In contrast, at least four studies of high-risk U.S. audiences have detected positive outcomes of exposure to television storylines about HIV or AIDS. These results are encouraging because the positive

EE findings from developing countries cannot be generalized to the United States.[4] New technologies such as satellite television are beginning to change the situation overseas, but developing countries have had few alternatives to single, government-sponsored media channels. It is not surprising that reasonably entertaining EE narratives reached large segments of these essentially captive audiences. In contrast, today's domestic media environment is an overwhelming banquet of channel options and U.S. audiences are highly fragmented. Moreover, existing character and plot frameworks may be far from ideal from an EE perspective, and health experts in the United States can only hope that their content recommendations will be followed.

## A Study of HIV/AIDS Information Seeking

The first storyline grew out of ongoing HH&S efforts to encourage inclusion of health messages in daytime soap operas. Although viewed by fewer people than popular evening network shows, soap operas reach many high-risk women. Compared to White women, African-American women have 24 times the annual rate of HIV/AIDS infection per 100,000 population members (CDC, 2005). Thirty-one percent of African-American respondents to the 1999 Healthstyles survey (Beck, Pollard, & Greenberg, 2000) reported watching soap operas at least twice a week, compared with 25% of Hispanics and 17% of Whites. Among regular viewers, minority women were more likely to say that they had learned something about diseases and how to prevent them from soap operas in the last year (Beck et al., 2000).

Writers of an afternoon soap opera, *The Bold and the Beautiful (B&B)*, asked HH&S to link them to behavioral scientists at the CDC who specialize in HIV. The resulting collaboration led to a show watched by 4.5 million households according to Nielsen ratings. Viewers watched handsome, young, Hispanic Tony get tested for HIV prior to his marriage to Kristen. He learns (on August 3, 2001) that he is HIV-positive, and tells his doctor that he has used condoms consistently with his recent sex partners, all of whom were women. He struggles with the reality of his diagnosis, but his beautiful female psychiatrist helps him see that he has access to the best new drugs and medical care, and has reason to expect many years of high-quality life. Tony discloses his serostatus first to his previous partners and then (on August 13, 2001) to his fiancée, who overcomes her own fear and her family's objections to marry him. Tony and Kristen seek counseling about safer sex, eventually visit Africa, and adopt an appealing 8-year-old AIDS orphan whose own serostatus is unknown. The child turns out to be HIV-seronegative.

As is typical in Hollywood, the storyline was developed just weeks before the show was taped; these short timelines create major evaluation constraints. In this case, there was insufficient time to plan, propose, obtain clearances and funding for, and execute an evaluation study involving a new data collection process. Calls to the National STD and HIV Hotline were used to measure information-seeking behavior because they were already being tallied. *B&B* executives agreed to have Tony appear in a PSA that followed the episodes on August 3 and 13; the PSA referred viewers to the Hotline for answers to questions about HIV and AIDS.

Although there were up to 15 trained Hotline staff members answering calls when the show aired, the Hotline capacity was overwhelmed by the number of calls received after these two *B&B* episodes. Most callers got a recorded message to call back at a later time, but it was possible to tally the numbers of call attempts during those time slots.

There were dramatic, statistically significant spikes in call attempts on both days just after the *B&B* timeslot as shown in Figure 9.1. The spike on the second day reached 1,840 attempts in a time slot when fewer than 100 call attempts are usually made (Kennedy et al., 2004).

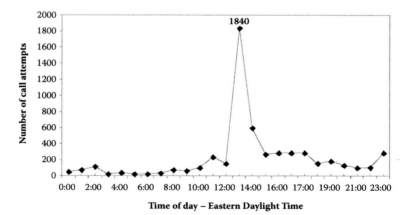

**FIGURE 9.1.** Originating call attempts to the CDC national STD and AIDS hotlines (800-342-2437) by time of day, August 13, 2001. (Reprinted from *Journal of Communication* with permission from Oxford Press.)

The average of the two spikes was significantly higher than the year's other peaks, some of which followed other types of television broadcasts with larger audiences (e.g., *60 Minutes*) or more message repetition (e.g., a weeklong "Rap it Up" PSA campaign).

## A Study of Intentions to Be Screened for Syphilis

The second study in this line of research examined intentions, a powerful predictor of behavior (e.g., Fishbein, Hennessey, Yzer, & Douglas, 2003). Obtaining testing and subsequently receiving treatment for syphilis would reduce the risk of HIV infection. Syphilis causes small, painless, sometimes internal sores that can be overlooked or misattributed, and the risk of HIV infection from a single sexual exposure is thought to be 10 to 300 times higher in the presence of open sores (Hayes, Schultz, & Plummer, 1995).

Syphilis was on the road to elimination in the United States in 1999, with the lowest annual number of cases in 40 years. But in 2000, several U.S. cities began to report outbreaks of the disease among men who have sex with men (MSM). Many of these cases were diagnosed among men who were already infected with HIV, so the rise in syphilis cases caused concern about the potential for parallel increases in HIV among MSM. In the spring of 2002, as prime-time shows started to plan for the next television season (September–May), the director of the CDC conducted a briefing with TV writers in Los Angeles, including writers and producers of *ER*, a top-rated evening series on a national network. Syphilis was one of the topics covered, and writers were encouraged to consider weaving it into their plans for story arcs during the next several months.

In March 2003, *ER* launched a storyline in which an elected city official visits the emergency room to be treated for what turned out to be a case of syphilis. Scriptwriters created a dramatic ethical dilemma in which the ER physician was asked by the official to protect his privacy by failing to record the treatment. A few days later, the official's young assistant (and sex partner) comes into the ER with similar symptoms. The assistant is diagnosed with syphilis, and given the standard antibiotic treatment. In a plot twist that heightened dramatic tension but deviated markedly from EE's prescribed consequences for role models, the young man dies from an allergic reaction to the antibiotic he was administered. As a result, exposure to this storyline could have had the unintended effects of discouraging viewers from obtaining screening for syphilis.

The effects of exposure were investigated in an online survey conducted by volunteers from a community-based organization (CBO) that serves gay men. Survey respondents were visitors to Internet chat rooms for gay men who accepted the CBO's invitation to take a survey on media and health. This strategy was chosen because men who frequent gay chat rooms seek sexual contacts there.

The chat rooms drew visitors from the eight major U.S. cities where outbreaks of syphilis were reported in 2003. The median age of the 500 participants was 35 (range = 15–63). Eighty-eight percent were Whites, 79% had had at least some college education, and 57% reported having seen the *ER* storyline about syphilis (Whittier et al., 2005).

Linear regressions were used to examine the independent effects of demographics, seeing the *ER* episode, regular *ER* viewership, and chatting about it online on two outcomes: (a) the intention to be screened for syphilis, and (b) the intention to tell others to be screened. Exposure to the *ER* storyline was a highly significant predictor of the intention to be screened, and a significant predictor of telling others to be screened.

Perhaps because of their relatively high educational level, respondents did not seem to have been confused or discouraged by the potentially mixed message sent by the allergy-related death of the younger gay man. And the show did reach a high-risk group; MSM who visit chat rooms may be at relatively high risk of syphilis and HIV infection, compared to other gay men (Chaisson et al., 2003). At least one syphilis outbreak has been traced to an Internet chat room (Klausner, Wolf, Fischer-Ponce, Zolt, & Katz, 2000).

The response rate in this study was only around 4%, and there is no way to know how the respondents differed from the majority of men who frequent chat rooms. Similarly, there is no way to know whether the good intentions of respondents were strong enough and lasted long enough to lead to actual screening; the screening venues that ask patients what prompted them to seek screening keep the information in-house. However, the results of this study suggest that there is more to be gained than lost from the modified, network television version of EE that is feasible in the United States. Health stories will be broadcast with or without expert consultation, and there is an argument to be made for providing accurate health information to script writers, even when health experts have no control over its ultimate form or context.

## A Study of Intentions to Be Tested for HIV

The third study in this line of research was conducted to examine the effects of viewing a show that attempted to increase HIV testing by reducing AIDS stigma. Stigmatizing attitudes toward HIV/AIDS increase the suffering of infected individuals and discourage them from seeking HIV testing, disclosing their positive serostatus to those who need to be informed, and adhering to treatment regimens that require public behavior (Chesney & Smith, 1999; Hutchinson, Corbie-Smith, Thomas, Mohanan, & del Rio, 2004). One component of HIV stigma, misconceptions about casual contagion of the disease, appears to be decreasing in prevalence over time. However, another component—victim-blaming—has been evident in approximately 20% of the U.S. population for the last decade (Herek, Capitanio, & Widaman, 2002).

Information dissemination, skills building, and counseling interventions have had partial success in decreasing HIV stigma in the short run, but none of these methods has reached deeply into the general population. Between January and May of 2003, an EE intervention that could help to fill this gap was mounted by collaborators from the KFF and writers from the situation comedy *Girlfriends*.

The previous year, Viacom, the then-parent company of the UPN network that broadcasts *Girlfriends,* had made a commitment to direct its resources toward fighting the HIV/AIDS epidemic. Although it was difficult to work such a serious topic into a comedy format, it did prove to be possible to preserve much of the classic EE formula.

The AIDS storyline was introduced into an already popular series about four African-American women who had been friends since college, 12 years earlier. The audience meets Reesie, a former college roommate of one of the girlfriends. During college, Reesie had "stolen" Brian, a boyfriend of one of the main characters, and had married him, prompting the girlfriends to vow to hate and shun her. When she surfaces as part of a wedding party for her old roommate (who had kept in touch despite the vow), the jilted girlfriend is furious until she learns that Brian infected Reesie with HIV. The feuding women reconcile, the four girlfriends overcome their fears of casual contagion, and there are some poignant scenes in which Reesie and other HIV-infected women talk about their fears and undiminished personhood. At the end of the storyline, Reesie dies and is memorialized in an independent film made by one of the girlfriends.

Members of a Web cohort were interviewed to assess the impact of viewing this storyline on African-American women, the primary audience of *Girlfriends*. The viewers were more likely to have considered an HIV test than other online survey respondents, even after the effects of age, race, and education were controlled statistically (Kennedy et al., 2007). This finding is impressive because the audience was composed primarily of young, educated, African-American women, a group with lower levels of HIV stigma than the general population to begin with, and thus less room for improvement.

## Study 4

A small pre/post pilot study of a Spanish-language radio soap opera broadcast in Nashville, Tennessee, demonstrates that EE broadcasts are possible when financial resources are limited. It also serves as a reminder that EE exposure may interact with individual factors such as level of cognitive development or acculturation.

Called *Enfrentate* (stop and think), the goal of the radio soap opera was delaying sexual initiation among Hispanic adolescents. It consisted of 10 episodes, each of which was 3 minutes long. It was broadcast twice each weekday on a local Spanish music station for 2 weeks during the 2003 school year. Developed with support from a small local grant, the soap opera portrays 15-year-old Margarita, a good student who wants to be a writer when she grows up. She lives in low-income housing and her home life is fraught with distractions, but she struggles to focus on her studies so that she can achieve her goal. Margarita agrees with her mother that early sex has the potential to derail her, and her wealthy, handsome boyfriend is supportive of her aspiration and decision, but other girls make active attempts to have sex with him. There are some rumors and misunderstandings about whether he succumbed, but he is vindicated. In a subplot, a gay friend of Margarita's is diagnosed with HIV, runs away, and considers suicide, but she convinces him to return home where he becomes an HIV prevention trainer. Listeners are exposed to negotiation and refusal skill training because they hear an HIV prevention workshop, and these skills are also modeled in the main plot. As the series concludes, Margarita wins a writing prize and is applauded by her boyfriend and mother.

This soap opera was translated from an earlier English version developed for African-American teens in Nashville (Strand, Rosenbaum, Hanlon, & Jimerson, 2000). Teens and adults from the local Hispanic community reviewed the translation for language and content appropriateness. Qualitative reactions to the series were collected from teens who listened to it on tape in focus groups, and pre/post quantitative data on theoretical predictors of delaying sexual initiation were collected from other teens ($N = 31$). After listening to the tape, the teens' knowledge about sexually transmitted diseases (STDs), beliefs that delay of sexual initiation is important, and levels of delay self-efficacy increased significantly.

Teens in the focus groups said that the storyline was realistic, but they wanted better actors, more "Spanglish," more music cues for the dramatic moments, and a plot that encompassed a wider range of issues that teens face (Kennedy, Clayton-Davis, McGuire, & Lund, 2005). Whether the latter revision would strengthen the effect of exposure or distract from the central theme is an empirical question, and its answer may vary with the cognitive developmental level of the teen or other individual factors. Recent young immigrants from Latin America may be attracted to the telenovela format because it is familiar, but may find it less appealing as they assimilate to standard American youth culture. Data that shed light on this issue would help program designers.

## Research Issues

Largely because of constraints on planning time and resources, the methodologies in each of the four studies summarized previously were marred by threats to validity. To name a few, the *B&B* hotline call attempt data contain unknown proportions of unique and repeat callers, the sample in the *ER* chat room study was self-selected, the complex construct of HIV stigma was not adequately measured in the *Girlfriends* study, and there was no way to estimate the effect of social desirability in the Nashville radio soap opera study. On the other hand, the methodological limitations varied across studies, and may compensate for each other to some degree in the bigger picture.

The available evidence triangulates around the conclusion that EE can help to prevent HIV not only in developing countries, but also in the United States. It is clear, however, that we have only scratched the surface of the EE research agenda. Questions for which research has not yet provided answers are listed in two reports from expert panels sponsored by CDC (see http://www.cdc.gov/communication/ eersrch.htm and http://www.learcenter.org/html/projects/?cm=hhs/ research). The first report set priorities for EE interventions that target general audiences; the priorities included:

- Identifying the most effective research techniques and methodologies, the mechanisms of EE effects, the exposure dosage levels needed, and the factors that prompt and minimize unintended, oppositional, or "boomerang" effects such as identification with the negative role model.
- Determining how EE can be used to generate community discussion (e.g., in chat rooms) and how that discussion mediates/moderates EE effects.
- Finding ways to extend beyond a few weeks the duration of positive EE effects on knowledge (Brodie et al., 2001) and other behavioral determinants.
- Finding out how often we can use the EE approach before audience resistance increases, and how to refresh the formula.

The second report dealt with research priorities for minority audiences. It stressed attention to the diversity between and within ethnic and racial categories, and working with community stakeholders. It urged researchers to ask if and when EE works differently across audiences. The report acknowledged that there is misunderstanding and distrust of the medical establishment in the African-American community, partly as a result of the infamous Tuskegee syphilis study (Freimuth et al., 2001). Consequently, panelists gave high priority to questions about the indigenous institutions and practices that can add credibility to EE offerings and amplify or reinforce EE effects among minority audiences. Finally, the report suggested finding out what kinds of scholarly products would be of interest to writers and producers.

Singhal and Rogers (2004) argue for "methodological pluralism" (i.e., supplementing quantitative survey findings with qualitative data) in answering outstanding EE research questions, and point to the letters and e-mail messages that highly involved audience members send to shows as good sources of qualitative data on health storylines.

Tracking exposure through ongoing, near-real-time ratings and rapid surveys is also recommended; with this information, strategies to promote viewership can be adjusted as necessary. Hotline data can be used to track exposure if messages include markers or tracers (i.e., references to health themes in project-specific language).

An efficient way to build the EE knowledge base would be to conduct small-scale experimental studies of the effects of manipulating specific narrative elements (e.g., putting health messages in a main plot or a subplot). It would be worthwhile to find out if and when the results of internally valid laboratory studies generalize to real-world audiences and whether or not the results would be convincing to writers and producers.

Of course, one cannot add methodological rigor to evaluations of nationwide EE broadcasts by using experimental designs (or randomized controlled trials). National television is "full coverage" and there is no really valid comparison area for the United States. Survey responses of individuals who are exposed to broadcasts must be compared to responses from the unexposed, an analysis that is subject to self-selection bias. To avoid claiming that EE exposure had outcomes that were really a function of the preexisting propensity to be exposed, evaluators should consider borrowing the technique of propensity scoring from econometrics (Yanovitzky, Zanutto, & Hornick, 2005).

Informing EE research and practice with a wider range of theories could be useful. For example, information-processing models may guide us in using dramatic devices to focus audience attention on important information and make it memorable (Kennedy et al., 2004). Singhal and Rogers (2004) pointed to narrative theory (Fisher, 1987) to explain how EE interventions work on a rhetorical level. Sood et al. (2004) argued that agenda setting theory and similar perspectives could put EE narratives into context, perhaps making it possible to predict differential reactions to EE over time and interactions between mass media and society. Cultural theories (e.g, Hong, Morris, Chiu, & Benet-Martinez, 2000; Oetting & Beauvais, 1990–1991) could help to predict differential EE outcomes across groups. Some resistance to or distortion of messages has been noted among some cultural subgroups (Singhal & Rogers, 2004), even though associations between EE and widespread increases in health behavior have been detected in more than a dozen studies spanning multiple cultural contexts.

Finally, additional theoretical work and empirical tests are needed to inform decisions about using alternatives to the mass-mediated serial drama format. Alternative formats are being employed at a pace that has outstripped that of relevant research. For example, the South African version of *Sesame Street* is using an HIV-positive puppet character to transmit antistigma messages to preschoolers (see p. 44 of the program pdf file at http://www.ee4.org/program.htm). Other information channels such as comic books, street theater, and the Internet have been used alone or in combination with radio and television in EE programs. New entertainment formats (e.g., music videos) have also been used (see http://www.ee4.org for examples).

## Conclusion

When barriers to adopting HIV prevention behaviors go beyond ignorance of the health benefits of the behaviors, communicating facts is obviously insufficient. Some of the additional barriers are emotional, and an EE narrative can touch emotion and help move audiences to action. But even though receptivity to a good story may be a universal human trait (Schank, 1990), artists, scientists, and advocates must work together to understand exactly what makes a story good from the perspectives of various at-risk audiences. With the extended attention of audiences provided by the EE format, it has been possible to address more than one complex issue (e.g., HIV/AIDS and family planning) successfully in a single series. This is good news and should be explored further. And even though the entertainment industry continues to air stories about HIV and AIDS, it would be wise to investigate topic fatigue—the perception on the parts of writers that a topic has "been done." Taking these next steps will help to leverage the vast potential of the modern entertainment industry to change the individual and collective attitudes and behaviors that perpetuate the AIDS epidemic.

## Notes

1. Letter read at the 1999 Soap Summit by Patricia Fili-Krushel, first head of daytime programming at ABC.
2. This research design feature is sometimes chosen for ethical reasons when a treatment is promising and the comparison or control group or area is in need of efficacious intervention.

3. Health profiles of Hispanics differ by country of origin. Puerto Ricans suffer disproportionately from HIV/AIDS, asthma, and infant mortality, whereas Mexicans are at high risk for diabetes. All Hispanic groups have barriers to care access. See http://www.cdc.gov/omh/Populations/HL/HL.htm for specific information.

4. Conversely, there was concern about unintended consequences overseas of the first U.S. show studied in this line of research. It is translated into numerous languages and shown in countries where HIV prevalence is many times that of the United States. It is reassuring that, despite the lack of cultural tailoring and contextual relevance of the broadcast, there is evidence that exposure to the show may actually be lowering HIV stigma in the one developing country for which data are available (O'Leary et al., 2007).

## References

Bandura, A. (1977). *Social learning theory.* Englewood Cliffs, NJ: Prentice-Hall.

Beck, V. (2004). Working with daytime and prime-time television shows in the United States to promote health. In A. Singhal, M. J. Cody, E. M. Rogers, & M. Sabido (Eds.), *Entertainment-education and social change: History, research, and practice* (pp. 207–224). Mahwah, NJ: Lawrence Erlbaum Associates.

Beck, V., Pollard, W., & Greenberg, B. (2000, November). *Tune in for health: Working with television entertainment shows and partners to deliver health information for at-risk audiences.* Paper presented at the meeting of the American Public Health Association, Boston.

Bouman, M. (2004). Entertainment-education television drama in the Netherlands. In A. Singhal, M. J. Cody, E. M. Rogers, & M. Sabido (Eds.), *Entertainment-education and social change: History, research, and practice* (pp. 225–242). Mahwah, NJ: Lawrence Erlbaum Associates.

Brodie, M., Foehr, U., Rideout, V., Baer, N., Miller, C., Flouroy, R., et al. (2001). Communicating health information through the entertainment media. *Health Affairs, 20,* 192–199.

Brown, W. J., & Singhal, A. (1999). Entertainment-education strategies for social change. In D. P. Demers & K. Viswanath (Eds.), *Mass media, social control and social change* (pp. 263–280). Ames: Iowa State University Press.

Centers for Disease Control and Prevention. (2005). *HIV/AIDS Surveillance Report, 2004, 16,* Atlanta, GA: Author.

Chaisson, M. A., Hirshfeld, S., Humberstone, M., DiFilippi, J., Newstein, D., Koblin, B., et al. (2003). The Internet and high-risk sex among men who have sex with men. In *Program and Abstracts of the 10th Conference on Retroviruses and Opportuinistic Infections*, Boston, Abstract 37.

Chesney, M. A., & Smith, A. W. (1999). Critical delays in HIV testing and care: The potential role of stigma. *American Behavioral Scientist, 42,* 1162–1174.

Cody, M. J., Fernandez, S., & Wilkin, H. (2004). Entertainment-education programs of the BBC and BBC World. In A. Singhal, M. J. Cody, E. M. Rogers, & M. Sabido (Eds.), *Entertainment-education and social change: History, research, and practice* (pp. 243–260). Mahwah, NJ: Lawrence Erlbaum Associates.

Fishbein, M., Hennessy, M., Yzer, M., & Douglas, J. (2003). Can we explain why some people do and some people do not act on their intentions? *Psychology of Health and Medicine, 8,* 3–18.

Fisher, W. (1987). *Human communication as narration.* Columbia: University of South Carolina Press.

Freimuth, V. S., Quinn, S.C., Thomas, S.B., Cole, G., Zook, E., & Duncan, T. (2001). African Americans' views on research and the Tuskegee syphilis study. *Social Science and Medicine, 52,* 797–808.

Galavotti, C., Pappas-DeLuca, K. A., & Lansky, A. (2001). Modeling and reinforcement to combat HIV: The *MARCH* approach to behavior change. *American Journal of Public Health, 91,* 1602–1607.

Hayes, R. J., Schultz, K. F., & Plummer, F. A. (1995). The co-factor effect of genital ulcers on the per-exposure risk of HIV transmission in sub-Saharan African. *Journal of Tropical Medicine and Hygiene, 98,* 1–8.

Herek, G. M., Capitanio, J. P., & Widaman, K. F. (2002). HIV-related stigma and knowledge in the United States: Prevalence and trends, 1991–1999. *American Journal of Public Health, 92,* 371–377.

Hong, Y., Morris, M. W., Chiu, C., & Benet-Martinez, V. (2000). Multicultural minds: A dynamic constructivist approach to culture and cognition. *American Psychologist, 55,* 709–720.

Hutchinson, A. B., Corbie-Smith, G., Thomas, S. B., Mohanan, S., & del Rio, C. (2004). Understanding the patient's perspective on rapid and routine HIV testing in an inner-city clinic. *AIDS Education and Prevention, 16,* 101–114.

Kennedy, M. G., Clayton-Davis, J., McGuire, A., & Lund, M. (2005). *A pilot cross-cultural adaptation of an HIV-prevention radio soap opera for teens.* Unpublished manuscript.

Kennedy, M. G., O'Leary, A., Beck, V., Pollard, K., & Simpson, P. (2004). Increases in calls to the CDC National STD and AIDS Hotline following AIDS-related episodes in a soap opera. *Journal of Communication, 54,* 287–301.

Kennedy, M. G., O'Leary, A., Wright-Fofanah, S., Dean, E., Chen, Y., & Baxter, R. (2007). *Effects on HIV stigma viewing of an HIV-relevant storyline in a television situation comedy.* Manuscript submitted for publication.

Klausner, J. D., Wolf, W., Fischer-Ponce, L., Zolt, I., & Katz, M. H. (2000). Tracing a syphilis outbreak through cyberspace. *Journal of the American Medical Association, 284,* 447–449.

Oetting, G. R., & Beauvais, F. (1990–1991). Orthogonal cultural identification theory: The cultural identification of minority adolescents. *International Journal of the Addictions, 25,* 655–685.

O'Leary, A., Kennedy, M., Pappas-Deluca, K. A., Nkete, M., Beck, V., & Galavotti, C. (2007). Association between exposure to an HIV storyline in "The Bold and the Beautiful" and HIV-related stigma in Botswana. *AIDS Education and Prevention, 19*(3), 209–217.

Pappas-DeLuca, K. (2004, August 25). *Results from a midterm assessment of an HIV/AIDS behavior change radio drama in Botswana.* Paper presented at the Centers for Disease Control and Prevention, Atlanta, GA.

Piotrow, P. T., & de Fossard, E. (2004). Entertainment-education as a public health intervention. In A. Singhal, M. J. Cody, E. M. Rogers, & M. Sabido (Eds.), *Entertainment-education and social change: History, research, and practice* (pp. 39–60). Mahwah, NJ: Lawrence Erlbaum Associates.

Poindexter, D. O. (2004). A history of entertainment-education, 1958–2000. In A. Singhal, M. J. Cody, E. M. Rogers, & M. Sabido (Eds.), *Entertainment-education and social change: History, research, and practice* (pp. 21–38). Mahwah, NJ: Lawrence Erlbaum Associates.

Rogers, E. M., Vaughn, P. W., Swalehe, R. M. A., Rao, N., Svenkerud, P., & Sood, S. (1999). Effects of an entertainment-education radio soap opera on family planning in Tanzania. *Studies in Family Planning, 30,* 193–211.

Sabido, M. (2004). The origins of entertainment-education. In A. Singhal, M. J. Cody, E. M. Rogers, & M. Sabido (Eds.) (2004). *Entertainment-education and social change: History, research, and practice* (pp. 61–74). Mahwah, NJ: Lawrence Erlbaum Associates.

Schank, R. (1990). *Tell me a story: Narrative & intelligence.* Evanston, IL: Northwestern University Press.

Singhal, A., Cody, M. J., Rogers, E. M., & Sabido, M. (Eds.). (2004). *Entertainment-education and social change: History, research, and practice.* Mahwah, NJ: Lawrence Erlbaum Associates.

Singhal, A., & Rogers, E.M. (1999). *Entertainment-education: A communication strategy for social change.* Mahwah, NJ: Lawrence Erlbaum Associates.

Singhal, A., & Rogers, E. M. (2004). The status of entertainment-education worldwide. In A. Singhal, M. J. Cody, E. M. Rogers, & M. Sabido (Eds.), *Entertainment-education and social change: History, research, and practice* (pp. 3–20). Mahwah, NJ: Lawrence Erlbaum Associates.

Singhal, A., Sharma, D., Papa, M. J., & Witte, K. (2004). Air cover and ground mobilization: Integrating entertainment-education broadcasts with community listening and service delivery in India. In A. Singhal, M. J. Cody, E. M. Rogers, & M. Sabido (Eds.), *Entertainment-education and social change: History, research, and practice* (pp. 351–376). Mahwah, NJ: Lawrence Erlbaum Associates.

Sood, S., Menard, T., & Witte, K. (2004). The theory behind entertainment-education. In A. Singhal, M. J. Cody, E. M. Rogers, & M. Sabido (Eds.), *Entertainment-education and social change: History, research, and practice* (pp. 117–152). Mahwah, NJ: Lawrence Erlbaum Associates.

Strand, J., Rosenbaum, J., Hanlon, E., & Jimerson, A. (2000). The PMI community demonstration sites project: Lessons in technical assistance. *Social Marketing Quarterly, 6*, 13–22.

UNAIDS. (2004). UNAIDS 2004 report on the global AIDS epidemic. Retrieved March 2, 2006, from http://www.unaids.org/bangkok2004/report.html

Vaughn, P. W., & Rogers, E. M. (2000). A staged model of communication effects: Evidence from an entertainment-education radio soap opera in Tanzania. *Journal of Health Communication, 5*, 203–227.

Vaughn, P. W., Rogers, E. M., Singhal, A., & Swalehe, R. M. A. (2000). Entertainment-education and HIV/AIDS prevention: A field experiment in Tanzania. *Journal of Health Communication, 5*(Suppl.), 81–100.

Whittier, D. K., Kennedy, M. G., St. Lawrence, J. S., Seeley, S., & Beck, V. (2005). Embedding health messages into entertainment television: Effect on gay men's response to a syphilis outbreak. *Journal of Health Communication, 10*, 251–259.

Yanovitzky, I., Zanutto, E., & Hornik, R. (2005). Estimating causal effects of public health education campaigns using propensity score methodology. *Evaluation and Program Planning, 28*, 209–220.

# 10

# The Agenda-Setting Process and HIV/AIDS

*James W. Dearing*
Kaiser Permanente Colorado

*Do Kyun Kim*
Ohio University

With publication of an epidemiologic note in the June 4, 1981, issue of the *Morbidity and Mortality Weekly Report,* the first five cases of what would become known as HIV/AIDS began. Now, 26 years later, HIV infects 21% of the Botswana population (UNAIDS, 2004) and more than 40 million people worldwide (UNAIDS & World Health Organization [WHO], 2005). More than 20 million people have died of AIDS. China is expected to have 10 million cases within 4 years (Ingham, 2004). In the United States, the issue of HIV/AIDS has become a part of everyday life even as the disease newly threatens gay male populations because of exploding rates of crystal methamphetamine use paired with instant Internet advertising for sex partners (Specter, 2005).

In this chapter, we first introduce the perspective of agenda-setting research, which centrally concerns mass media, public opinion, and policymaking as a way in which society can be understood. Scholars who contribute to this literature define themselves as mass communication researchers, political scientists, or scholars of social movements and collective behavior. Then, we review the history of HIV/AIDS as a public issue in the United States through an agenda-setting lens.

What is the Agenda-Setting Process?

An *agenda* is a set of issues that is communicated in a hierarchy of importance at a point in time. Political scientists Roger Cobb and Charles Elder defined an agenda in political terms as "a general set of political controversies that will be viewed at any point in time as falling within the range of legitimate concerns meriting the attention of the polity" (Cobb & Elder, 1972, p. 14). Though we conceptualize an agenda as existing at a point in time, agendas are the result of dynamic interplay. As different issues rise and fall in importance over time, agendas provide snapshots of this fluidity.

The *agenda-setting process* is an ongoing competition among issue proponents to gain the attention of media professionals, the public, and policy elites. Agenda setting offers an explanation of why information about certain issues, and not other issues, is available to the public in a democracy; how public opinion is shaped; and why certain issues are addressed through policy actions whereas other issues are not.

Conflict is a means by which a condition can become understood as a problem, and then achieve the status of an issue. Relatively objective conditions such as the epidemiology of avian flu or Hurricane Katrina are not inherently conflictual. Conflict is a quality brought to prolonged social conditions through the responses by organized interests as they work to socially construct what a condition such as a disease or a disaster means to us as a society. Is a hurricane and its aftermath to be understood as a problem of disaster preparedness, or inattention to poverty, or inept federal agency response, or global warming? Problem definition, whether by people in discussion with one another, by media professionals, or by elected officials, is a process of *framing*, the giving of meaning to particular conditions (Pan & Kosicki, 2001). Framing, in providing advantage to certain organized interests, is often decided through conflict.

Cobb and Elder (1972) defined an *issue* as "a conflict between two or more identifiable groups over procedural or substantive matters relating to the distribution of positions or resources" (p. 32). An issue is whatever is in contention (Lang & Lang, 1981). The two-sided nature of an issue is important in understanding why and how an issue climbs up an agenda. The potentially conflictual nature of an issue helps make it newsworthy as proponents and opponents of the issue battle it out in the shared "public arena," which, in modern society, is mass and specialty media.

The perspective of Cobb and Elder (1972) and Lang and Lang (1981) that an issue embeds conflict reminds us that agenda setting is inherently a political process. At stake is the relative attention given by the media, the public, and policymakers to some issues *and not to others* (Hilgartner & Bosk, 1988). We can think of issues as "rising or falling" on the agenda, or "competing with one another" for attention. *Issue proponents,* individuals or groups that advocate for attention to be given to an issue, help determine the position of an issue on an agenda, sometimes at the cost of another issue or issues. Agenda setting can be a "zero-sum game" because space and time on the media agenda are scarce resources (Zhu, 1992). But sometimes a hot issue does not supplant coverage of other issues, especially related issues (Hertog, Finnegan, & Kahn, 1994).

This is the agenda-setting *process,* modeled as the media agenda, the public agenda, and the policy agenda, and the interrelationships among these three elements, where conditions may be framed as problems and become public issues (see Fig. 10.1). A scholarly research tradition exists for each of these three types of agendas. The first research tradition is called *media agenda setting* because its main dependent variable is the importance of an issue on the mass media agenda. The

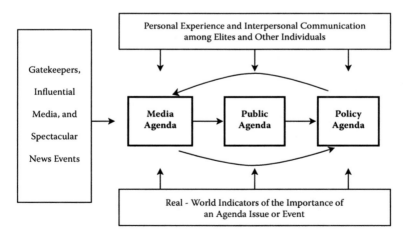

**FIGURE 10.1.** Three main components of the agenda-setting process: the media agenda, public agenda, and policy agenda. From Agenda-setting research: Where has it been, where is it going? by E. M. Rogers and J. W. Dearing. In J. A. Anderson (Ed.), *Communication Yearbook 11* (pp. 555–594), 1988, Thousand Oaks, CA: Sage. Copyright 1988 by International Communication Association. Reprinted with permission.

second research tradition is called *public agenda setting* because its main dependent variable is the importance of a set of issues on the public agenda. The third research tradition is called *policy agenda setting* because the distinctive aspect of this scholarly tradition is its concern with policy actions regarding an issue, in part as a response to the media agenda and the public agenda (Rogers & Dearing, 1988).

Individuals engage in active psychological sensemaking about public issues (Gamson, 1992; Liebes & Katz, 1990; Neuman, Just, & Crigler, 1992), as well as active organized activities that are intended to influence the outcomes of public issue debates (Blumer, 1971; Dearing & Rogers, 1996; Downs, 1972; Kingdon, 1984). For most issues, the vast majority of people are inattentive rather than attentive, more passive than active. But occasionally, even inattentive members of the public can, driven by perceived relevance and interest, become very active and take charge of their information environment and organize for action, which is a key means by which public opinion exerts itself on policymakers and their sources of information, such as congressional staff and consultants (Blumer, 1948). When considered at the higher order aggregate of a system, this view of small intensely interested groups of citizens efficaciously pushing for redress or change means that society as a whole is, through the diffusion of issues and governmental responses to them, a complex type of information processor (Baumgartner & Jones, 1993).

## The Issue of HIV/AIDS in the 1980s[1]

Although the first HIV/AIDS cases were diagnosed in the United States in 1981, this issue did not attract much media attention until 4 years later, in mid-1985. By that time, more than 10,000 individuals had been diagnosed with AIDS, and about half that number had died. Why were the media so slow in discovering the issue of HIV/AIDS? What finally put it on the agenda? Dearing collaborated in several studies of HIV/AIDS as a public issue in the 1980s; we base this section on those accounts (Dearing, 1989, 1992; Dearing & Rogers, 1992, 1996; Rogers, Dearing, & Chang, 1991).

The media agenda was measured by the number of news stories about HIV/AIDS in the *New York Times,* the *Washington Post,* the *Los Angeles Times,* and the network evening newscasts of ABC, NBC, and CBS. From June 1981 through December 1988 (a period of

91 months), the six media of study carried 6,694 news stories about HIV/AIDS. Because media coverage of HIV/AIDS in each of the six media of study were highly intercorrelated across time, we combined the coverage by all six media into a variable indexing total mass media coverage of HIV/AIDS, which we utilized to measure the media agenda.

For the first 4 years of the epidemic, a point at which 9,944 individuals had AIDS, the issue was quite low on the mass media agenda. U.S. national mass media were slow to respond to the issue because of the lack of involvement of two traditional agenda-setting influences: the White House and the *New York Times.* President Reagan chose not to give a talk about AIDS until May 1987, 72 months into the epidemic, a point at which 35,121 AIDS cases had been reported by the Centers for Disease Control and Prevention (CDC).

The *New York Times* published its first Page 1 story about HIV/AIDS on May 25, 1983, 12 months later than the *Los Angeles Times,* and 10 months later than the *Washington Post.* The *New York Times* management did not consider HIV/AIDS to be newsworthy from 1981 to mid-1985. Moreover, the newspaper's key medical writer broke his leg and was physically unable to cover breaking stories during this time. When a new executive editor was appointed in late 1985, coverage of HIV/AIDS expanded dramatically.

The number of news stories about HIV/AIDS escalated from an average of 14 per month prior to July 1985, to 143 per month after that date. Most scholars at the time credited this tenfold increase in news coverage to the announcement that film actor Rock Hudson had AIDS. Our analysis showed that it was actually a concomitant news story of a young boy with AIDS, Ryan White, more so than Hudson, that propelled this issue up the media agenda. Although the White and Hudson disclosures together represented only 3% of our 6,694 news stories of study, the personification of HIV/AIDS by White and Hudson reframed the issue for news people, who responded by giving more attention to HIV/AIDS. Even before July 1985, the rather limited AIDS coverage by the U.S. media had created a sharp increase in public awareness during 1983 and 1984 of the disease, and had begun to correct the widespread misperceptions about methods of HIV transmission such as toilet seats and mosquito bites.

How was HIV/AIDS framed in the mass media? We identified four eras in the media coverage of AIDS: an initial era, a science era, a human era, and a political era (see Fig. 10.2). The initial era of

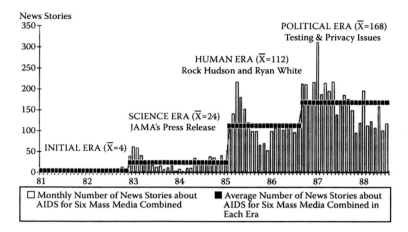

**FIGURE 10.2.** Four eras of media salience and framing for the issue of HIV/AIDS in the 1980s. From "AIDS in the 1980s: The agenda-setting process for a public issue," by E. M. Rogers, J. W. Dearing, and S. Chang, 1991, *Journalism Monographs, 126.* Copyright 1991 by the Association for Education in Journalism and Mass Communication. Reprinted with permission.

HIV/AIDS media coverage was marked by only 59 new stories, most of which concerned the mystery of this new disease.

Media coverage during the second phase of 26 months through June 1985 depended on scientific sources. Forty percent of the 606 news stories in the science era were based on scientific sources as researchers began to unravel the mystery.

The third phase of 19 months through January 1987, the human era, was characterized by personalizing the issue of HIV/AIDS. It was during this period that the Rock Hudson and Ryan White news events helped convince the U.S. public that HIV/AIDS was not just an epidemic among a unique category of people. These two events created the major turning point for the issue of HIV/AIDS on the U.S. media agenda.

The fourth phase of 23 months, February 1987 through December 1988, was a political era for the issue of HIV/AIDS. Public controversies emerged about certain aspects of the epidemic, especially public policy concerning mandatory testing and individual privacy. The government thus became deeply involved, and so HIV/AIDS became a political issue.

When interaction among the time-series data is analyzed for each of the four eras, the general model of the agenda-setting process (see Fig. 10.1) was supported. During the initial era, the science agenda and the real-world indicator affected the media agenda. Many of the news stories were rewrites of science and medical journal press releases. During the science era, when scientific information about disease transmission dominated news content, the media agenda affected the polling agenda (pollsters asked questions in response to media coverage about AIDS). During the (third) human era, the media agenda and the polling agenda influenced each other. This relationship occurred because media organizations sponsored polls that asked questions about HIV/AIDS and then created news stories based on the poll results. During the (fourth) political era, both the science agenda and the media agenda influenced the policy agenda. The media agenda–policy agenda relationship during this fourth era contradicts the results from the full 91-month time-series analysis.

These results suggest that the framed and reframed public issue of HIV/AIDS, when studied over time, comprised a natural history or "issue-attention cycle." Both Herbert Blumer (1971) and Anthony Downs (1972) suggested that a condition that achieves the status of a social problem and then a public issue follows a more or less regular process that consists of a series of stages. This is precisely what our early studies of HIV/AIDS showed. Additionally, our analyses showed that an issue becomes important on multiple agendas, and that it is this interaction that leads to social change as an issue becomes institutionalized through government, private, and nonprofit responses to it.

Public policies, in particular, often function not to solve difficult societal problems but to institutionalize a response to those problems. The policy institutionalization of responses to public issues is how governments grow (Baumgartner & Jones, 1993). It is to this topic that we now turn our attention in analyzing the more recent history for the issue of HIV/AIDS.

## HIV/AIDS in the 1990s and Beyond

Much has happened with the problem of AIDS and the continuing public issue of what to do about it since 1992 when the first version of the present chapter appeared. President Clinton promised full funding of the Ryan White CARE Act, established the White House Office of National AIDS Policy, convened the first White House Conference on AIDS, and established the Presidential Advisory Council on HIV/

AIDS. Federal and state spending on AIDS testing, treatment, and prevention soared. Rights were extended to people living with HIV/AIDS through multiple programs, acts, and court cases. By 1998, large-scale human trials began for an HIV vaccine (Gostin, 2004). Combinations of treatment protocols, behavior modifications, and medications have led to vastly longer time periods between onset of HIV and full-blown AIDS. In America, tens of thousands of HIV-positive people live long lives just as do many people with diseases such as diabetes.

During the 1990s, federal agencies such as the National Institutes of Health (NIH; primarily in terms of biomedical research) and the CDC (mostly for epidemiological research and behavioral interventions including public communication campaigns) were progressive and responsive to the moving epidemic. These and other federal agencies established important offices to jump-start AIDS research and prevention programs, such as the NIH Office of AIDS Research. Nationwide, the CDC awarded block grants to states, territories, and major cities each year as long as they engaged their citizens in community-based prevention planning (Dearing, Larson, Randall, & Pope, 1998). AIDS overtook cancer in federal spending. Academic journals devoted to HIV/AIDS began. In the 1990s, it was not unusual to peruse an academic journal in any discipline and find one or more articles reporting the results of a study concerning HIV/AIDS. This prominence reflects how high the issue of AIDS has risen in the federal government, where spending was estimated at $19.7 billion for fiscal year 2005, for treatment (65%), research (15%), income support (10%), and prevention programs (10%) (Johnson & Coleman, 2005).

How have the mass media responded to this massive, recurring investment and prominence? Mass media stories that are solely devoted to HIV/AIDS have declined in number and length, and have become more event-dependent, relying on celebrities and press conferences to break through the routinization or "compassion fatigue" that characterizes the response of many people now to this issue (Kaiser Family Foundation, 2004; Swain, 2005). Mass media journalists have a more difficult time now convincing their editors that a story about HIV/AIDS is newsworthy (Brodie, Hamel, Kates, Altman, & Drew, 2004). And with this sense of complacency and institutionalization of the issue has come the belief that the problem of AIDS is waning. New discoveries in prevention and, especially, treatment, have signaled that its end is in sight or, at least, manageable for life even as the disease itself has moved into new populations of Latinos, African Americans, incarcerated youth and adults, and the poor in inner cities (Gostin, 2004), even as new generations of young gay men in America's cities assert their own sexual freedom with the lessened sense of personal responsibility brought about by rampant use of designer drugs (Specter, 2005). Most ominously, AIDS is surging worldwide in countries without the medical, pharmacological, organizational, and political infrastructure of the United States. It is worth remembering that the first U.S. populations infected with HIV—gay men—though highly stigmatized, nevertheless were highly educated, middle and upper class, White, and politically active, and still the virus exhibited rapid spread.

Yet does decline really capture what has happened to mass media coverage of the issue of AIDS? AIDS has become the subject of comics, hundreds of public service announcements, workplace discrimination training, many hundreds of school-based interventions, and hundreds of thousands of hours of community-planning group discussions across the nation. AIDS has become firmly entrenched in popular culture. AIDS was prominently featured in 81 motion pictures from 1985 through 1998 (Fuller, 2003).

One of the common responses of journalists, editors, and indexing staff inside media organizations to issues that become large, multifaceted, and, thus, no longer very newsworthy, is to still give coverage to them but in the context of other frames and issues. That is, a very large issue that persists (like AIDS) loses its informational value to journalists. It retains its importance, but its omnipresence means that it is subsumed into more event-driven, newer issues about which viewerships and readerships are not tired. AIDS gets mentioned in a story about worker rights. AIDS is mentioned as a part of the president's foreign relations strategy. AIDS becomes a charity of major league baseball. AIDS becomes an example in a story about a new model for nursing care.

We tested this notion that AIDS has not declined in mass media coverage as much as it has filtered into stories about many other issues. To do this in a way consistent with our perspective on the agenda-setting process (see Fig. 10.1), we constructed new time-series of data representing the media agenda, the public agenda, and the policy agenda for the issue of HIV/AIDS in the U.S. for the years 1983 to 2003. Our expectation that the media and public agendas will affect the policy agenda for this issue is based on the democratic theory that governments respond to citizens (including the interpretation by government officials that media coverage is evidence of citizen interest), strong empirical results demonstrating that public opinion is the dominant influence on policy making in the United States (Erikson, Wright, & McIver, 1993, p. 244), and our earlier reported empirical results showing how these same variables were related to each other during the 1980s (Rogers et al., 1991).

Because we wanted to capture the range of articles in which AIDS was mentioned even when it was not the focus of the story, we selected all news articles in the *New York Times* mentioning HIV or AIDS either in the title or in the content of the article. Besides being the premier agenda-setting newspaper for other U.S. newspapers, the *Times* has been shown to covary closely to other large metropolitan newspapers as well (Rogers et al., 1991). Thus in this analysis, we purposely created a very inclusive version of the media agenda for the issue of AIDS.

We represented the public agenda as the annual proportion of respondents to Gallup public opinion polls responding that HIV/AIDS was the most important problem facing the United States. We used the annual total U.S. Department of Health and Human Services (HHS) spending on HIV/AIDS to represent the policy agenda. In addition, because policy decision makers especially can be expected to respond to long-term social conditions for which clear incontrovertible data exist, we created a fourth time-series, representing the real-world problem of HIV/AIDS, using the annual number of new HIV cases combined with deaths due to AIDS in the United States.

As an example of these data, for our most recent year, 2003, in the 20-year time-series, the number of stories mentioning HIV or AIDS in the *New York Times* was 1,212 (the 18th year in a row in which the annual number of such articles had topped 1,000 in the *Times*); well less than 0.2% of respondents in Gallup polls picked HIV/AIDS as the nation's most important problem; HHS spending on HIV/AIDS was $6,093,846,000; and the number of new HIV cases and AIDS deaths in the United States was 65,614. We show the 20-year time-series for each of these four variables of interest in Figure 10.3 through Figure 10.6.

With the four time-series, we conducted two types of analysis: first, an analysis of the overall agenda setting process over time, and second, a finer-grained look to investigate relationships among each variable. For the overall agenda-setting process, we constructed a multiequation model with all four time-series:

$$Y_p = -1679127 + 17.23 \ X_r + 4034.42 \ X_m - 1483441 \ X_{pu} + ei$$

where $Y_p$ = policy agenda; $X_r$ = real-world indicator; $X_m$ = media agenda; $X_{pu}$ = public agenda.

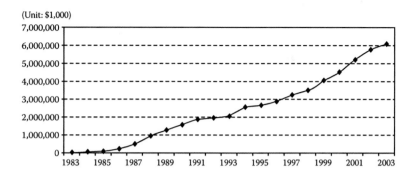

**FIGURE 10.3** The annual amount of U.S. Department of Health and Human Services funding in the United States for HIV/AIDS.

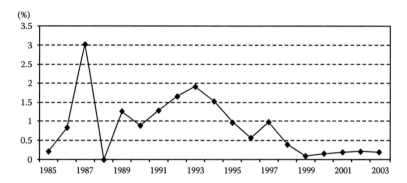

**FIGURE 10.4** The annual percentage of Americans responding that HIV/AIDS was the most important problem facing the nation in Gallup Organization public opinion polls.

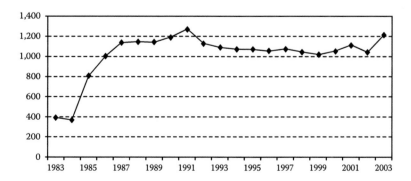

**FIGURE 10.5** The annual number of articles in the *New York Times* mentioning HIV, AIDS, or HIV/AIDS.

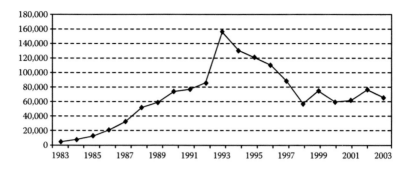

**FIGURE 10.6.** The annual number of new HIV cases and AIDS deaths in the United States.

Results from this test produced an $R^2 = .536$ (Adj. $R^2 = .454$), $p < .05$. The public agenda ($t = -3.328$) and media agenda ($t = 2.385$) were statistically significant predictors of the policy agenda. After running this initial regression, we dropped the insignificant real-world indicator variable from the equation and reran the reduced regression. Even though the exclusion of the real-world indicator resulted in statistically significant outcomes for the other variables, this exclusion reduced the $R^2$ value ($R^2 = 0.447$, Adj. $R^2 = 0.386$). A reduced $R^2$ is expected with the removal of a variable (Pindyck & Rubinfeld, 1998).

Empirically, this result can be interpreted in one of two ways. Either there is a model specification problem after eliminating the real-world indicator, or the media agenda and public agenda are stronger influences on the policy agenda compared to the real-world indicator. This latter interpretation is consistent with our prior model of the agenda-setting process and prior empirical results (Fig. 10.1; see also Dearing & Rogers, 1996). Even though incontrovertible facts such as the mounting number of deaths due to AIDS can be levers for policy change, especially when paired with trigger events, over a long time period their effect may wash out because attention by the media, the public, and policymakers goes elsewhere, often driven by coverage of spectacular events.

Next, we considered the separate interrelationships between variables. We included the real-world indicator in these analyses because it may influence the policy agenda, the media agenda, or the public agenda separately though still not contributing to variance explained in the simultaneous model test.

With the three main components of the agenda-setting process presented in Figure 10.1 and prior agenda-setting research in mind, we constructed a diagram explaining the interconnectivity among these components and the real-world indicator (see Fig. 10.7). Based on this design, nine single-equation regression models were constructed:

$$\text{Model 1: } Y_{poi} = \alpha_{po} + \beta X_{ri} + \varepsilon_i$$

$$\text{Model 2: } Y_{mi} = \alpha_m + \beta X_{ri} + \varepsilon_i$$

$$\text{Model 3: } Y_{pui} = \alpha_{pu} + \beta X_{ri} + \varepsilon_i$$

$$\text{Model 4: } Y_{poi} = \alpha_{po} + \beta X_{mi} + \varepsilon_i$$

$$\text{Model 5: } Y_{mi} = \alpha_m + \beta X_{poi} + \varepsilon_i$$

$$\text{Model 6: } Y_{pui} = \alpha_{pu} + \beta X_{poi} + \varepsilon_i$$

$$\text{Model 7: } Y_{poi} = \alpha_{po} + \beta X_{pui} + \varepsilon_i$$

$$\text{Model 8: } Y_{pui} = \alpha_{pu} + \beta X_{mi} + \varepsilon_i$$

$$\text{Model 9: } Y_{mi} = \alpha_m + \beta X_{pui} + \varepsilon_i$$

where $Y_{po}$ = policy agenda; $Y_m$ = media agenda; $Y_{pu}$ = public agenda, $X_r$ = real-world indicator; $X_m$ = media agenda; $X_{po}$ = policy agenda; and $X_{pu}$ = public agenda.

After running the nine recursive ordinary least squares regression equation models, five relationships proved to be statistically significant, described by the five regression model results that follow:

$$\text{Model 1: } Y_{poi} = 1133871.7 + 0.41 X_{ri} + ei$$

$$\text{Model 2: } Y_{mi} = 801.9 + 0.556 X_{ri} + ei$$

$$\text{Model 4: } Y_{poi} = -1234498 + 0.441 X_{mi} + ei$$

$$\text{Model 5: } Y_{mi} = 888.205 + 0.441 X_{poi} + ei$$

$$\text{Model 8: } Y_{pui} = -0.652 + 0.413 X_{mi} + ei$$

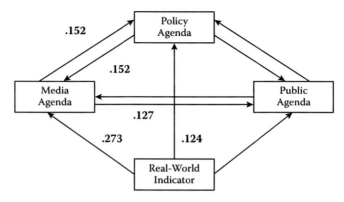

**FIGURE 10.7.** Summary of separate relationships among the policy agenda, the media agenda, the public agenda, and the real-world indicator. Adjusted $R^2$ results are indicated in the paths.

**TABLE 10.1   Summary of Valid Models**

| Models and Variables | B | SE B | β |
|---|---|---|---|
| Model 1 AIDS cases | 19.377 | 9.903 | 0.410* |
| Model 2 AIDS cases | 0.003361 | 0.001168 | 0.556** |
| Model 4 Number of *NYT* articles | 2.318 | 7.787 | 0.441* |
| Model 5 HHS funding for AIDS | 0.000 | 0.000 | 0.441* |
| Model 8 Number of *NYT* articles | 0.001 | 0.001 | 0.413* |

Note. Adjusted $R^2$ = .124 for Model 1; adjusted $R^2$ = .273 for Model 2; adjusted $R^2$ = .152 for Model 4; adjusted $R^2$ = .152 for Model 5; adjusted $R^2$ = .127 for Model 8.
*$p < .05$
**$p < .01$

Statistical results for these models appear in Table 10.1; each model number corresponds to a bolded number in Figure 10.7, summarizing the significant relationships among the four time-series.

As Models 1 and 2 show, the number over time of HIV infections and deaths is a real-world indicator that directly affects editorial decisions about what is important. With cumulative infections in well over 900,000 Americans, the problem has become a constant influence on the media agenda. This continuing, normalized extent of coverage by journalists has cued members of the general public that AIDS is a continuing problem (Model 8).

Once the issue of HIV/AIDS emerged on the media agenda, reciprocal interactions between media coverage and the policy agenda (i.e., federal funding) became and continued to be very active (Models 4 and 5). These findings support the idea that when confronted with incontrovertible, conclusive data about problem severity and prevalence, the media agenda and the policy agenda will mutually affect one another. Stated differently, what began as a one-way causal relationship in which media coverage led to policy decisions and resource allocations evolved into a symbiotic relationship in which high levels of funding and new programs to spend those dollars are reported because they are large amounts and new programs; later media coverage of people affected and high numbers of infected Americans serve as rationale for further high funding levels and new programs.

There is little doubt that circularity better defines the total agenda-setting process than does a linear and directional media–public policy model. Kingdon (1984), Linsky (1986), Rogers and Dearing (1988), Baumgartner and Jones (1993), and Trumbo (1995), among others, argue for circular models of the agenda-setting process that include certain general directional relationships (such as media to public). Even those scholars who present their ideas as stage models, such as Blumer (1971), Downs (1972), and Nelson (1984), include recursive feedback loops. Recursivity means that the policy agenda, for example, has influence on the public agenda and public behavior. But just as directionality in effects appears to be contingent on issue type (Manza & Cook, 2002), so too might recursivity depend on certain issue parameters. In the present study, and based also on our prior research about the issue of HIV/AIDS, we believe that recursivity is time-dependent. In the first decade of the issue of AIDS in our whole-model test, the real-world indicator contributed to the overall ascendancy of the issue. Now, perhaps due to the effects of a perceived satisfactory institutional response, lowered public opinion in terms of issue salience as well as changes in problem severity (at least in the short term) do not much affect continued rates of media coverage and funding allocation.

## Conclusion

We conclude that the contemporary issue of HIV/AIDS in the United States is institutionalized. The issue has not just persisted in media coverage, but become integrated into articles in all sections of a newspaper like the *New York Times,* appearing in arts, entertainment, sports, international news, metro coverage, and so on, as well as in national news stories. This is a reflection that the issue has become a normalized part of the American social ecological context.

Among the general public, the issue has been supplanted by others that are more topical (and ephemeral) such as most international conflicts, corporate scandals, and natural disasters. Perhaps the point is not that people are unconcerned with HIV/AIDS; it is, perhaps, rather that they know that our multiple levels of government and thousands of nongovernmental organizations have responded to AIDS in many ways, in what is now an institutionalized response (Baumgartner & Jones, 1993). Perhaps we as a polity are more or less comfortable that the issue is being effectively addressed, which when tracked produces what may appear as a pattern of declining intrigue or "boredom" consistent with other research about the history of public attention (Henry & Gordon, 2001). Such reasoning suggests an example of representative democracy, in which members of the public believe in the severity of the problem that continues to affect a minority of residents, but also cede real attention to their representatives in resource allocation decisions—elected officials and professional bureaucrats—who respond to and affect media coverage of the institutionalized issue. Presumably, this state of institutionalization embeds many opportunities for priming—cues that elicit prior frames for people to reorient them to the issue at hand as a heuristic—of public salience and meaning when spikes in issue attention occur, driven either by policymakers or by media personnel (Sheafer & Weimann, 2005).

A state of institutionalization is not characterized by declines in media attention that precipitate declines in policy attention, an effect pattern that characterizes the agenda-setting process (Dearing & Rogers, 1996; Yanovitzky, 2002). Rather, institutionalization implies steady states of attention: persistent if not spectacular coverage; continuing and predictable levels of funding. This is the state of affairs for the issue of HIV/AIDS reported here.

The challenge, we submit, for the United States as a country, is to not let responses to HIV/AIDS become sedentary. Funding can remain consistent while target audiences and strategies to reach them change. Innovative and effective solutions to what remains a shifting epidemiology will always be needed at multiple levels in society (Curtis, 2004). New means of reaching and affecting individuals at high risk of infection must be pursued through new partnerships and new technologies (Freimuth & Quinn, 2004). Especially for high-risk unique populations, the traits or cultural characteristics that are common across a family of such groups (such as preservation of face, importance of context in communication, and respect for the elderly among Asian Americans) must be highlighted and used in the political battles ahead and in the staging of news events to convince journalists of the newsworthiness of AIDS as an issue, while at the same time, outreach activities and communication campaigns for Asian Americans need to take into account the specific cultural and linguistic differences that distinguish Burmese, Cambodian, Chinese, Filipino, Japanese, Korean, Samoan, Thai, Tongan, Vietnamese, and others from one another (Yep, 2003).

Groups seeking media attention for AIDS-related issues must find new ways of attracting attention and new ways of portraying their cause or they will not receive coverage (Dearing, 1989; Gillett, 2003). In such ways, our society can reap the benefits of a professional and institutionalized response to HIV/AIDS, while at the same time not risking complacency as new population segments come to define the disease.

## Note

1. This section draws heavily on a previous version of this chapter (Dearing & Rogers, 1992). We wish to acknowledge the late Everett M. Rogers as an important contributor to our thinking about the agenda-setting process as a type of issue diffusion, and its application to the problem of HIV/AIDS in particular.

## References

Baumgartner, F. R., & Jones, B. D. (1993). *Agendas and instability in American politics.* Chicago: University of Chicago Press.

Blumer, H. (1948). Public opinion and public opinion polling. *American Sociological Review, 13*(5), 542–554.

Blumer, H. (1971). Social problems as collective behavior. *Social Problems, 18*(3), 298–306.

Brodie, M., Hamel, E. B., Kates, L. A., Altman, J., & Drew, E. (2004). AIDS at 21: Media coverage of the HIV epidemic 1981-2002. *Columbia Journalism Review, 45*(6), A1–A8.

Cobb, R. W., & Elder, C. D. (1972). *Participation in American politics: The dynamics of agenda-building.* Boston: Allyn & Bacon.

Curtis, D. (2004). Looking for strengths in response to AIDS: Individual, group, and public authority roles in strategy. *Public Administration and Development, 24,* 51–59.

Dearing, J. W. (1989). Setting the polling agenda for the issue of AIDS. *Public Opinion Quarterly, 53*(3), 309–329.

Dearing, J. W. (1992). Foreign blood and domestic politics: The issue of AIDS in Japan. In E. Fee & D.M. Fox (Eds.), *AIDS: The making of a chronic disease* (pp. 326–345). Berkeley: University of California Press.

Dearing, J. W., Larson, R. S., Randall, L. M., & Pope, R. S. (1998). Local reinvention of the CDC HIV prevention community planning initiative. *Journal of Community Health, 23,* 113–126.

Dearing, J. W., & Rogers, E. M. (1992). AIDS and the media agenda. In T. Edgar, M. A. Fitzpatrick, & V. Freimuth (Eds.), *AIDS: A communication perspective* (pp. 173–194). Hillsdale, NJ: Lawrence Erlbaum Associates.

Dearing, J. W., & Rogers, E. M. (1996). *Agenda-setting.* Thousand Oaks, CA: Sage.

Downs, A. (1972). Up and down with ecology: The issue-attention cycle. *Public Interest, 28,* 38–50.

Erikson, R. S., Wright, G. C., & McIver, J. P. (1993). *Statehouse democracy: Public opinion and policy in the American states.* New York: Cambridge University Press.

Freimuth, V. S., & Quinn, S. C. (2004). The contributions of health communication to eliminating health disparities. *American Journal of Public Health, 94*(12), 2053–2055.

Fuller, L. K. (2003). Filmic fictions: Depictions of AIDS in motion pictures. In L. K. Fuller (Ed.), *Media-mediated AIDS* (pp. 117-134). Cresskill, NJ: Hampton Press.

Gamson, W. (1992). *Talking politics.* New York: Cambridge University Press.

Gillett, J. (2003). The challenges of institutionalization for AIDS media activism. *Media, Culture & Society, 25,* 607–624.

Gostin, L. O. (2004). *The AIDS pandemic.* Chapel Hill: University of North Carolina Press.

Henry, G. T., & Gordon, C. S. (2001). Tracking issue attention: Specifying the dynamics of the public agenda. *Public Opinion Quarterly, 65,* 157–177.

Hertog, J. K., Finnegan, J. R., Jr., & Kahn, E. (1994). Media coverage of AIDS, cancer, and sexually transmitted diseases: A test of the public arenas model. *Journalism Quarterly, 71*(2), 291–304.

Hilgartner, S., & Bosk, C.L. (1988). The rise and fall of social problems: A public arenas model. *American Journal of Science, 94*(1), 53–78.

Ingham, R. (2004, September 10). China, India at the tipping point in AIDS crisis. *Agence France-Presse.* Retrieved June 6, 2006, from http://www.globalhealth.org/news/article/5049.

Johnson, J. A., & Coleman, S. (2005). *AIDS funding for federal government programs: FY1981–FY2006* (CRS Report for Congress, No. RL30731). Washington, DC: Congressional Research Service.

Kaiser Family Foundation. (2000). AIDS at 21: Media coverage of the HIV epidemic, 1981–2002. *Columbia Journalism Review* (Suppl.).

Kingdon, J. W. (1984). *Agendas, alternatives, and public policies*. Boston: Little, Brown.

Lang, G. E., & Lang, K. (1981). Watergate: An exploration of the agenda-building process. In G. C. Wilhoit & H. DeBock (Eds.), *Mass communication review yearbook 2* (pp. 447–468). Newbury Park, CA: Sage.

Liebes, T., & Katz, E. (1990). *The export of meaning*. New York: Oxford University Press.

Linsky, M. (1986). *How the press affects federal policy making*. New York: Norton.

Manza, J., & Cook, F. L. (2002). A democratic polity? Three views of policy responsiveness to public opinion in the United States. *American Politics Research, 30*(6), 630–667.

Nelson, B. J. (1984). *Making an issue of child abuse: Political agenda setting for social problems*. Chicago: University of Chicago Press.

Neuman, W. R., Just, M. R., & Crigler, A. N. (1992). *Common knowledge: News and the construction of political meaning*. Chicago: University of Chicago Press.

Pan, Z., & Kosicki, G. M. (2001). Framing as a strategic action in public deliberation. In S. D. Reese, O. H. Gandy, & A. E. Grant (Eds.), *Framing public life* (pp. 35–65). Mahwah, NJ: Lawrence Erlbaum Associates.

Pindyck, R. S., & Rubinfeld, D. L. (1998). *Econometric models and economic forecasts* (4th ed.). Boston: Irwin/McCraw-Hill.

Rogers, E. M., & Dearing, J. W. (1988). Agenda-setting research: Where has it been, where is it going? In J. A. Anderson (Ed.), *Communication yearbook 11* (pp. 555–594). Thousand Oaks, CA: Sage.

Rogers, E. M., Dearing, J. W., & Chang, S. (1991). AIDS in the 1980s: The agenda-setting process for a public issue. *Journalism Monographs, 126*.

Sheafer, T., & Weimann, G. (2005). Agenda building, agenda setting, priming, individual voting intentions, and the aggregate results: an analysis of four Israeli elections. *Journal of Communication, 55*(2), 347–365.

Specter, M. (2005, May 23). Higher risk. *The New Yorker,* pp. 38–45.

Swain, K. A. (2005). Approaching the quarter-century mark: AIDS coverage and research decline as infection spreads. *Critical Studies in Media Communication, 22*(3), 258–262.

Trumbo, C. (1995). Longitudinal modeling of public issues: An application of the agenda-setting process to the issue of global warming. *Journalism and Mass Communication Monographs, 152*.

UNAIDS. (2004). *UNAIDS global report 2004*. New York: Author.

UNAIDS & World Health Organization. (2005, December). *AIDS epidemic update: Special report on HIV prevention*. New York: Author.

Yanovitzky, I. (2002). Effects of news coverage on policy attention and actions: A closer look into the media-policy connection. *Communication Research, 29*(4), 422–451.

Yep, G. A. (2003). "See no evil, hear no evil, speak no evil": Educating Asian Americans about HIV/AIDS through culture-specific health communication campaigns. In L. K. Fuller (Ed.), *Media-mediated AIDS* (pp. 223–236). Cresskill, NJ: Hampton Press.

Zhu, J. (1992). Issue competition and attention distraction in agenda-setting: A zero-sum perspective. *Journalism Quarterly, 69*(4), 825–836.

# 11

# The Rhetoric of Science versus Politics in U.S. HIV Testing and Prevention Policy

*J. Blake Scott*
University of Central Florida

In April 2003, the Centers for Disease Control and Prevention (CDC) announced a new initiative—Advancing HIV Prevention: New Strategies for a Changing Epidemic (AHP)—that shifted the focus of prevention funding to the identification and prevention case management of persons living with HIV. HIV antibody testing is the centerpiece of the new initiative's four key strategies: (a) making HIV testing or screening a routine part of medical care, (b) implementing new models of testing outside of medical settings (through the use of rapid tests), (c) providing prevention services to persons living with HIV, and (d) ensuring the routine HIV screening of all pregnant women (CDC, 2003a, p. 331).

Much of the media response to the new initiative characterized it as a marked shift in the CDC's focus; "Federal Spending on HIV Prevention to Shift Course" read one newspaper headline, and "U.S. Shifts Strategy to Curb HIV's Spread" read another (Ornstein, 2003; Wahlberg, 2004). Some of these reports focused on a new emphasis on and dramatic expansion of HIV testing. Although AHP certainly called for expanded testing, the emphasis on HIV testing in prevention efforts was not a new one; as I document in my book *Risky Rhetoric,* "HIV testing has historically been the *keystone* public health response to HIV-AIDS prevention," overshadowing education, treatment, and other approaches (Scott, 2003, p. 2).

In justifying its initiative, the CDC argued that earlier prevention efforts had been less than effective and that the new strategies were based on sound science and proven public health approaches. Although some welcomed the initiative as a long-overdue move toward science, many HIV organizations and activists interpreted it as the dangerous narrowing of prevention policy driven not by science but by politics. Their response to the CDC's initiative entered into and helped fuel a larger debate about the role of science in the Bush administration's HIV/AIDS policies and approach to policy-making more generally.

Rhetors on both sides of the debate over HIV prevention policy aligned themselves with sound, effective science and the goal of protecting the public health, and both accused competing arguments and approaches as being invalid, inaccurate, ineffective, and, most of all, motivated by political, nonscientific goals. Each side argued that its prevention approaches were good, effective, beneficial, or promising because they were driven by science whereas the approaches of their opponents were bad, ineffective, harmful, or dangerous because they were driven by politics or ideology. In rhetorical terms, we might identify this opposition of science versus politics as a topos or a conceptual vantage point that framed the debate and made certain lines of argument possible and others less possible. Borrowing from Paula Treichler (1999), we might call the trajectory of arguments employing this topos an "epidemic of argumentation," that is, an outbreak of arguments about the roles of science and politics in prevention policy (p. 39). Indeed, both sides' attempts to use science and its discursive traditions to control this "epidemic" only further contributed to it, spawning new, often problematic claims about the science behind their arguments and those of their opponents.

This chapter critically examines the arguments around AHP, focusing on the use of the science versus politics topos. My analytic lens moves in and out of a variety of interconnected texts, from CDC recommendations to media reports to activist letters. In discussing my assessment of the current trend in HIV prevention policy—with its emphasis on testing, prevention management of infected persons, and abstinence-only education—as shortsighted and risky, I explain the limitations of the science versus politics topos and offer an alternative framework for responding to problematic policy.

## The Science Behind Advancing HIV Prevention

The CDC (2003a) began its announcement of the AHP initiative by explaining the exigencies behind it: recent increases in new HIV infections in the United States, especially among men who have sex with men (MSM); the leveling of AIDS cases and deaths since 1998, following a decline; the estimated 40,000 new HIV infections per year since the early 1990s; and the estimated 180,000 to 280,000 infected people who are unaware of their serostatus (approximately 25% of the total number of infected). According to CDC officials, these statistics suggested that existing prevention efforts focusing on those at high risk—including targeted testing and community-based preventive education—had stalled and that new, more "proven" public health approaches—such as routine testing, partner notification, and the prevention management of infected individuals—were needed (CDC, 2003a, p. 331).[1]

In addition to the changing epidemic and stalled prevention efforts, the CDC's announcement of AHP emphasized another exigency: the development and approval of a new rapid HIV test—OraQuick—that could generate results in 20 minutes and that could be administered by nonmedical personnel in nonmedical settings (e.g., testing vans on the street, bars, prisons). The CDC would fund programs by community-based organizations and health departments using OraQuick in order to increase access to testing in high-prevalence community settings and to better ensure that testees receive their results.[2] Thus, the CDC described its initiative as drawing on advances in HIV-testing technology as well as proven prevention approaches to regain control of a changing, indeterminate, and threatening epidemic.

Although the CDC's new initiative came as a surprise to some prevention workers, the emphasis on primary prevention efforts to target people living with HIV was not without precedent. A group of CDC researchers and officials had previously proposed what they called the "Serostatus Approach to Fighting the Epidemic" (known as SAFE) in 2001 (Janssen et al., 2001). Like AHP, SAFE prioritized prevention strategies for infected individuals. SAFE was more comprehensive, however, as it called for increasing high-quality care and treatment, increasing efforts to help infected individuals adhere to treatment, extending prevention services, and offering training for those who provide such services. Notably, the authors of the SAFE article stressed that their approach should be added to rather than replace existing approaches and that it would require a massive increase in funding for both prevention and treatment-related services.

In contrast to SAFE, AHP was not accompanied by a call for dramatic increases in funding for comprehensive prevention and treatment. A CDC official explained that, with basically flat funding year after year, the agency just didn't have the resources for prevention efforts (besides testing, that is) aimed at the full range of at-risk populations (Roth, 2003). From a cost standpoint, HIV testing is certainly cheaper than other prevention efforts, especially those that involve longer-term approaches.[3] Testing also made sense from an ideological standpoint, as one of its sociocultural functions is to reassure the general public by identifying risky persons and reinforcing comforting healthy–risky, us–them boundaries (Scott, 2003, p. 88).

Also unlike SAFE, the CDC's testing initiative focused mainly on the testing and identification of infected persons (both directly and through partner notification), largely overlooking the challenges of ensuring ongoing prevention and connecting these people to treatment and other needed services. Indeed, the CDC proposed passing these crucial efforts on to mostly unprepared and often unwilling physicians and other regular health care providers. To encourage their participation, the CDC (2003a) proposed simplified HIV-testing procedures that do not require prevention counseling; such counseling "should not be a barrier to testing," the announcement stated (p. 331).

To its credit, the CDC (2003a) connected the impact of HIV testing to other prevention efforts in its AHP announcement, stating that "an emphasis on greater access to testing and on providing prevention and care services for persons infected with HIV can reduce new infections" (p. 331). But other CDC-issued statements and arguments regarding the new initiative would collapse this connection and seemingly attribute the power of prevention to testing alone, a move, in part, made possible by the legitimating power of science. Rob Janssen, director of the CDC's Division of HIV/ AIDS Prevention, flatly stated that "[HIV] testing itself and learning that one is positive is an important HIV intervention" (Wahlberg, 2004). CDC Director Gerberding made the unqualified claim that "most people who know they're HIV-positive take appropriate steps to protect their partners" (Sternberg, 2003a), a claim echoed in other CDC publications. For example, the *CDC's New Initiative: Questions and Answers* claims that "many studies have shown that receiving a positive HIV test result reduces risk behavior by 60–80 percent" (CDC, 2003b). Such claims were loosely supported with references to scientific studies, studies that actually present much more nuanced and qualified conclusions. By looking past many factors that can shape prevention, such claims exaggerate the power and benefits of testing and the knowledge that it produces.

But such claims have been common in the rhetoric of HIV testing. In *Risky Rhetoric,* I explain how the line of argument that I call "the knowledge enthymeme" shaped public health responses to testing throughout the epidemic (Scott, 2003). An enthymeme can be defined as a body of persuasion whose force comes from a movement through a chain of premises and surrounding cluster of appeals. In its most basic form, the knowledge enthymeme posits that testing produces knowledge that leads to beneficial effects. Though defined in various ways, the knowledge produced by testing is the main source of agency. The knowledge enthymeme's argumentative chain depends on a web of appeals, including the notion of the epidemic as out of control, the belief that technology can help us manage and control an uncertain and threatening future, and, of course, the commonplace of "knowledge = power." In its manifestations in the rhetoric surrounding the CDC's testing initiative, the knowledge enthymeme can be encapsulated like so: Expanded testing will produce knowledge that will, in the case of those who test positive, lead to individual empowerment, preventive actions, and an overall reduction in transmission. The diagram in Figure 11.1 shows the movement of the enthymeme's chain of premises.

In this enthymeme, the main exigency for testing is the threat of infected individuals unknowingly transmitting HIV to others, and "knowledge" can be defined as knowledge of serostatus and, possibly, of how to prevent transmission. The technologically produced knowledge of one's serostatus, in particular, is given an almost magical quality, empowering the infected person to take self-evident preventive actions.

The assumptions made by the movement of the knowledge enthymeme are questionable. First, the enthymeme assumes that testing will lead to knowledge of serostatus, not a certainty given that approximately 30% of testees do not return for their test results. With

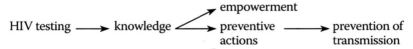

**FIGURE 11.1.**   The knowledge enthymeme's chain of premises.

rapid HIV testing, which can provide results in 20 minutes, the movement from testing to this knowledge is more likely, but even in this case the testee must take a confirmatory test that requires the typical 1- to 2-week waiting period.

Second, some versions of the knowledge enthymeme assume that knowledge of one's serostatus is enough to ensure behavior change, an assumption explicitly articulated in CDC statements. Again, this is not a new idea, as CDC testing and counseling guidelines have consistently named behavior change as a primary goal of testing. But now the assumption is less tied to counseling, as CDC (2003f) recommendations around the new initiative make counseling optional and propose more expedient versions of it. Pretest counseling, in particular, is often replaced with brochures or other stand-alone media. The same goes for rapid HIV testing—many of the protocols for it, too, are built around a brief one- or two-session model that treats counseling as little more than a quick information stop (see CDC, 2002). The provider administering the test might briefly deliver "science-based," one-size-fits-all messages about HIV transmission and how to prevent it (see Attachment 1 of CDC, 2003d), but in many cases this counseling falls far short of the contextualized, client-based counseling that the CDC has recommended for several years.[4] Client-based testing should be culturally and linguistically tailored to the client and must center on the client's in-depth, contextualized consideration of risk and negotiation of risk reduction strategies (CDC, 2001). In addition, some of the testing procedures encouraged by routine and rapid testing only bother to "counsel" those who test positive, leaving high-risk clients who test negative to acquire prevention messages on their own.

Even more detailed protocols that make a gesture to be client centered are too streamlined to be practical. A two-session protocol for rapid testing developed for a CDC study, for example, assigns 2 to 4 minutes to discuss the client's previous risk reduction experiences and obstacles and 4 to 5 minutes to develop concrete risk reduction strategies (CDC, 2002). Such a protocol forecloses an in-depth exploration of risk and prevention. The CDC's (2003d) recommendations for *Prevention in Medical Care Settings* similarly overdepends on general print messages and proposes only two brief moments (3–5 minutes) of counseling around the test. Despite these recommendations, many physicians and health care providers may not be comfortable with, trained in, or compensated for prevention counseling, and therefore may not offer it at all, even in an abbreviated, information-giving version (see Gorner, 2003; "HIV Education," 2003). Organizations offering rapid testing have expressed concern that those administering the tests in the field will be too overwhelmed to provide adequate counseling (Sherry, 2003).

Although critics of the new testing initiative would challenge several of its argumentative moves, few would directly challenge the CDC's claim that infected individuals are more likely to take preventive action upon learning their serostatus. Yet the evidence offered to support this claim is shaky. The studies cited by the CDC involved substantial counseling and, in some cases, enhanced, longer-term prevention case management (see, e.g., Colfax et al., 2002). The studies that showed risk reductions among infected individuals receiving prevention counseling focused on particular groups of people and did not assess the sustainability of these reductions after 1 year. More comprehensive meta-analyses of such studies have yielded mixed findings about the effects of testing and counseling on risk behavior, one stating that the inconclusive "pattern of results varied substantially across, and within, study populations" and that the studies "were often limited by considerable methodological weaknesses" (Wolitski, MacGowan, Higgins, & Jorgensen, 1997, p. 52; see also Higgins et al., 1991).

Other CDC recommendations seemed to better recognize the limitations of testing and to problematize the assertion that knowledge of one's serostatus will lead to sustained behavior change. The recommendation report *Incorporating HIV Prevention into the Medical Care of Persons Living with HIV,* for example, recognizes that risk reduction "behavior changes often are not maintained and that a substantial number of HIV-infected persons continue to engage in behaviors that place others at risk for HIV infection" (CDC, 2003c, p. 1). But in calling for ongoing prevention services to persons living with HIV, this report pins its hopes on brief clinician-delivered "interventions," such as those used with smoking, despite the lack of evidence suggesting that these approaches would be effective with HIV (p. 10). Although this CDC report provides more detailed and comprehensive guidelines for risk assessment, counseling, referral, and partner notification, it, too, seems more concerned with making testing and prevention more efficient and convenient for health care providers than with ensuring that infected persons have access to client-centered counseling and robust, ongoing prevention and other services.[5]

In claiming that knowledge of serostatus accompanied by brief prevention messages will lead to sustained behavior change and better health care, the knowledge enthymeme further assumes that infected individuals are empowered to make the "right" choices and that they have ready access to ongoing medical care (from regular checkups to drug treatment) and prevention services. Like the counseling protocols that they support, such assumptions mostly ignore the complex contexts of people's lives, including the power they have in their relationships, the power they have over any personal struggles (e.g., drug addiction), the conflicting cultural messages they might face, and their access to regular medical care.[6] Instead, ignorance is assumed to be the only major barrier to preventive actions.

The knowledge enthymeme's assumptions, which gloss over the contingencies of testing and prevention, are supported by appeals to the power of science and technology to identify infected individuals, enable them to take preventive actions, and thereby better contain the larger epidemic. Viewed this way, the knowledge enthymeme could be considered a "disciplinary rhetoric," or body of persuasion that works with other cultural forces to shape subjects and manage populations, though not always in the intended ways. Infected individuals are viewed as the sources of risk, whereas testing and the knowledge associated with it are viewed first and foremost as the tools needed to contain this risk. The CDC's (2003b) *Questions and Answers* publication explains that attention to infected persons must come first "because of their great potential to transmit HIV." Here the goal of identifying and containing risky bodies is blatant, whereas the goal of connecting these bodies to treatment is not mentioned. Instead of seeking to be fully responsive to the various needs of those who test positive, the initiative charges them with the primary responsibility to contain HIV.[7]

In the case of the AHP initiative, the knowledge enthymeme has helped fuel testing policy and procedures that seem shortsighted in their approaches to counseling and to linking (infected and uninfected) individuals to client-centered prevention, medical care, and other services. The current trend of testing policy may indeed identify more infected individuals, and, in some cases, this may lead to crucial treatment (especially for pregnant women) and preventive actions. In other cases, however, such policy might leave many individuals with little more than the knowledge of their serostatus.

## Science versus Politics in the Intertext
## of the HIV Prevention Debate

Although the CDC's announcement of AHP contributed to a lively debate about testing's role in the nation's HIV prevention policy, this debate was part of a larger, ongoing one about the direction of and role of science in U.S. HIV/AIDS policy under the Bush administration. Like those responding to the testing initiative, the arguments in the larger debate were framed largely by the science-versus-politics binary.

After taking office in 2001, President Bush began laying the groundwork for a national HIV prevention policy that privileged not only testing but abstinence-based education, appointing proponents of this approach, including former U.S. Representative Tom Colburn, to his Presidential Advisory Council on HIV and AIDS (PACHA).[8] The CDC began channeling a sizable portion of its budget for domestic prevention programs to abstinence-only programs, most run by faith-based organizations. Along with testing, abstinence education increasingly became a cornerstone of government-funded prevention efforts.

Around the same time, the U.S. Department of Health and Human Services (HHS) and CDC joined what some have described as a "war against condoms" and, by extension, the science showing their efficacy. In 2001, HHS pulled the CDC's condom fact sheet from its Web site for more than a year; the new fact sheet that later appeared emphasized abstinence and lacked important information about condom use and efficacy. The CDC was also pressured to remove a description of "Programs that Work" from its Web site (U.S. House, 2003, pp. 6, 11–12). Most of these programs focusing on sexually transmitted diseases (STDs), HIV, and pregnancy prevention among adolescents took comprehensive rather than abstinence-only approaches to sex education.

Information about condoms' efficacy was also removed from the Web site of the U.S. Agency for International Development (USAID), signaling a shift toward abstinence-centered approaches in the nation's global prevention aid (U.S. House, 2003, p. 12), and U.S. officials attempted to restrict references to the efficacy of condoms and comprehensive prevention in United Nations documents. Because of an amendment introduced by conservative members of Congress, the President's Emergency Plan for AIDS Relief devotes a third of its global prevention spending to "abstinence until marriage" programs.

Conservative activists, lawmakers, and others supporting the government's shift toward abstinence-only education argued that science was on their side (Medical Institute for Sexual Health, 2003). Foreshadowing the CDC's argument in its AHP announcement, supporters argued that stalled prevention progress indicated that existing prevention approaches had not been working. In defending himself against charges that the government had replaced science-based prevention strategies with unproven abstinence-based ones, U.S. Global AIDS Coordinator Randall Tobias responded with the causal argument that "the rising infection rates in the world prove that existing approaches relying on condoms have not been effective" (Human Rights Watch, 2004).[9]

Critics disputed all of these arguments, attacking the studies and interpretations cited by their opponents and citing studies showing the efficacy of condoms and comprehensive sex education. As the Human Rights Watch (2004) pointed out, the same National Institutes of Health (NIH) study cited by conservatives backing abstinence education showed an 85% decrease in risk of HIV transmission among consistent condom users versus nonusers (see HHS, 2001). In its document policy report *HIV Prevention Saves Lives,* the HIV Prevention Defense Working Group (2002) cited scientific reviews by the NIH, CDC, and the United Nations that confirmed the efficacy of existing prevention programs, including those involving condoms. Critics also countered that the biggest reason for stalled prevention success in the United States and the world was the gross underfunding of such efforts.

In their attempts to shift funding away from controversial programs, conservative lawmakers pressured HHS and the CDC to scrutinize the legality and efficacy of such programs. In 2001, U.S. Representative Marc Souder began pressuring HHS to audit government-funded safer-sex workshops targeting MSM by San Francisco's STOP AIDS Project, claiming that the workshops were obscene and promoted sexual activity, in violation of the Public Health Service Act. HHS Secretary Tommy Thompson and his inspector general began auditing the STOP AIDS workshops and similar programs by other organizations, and audits continued after Julie Gerberding became head of the CDC. The targeted organizations explained that their programs were based on CDC guidelines for community-level interventions and were approved by local review boards. After completing an audit of STOP AIDS, Gerberding notified the organization and Representative Souder that the CDC and HHS inspector general agreed that the workshops were in line with government policy and "based on current accepted behavioral science theories in the area of health promotion" (cited in Connolly, 2003). But Souder, a House committee chair, wasn't satisfied and demanded to see proof that the programs in question were effective, thereby challenging the science behind them. In issuing such a challenge, Souder invoked what Lawrence Prelli (1989) calls the scientific topos of skepticism, which suggests lines of argument about the "emotional attachment and systematic doubt" of those doing or using science. Souder suggested that STOP AIDS and the CDC were not skeptical enough about the efficacy of funded prevention programs.

In what one journalist called a "blatant victory of politics over public health," Gerberding soon reversed her position, notifying STOP AIDS that its workshops did indeed appear to promote and encourage sexual activity and must be changed or the group would lose federal funding (Block, 2003). Gerberding also stated the local review board process on which the CDC had been relying was insufficient. Despite the agency's stricter stance and even a federal court ruling that found the state of Louisiana had illegally used its federal prevention money to promote religion in abstinence programs, the CDC refused to audit abstinence-only programs (Meckler, 2002). In pointing this out, critics of the CDC's scrutiny also invoked the topos of skepticism, arguing that the CDC and conservative lawmakers pressuring it were only selectively skeptical, which proved they cared less about the efficacy of prevention programs than their political correctness.

STOP AIDS was joined by other organizations in expressing outrage at the CDC's about-face. Terje Anderson, executive director of the National Association of People with AIDS, warned that the decision would have a chilling effect on prevention organizations across the country; the decision's message, she argued, was that a "group of right-wing jihadists with political power will be looking over their shoulders as they attempt to meet the prevention needs of their communities" (Connolly, 2003).[10] Marsha Martin (2003) of AIDS Action protested in a letter to HHS Secretary Thompson that the audits of STOP AIDS and similar organizations suggested "an unacceptable shift away from scientifically based programs that deal realistically with sexual activity." In charging conservative policymakers with politically motivated censorship, including the censorship of science, these critics argued, in part, from the scientific topos of disinterestedness, which enables the rhetor to challenge the legitimacy of science based on the nonscientific motives of those producing or advocating it (see Prelli, 1989, p. 132).

In another case of political pressure and government scrutiny, U.S. Representative Joseph Pitts and 23 other members of Congress pressured the CDC and General Accounting Office to review organizations offering comprehensive sex education programs to youth, including Advocates for Youth, for possibly illegally using federal funds to lobby Congress via their Web sites.[11] Advocates of Youth spokesman Bill Barker accused the CDC of using audits politically to "impose a kind of censorship" (Kaufman, 2003). In this case, both Pitts and Barker argued from the topos of disinterestedness, each accusing the other of being politically motivated.

Prevention-related research was under attack as well. In April 2003, the *New York Times* revealed that scientists were being advised to avoid "controversial" terms such as "sex workers," "men who have sex with men," and "needle exchange" in their NIH grant applications (Goode, 2003). Another New York newspaper pointed out that studies of these topics were politically, not scientifically, controversial because they dealt with what conservatives thought to be unacceptable modes of transmission ("Mixed Signals," 2003). Later, a coalition of conservative church groups called the Traditional Values Coalition, along with conservative U.S. House members, pressured HHS to investigate how certain sex-based research studies won funding through the NIH, which uses a scientific peer review process. The executive director of the conservative coalition called the topics of the research, which included the sex practices of Mexican immigrants, truckers, and African-American teenage girls, "smarmy" and "prurient," adding that "reasonable people" would find them inappropriate for taxpayer funding (Wahlberg, 2003). Although these conservatives questioned the NIH's peer review process and public health importance of "controversial" topics, they primarily protested the studies on explicitly moral grounds. In arguing that taxpayer-funded prevention programs should be assessed by moral as well as scientific criteria, these conservatives illustrated what Sharon Crowley (2006) calls "ideologic" at work. Crowley coins this term to name "connections that can be forged [and disconnected and reconnected] among beliefs within a given ideology and/or across belief systems," in this case among values coming out of the authoritative traditions of science and religion (p. 75).

This and previous efforts at censorship prompted another round of accusations of politics and ideology driving public health policy. U.S. Representative Henry Waxman fired off an angry letter to HHS Secretary Thompson, calling the church coalition group's efforts "scientific McCarthyism," a witch hunt driven by political motives rather than scientific ones. Alan Leshner of the American Association for the Advancement of Science echoed this response, arguing that "we can't have moralizing and ideology trump science when it comes to protecting the public health" (Weiss, 2003).

The government's scrutiny of "controversial" prevention programs and studies mobilized the HIV Prevention Defense Working Group (2002), comprising more than 80 AIDS-related organizations, to respond with the policy paper *HIV Prevention Saves Lives*, circulated on Capitol Hill. Like earlier responses, this document accused the CDC of allowing policymakers "driven by political agendas rather than scientific imperative" to hold the "nation's commitment to prevention ... hostage to politics." The science-versus-politics binary pervades the entire paper, which first presents scientific studies that show the efficacy of existing HIV prevention approaches and then goes on to critique the government's shift toward abstinence-only education and increased scrutiny of sex-based prevention research as motivated by politics rather than based on scientific evidence and analysis.

## Science versus Politics in the Response to AHP

The CDC's announcement of AHP drew a flurry of responses that were fueled by and, in turn, helped shape the larger, ongoing controversy over HIV prevention policy. Although many responses met the initiative with caution, skepticism, or outright disapproval, a few wholeheartedly endorsed the policy shift. For example, Joe McIlhany (2003), president of the Texas-based Medical Institute for Social Health (which received federal prevention funding for abstinence-only education) and Bush appointee to the Advisory Committee to the CDC's Director, published a newspaper commentary titled "AIDS a Disease, Not a Political Issue." McIlhany argued that, throughout the epidemic, "traditional infectious disease control methods" (including routine testing) have been in "direct conflict" with the individual rights of gay men and others, with the latter prevailing. He goes on to hail the CDC's prevention initiative as a "bold and important policy change," and a desperately needed "first step toward treating HIV/AIDS like a public health challenge, not a political issue." Here the science of epidemiology and its "proven" disease control methods are contrasted to the exceptional, ineffectual responses motivated not by science but by politics, not by public health but by individual rights.

Many of the responses from community-based organizations, politicians, and other stakeholders took a strikingly different stance toward the CDC's initiative. These responses accused the CDC of not seeking the input of HIV/AIDS groups in developing the initiative, of usurping local control of prevention programs, of privileging expedient but less effective forms of testing, of taking an overly narrow approach to prevention efforts, of not calling for additional funding for prevention and treatment services, and, above all, of being driven not by science but by politics.

Some organizations, including recipients of federal prevention money, expressed surprise at the new initiative and dismay about not being consulted in its development. They saw the initiative as retreating from the CDC's earlier efforts to form partnerships with communities in prevention planning (indeed, community-planning partnerships have since lost federal funding in many areas). In its response to AHP and federal prevention policy more generally, the AIDS Project Los Angeles (APLA) called on policymakers to "honor local knowledge by protecting local control over how HIV prevention strategies are developed and prioritized" (Ayala, 2003). One head of a South Florida–based prevention program worried aloud that "the CDC has been promoting community involvement and leadership in HIV prevention efforts, and what I see now is that [this] is all gone," adding, "This seems to be political and ideological rather than scientifically based" (Wyman, 2003).

Community-based organizations and other groups complained that the new initiative would take funding away from locally developed, culturally relevant prevention approaches (e.g., social marketing campaigns, peer outreach and counseling, and safer sex education workshops), especially those targeting minority and MSM communities. In their place, the CDC would fund simplified, streamlined, and standardized versions of testing and of prevention counseling and case management. As the head of one community-based organization put it, the initiative would impose "prefab national solutions, overruling local agencies that have their finger on the pulse of their communities' needs and values" (Wyman, 2003). Such critiques argued that local expertise and experience were necessary to ensure the validity and efficacy of science-based prevention programs. In arguing that prevention approaches must be developed locally, these arguments invoked what Prelli (1989) has identified as the scientific topos of observational competence, used to argue that a scientist must have knowledge about and experience in a specific field or context, in this case the sociocultural contexts of specific communities. Thus, this argument about local expertise and empowerment was also framed by the science-versus-politics topos; in moving away from local, community-developed prevention programs, the argument went, the CDC was also moving away from sound science.

Those wary of the new initiative also protested the CDC's either–or argument for choosing one set of prevention approaches over another; the CDC should be adding to existing approaches rather than cutting them, they argued, as HIV prevention requires a full, varied range of approaches that target both infected and at-risk individuals. U.S. Senator Richard Durbin (2003), for example, wrote a letter to HHS Secretary Thompson, arguing that "a more comprehensive approach is essential, one that is mindful of the unique prevention needs of diverse communities across the United States" (see also San Francisco AIDS Foundation, 2003). To some extent, this response also rejected the CDC's exaggeration of testing's benefits, arguing instead that testing should be just one more component of prevention efforts rather than their cornerstone. A few critics further accused the CDC of privileging testing not in the interest of public health but in response to pressure from conservative politicians critical of safer-sex programs (Ornstein, 2003). As one activist leader put it, expanded testing would function "as a backdoor way of defunding" more controversial efforts (Ornstein, 2003).

In arguing for a more comprehensive prevention approach, some critics of the CDC took issue with its causal argument that existing efforts had not been working. (Of course, one irony of this assumption is that testing has played a major role in many of these efforts.) In addition to arguing that prevention efforts have indeed worked, critics of the CDC's initiative offered other explanations, some of which CDC officials also recognized, for the stable overall HIV incidence rate and the increase among MSM: lack of adequate prevention funding, an increase in people getting tested, complacency about HIV, and a spike in drug use.

In its *Questions and Answers* response to concerns about AHP, the CDC (2003b) clarified that the initiative "represents science-based public health principles and practices, not a political agenda" and described the initiative less as a dramatic shift than a refocusing, stating that it would continue to fund prevention efforts aimed at high-risk HIV-negative persons. At the same time, however, the CDC also explained that programs by community-based organizations would need to change their emphases to testing and prevention for positives in order to get future funding and that it would grant fewer but larger awards. The fears of community-based organizations were confirmed in the next funding cycle, when only about one third of the programs receiving CDC grants were awarded new grants (Russell, 2004).

In June 2003, not long after the CDC's AHP announcement, more than 150 AIDS organizations (led by the Whitman-Walker Clinic, Treatment Action Group, Title II Community AIDS National Network, and Gay Men's Health Crisis [GMHC]) sent a letter to President Bush, the 2004 Democratic presidential candidates, and members of Congress. The letter complained about the new initiative's shift of already inadequate resources away from community-based strategies, strategies proven effective by "overwhelming scientific data" (Arnold, Harrington, & Baker, 2003). The letter also put the initiative in the larger context of "a series of events which appear to prioritize political ideology over sound science and public health policies," events that included the shift toward abstinence education, political censorship of prevention programs and research deemed controversial by conservatives, and continued flat funding for U.S. prevention efforts. Beyond decrying what they characterized as a "troubling trend" in politically motivated policymaking, the letter's authors emphasized the stakes of this trend: "the health and safety of all citizens." In response to the CDC, the authors thus make a cause-and-effect argument of their own. The letter ends by calling on the president to "protect science" and public health policy from the "divisive politics of a few politicians." In addition to attacking the motives of conservative politicians, the authors position their comprehensive prevention efforts as benefiting the larger public health.

The week before World AIDS Day, on November 24, 2003, a related group of activists representing ACT UP, Health GAP, and other advocacy organizations marched on the White House to protest Bush's global and domestic AIDS policies. Marchers carried a banner that read "Voters Want AIDS Action, Not Weapons of Mass Deception," alluding to divestment in global and domestic "science-based prevention policies" as a betrayal of President Bush's stated commitment to fighting AIDS. "Rather than a war on AIDS, we're seeing a war on AIDS programs," stated one activist, going on to mention attacks on condom efficacy and programs that serve gay men and people of color (ACT UP, 2003). The group later released and circulated a report titled "HIV/AIDS Federal Policy Year in Review" (2003) that called for the Bush administration to "adequately invest in [U.S.] HIV treatment, care and prevention infrastructure" and to "prioritize sound science and public health ... strategies" over "conservative religious values" in this investment. In addition to recommendations about prevention efforts, the report goes on to make recommendations for the CDC, NIH, Ryan White CARE Act, AIDS Drug Assistance Program, and global AIDS efforts, thus broadening the science-versus-politics critique.

With the presidential election around the corner, the end of 2003 and 2004 would see more critiques of federal AIDS policy by politicians. The news that the CDC planned to revise its guidelines for the content of HIV prevention programs and add another layer of review of this content by state or local health departments prompted U.S. Representatives Waxman, Pelosi, and Hoyer to protest the "politicizing of prevention" in a letter to HHS Secretary Thompson, which spurred a back-and-forth interchange that included conservative politicians as well (see Sternberg, 2003b). Representative Dave Weldon (2003) wrote an editorial for *USA Today* that called existing HIV prevention programs "abject failures" and argued that the claims of Democratic politicians "don't appear to be supported by the facts."

A frequent critic of prevention policy under the Bush administration, Waxman extended his criticism of the administration's "attack" on science in a report published by the House Government Reform Committee and titled *Politics and Science in the Bush Administration* (U.S. House, 2003). Embodying perhaps the most striking use of the science-versus-politics binary, the report documents "numerous instances where the Administration has manipulated the scientific process and distorted or suppressed scientific findings" about a wide range of issues, including abstinence-only education and condom efficacy and also reproductive health, stem cell research, global warming, wetlands policy, oil and gas energy policy, and workplace safety (p. i). In its executive summary, the report states that, "The Administration's political interference with science has led to misleading statements by the President, inaccurate responses to Congress, altered web sites, suppressed agency reports, errone-ous international communications, and the gagging of scientists." In addition to their treatment of science, the report goes on to explain, these actions share another attribute: "The beneficiaries of the scien-tific distortions are important supporters of the President, including social conservatives and powerful industry groups" (p. i). Thus, the report accuses those attacking science of being motivated by eco-nomic gain as well as ideology. The report concludes by contrasting the necessity of "objective input of leading scientists and the impar-tial analysis of scientific analysis" with the suppression, distortion, and obstruction of science "to suit political and ideological goals" (p. 32). In addition to shutting science down, the report argues, the Bush administration perverted it and lied to the public about it—the ultimate acts of dogmatism.

The president has the prerogative to appoint leaders of federal agencies and help shape the agenda of these agencies, the report acknowledges, but "this prerogative should not extend to manipulat-ing scientific research, controlling the advice provided by scientific advisory committees, or distorting scientific information presented to decision makers and the public" (p. 1). Although the report rec-ognizes that politics cannot be totally absent from policymaking, it argues that such policymaking should be shaped by Science with a big "S" and politics with a small "p."[12]

In critiquing lawmakers' political interference with policymak-ing, the report draws on the scientific topos of communality, used to value research that comes out of established scientific networks and used to demarcate true science from sham science (Prelli, 1989, pp. 131–132). The report also aligns its critique about the interference with and suppression of science with similar critiques by the edi-tors of the most important scientific journals (e.g., *Science, Nature,* and *Lancet*), emphasizing that, in contrast, the administration's poli-cymaking moves come from outside of science, from nonscientists with "industry ties."[13]

## The Risky Rhetoric of Science versus Politics

The mostly sharp but occasionally more nuanced distinctions between science and politics in the arguments I've been discussing illustrate how a rhetorical topos can be disabling as well as generative. In framing their arguments with the science-versus-politics topos and grounding these arguments almost solely in scientific values, reasons, and evidence, critics of the shifts in prevention policy relied on what Crowley (2006), via William Connolly, might call a fundamentalism or "imperative to assert" an unquestionable source of authority, even as they accused their opponents of doing the same (p. 12).

The line of arguments framed by the science-versus-politics topos depended on narrow views of the political and ideological as nonscientific and even antiscientific, as hindrances to scientific validity and effectiveness. Instead of referring to power relations more generally, the political is described as the influence of politicians and/or activists seeking to shape policy for partisan, often economic, gain. Rather than a network of interpretation, ideology is described as a limited, usually irrational viewpoint. Both politics and ideology are linked to closed, limiting perspectives and already-set, nonnegotiable agendas; as a result, they contaminate and compromise science's objective search for knowledge and the policymaking process of determining the most effective applications of scientific knowledge and technology.

The idealized notions of prevention science made possible by the science-versus-politics topos are similarly limited and limiting. Science is often presented as an objective source of truth or knowledge, as the most important or even only set of knowledges on which to base prevention policy. In the words of a prominent scientist and critic of Bush administration policy, "As a scientist, the answer has to be *I believe in data*" (Specter, 2006, p. 64). Science and policy are also presented as discrete activities that should be shielded from ideological and political influences, at least as much as possible. To borrow a term from Bruno Latour (1987), the science-versus-politics binary black-boxes science, covering up the messy practices of science-in-the-making to make it appear clean, coherent, and ready-made. But science is not a pure, stable, and separate cultural domain free of politics or ideology, and viewing it as such can overlook the full range of cultural actors and forces that shape it.[14] Neither is science free of ambiguity, contradiction, or disputes; scientists often disagree about how to interpret data and conduct, evaluate, and apply research. For example, scientists at the CDC and their critics both interpreted the stalled prevention progress differently, even though both groups recognized that several factors contributed to the stable numbers of HIV and AIDS cases. Scientists have not reached a consensus about the effects of HIV testing and counseling on prevention behavior, even though the knowledge enthymeme assumes that they have.

Even positions that acknowledge the impossibility of politics-free science, such as the Waxman-sponsored report, still depend on a binary that limits the rhetor's repertoire of appeals and can lead to the additional challenge of arguing what the ratio should be or where the line should be between acceptable political influence and what one renowned scientist and Bush administration critic called "religious zealotry" (Specter, 2006, p. 61). And such distinctions can be wielded in the other direction, too, as illustrated by conservatives who argued that science-based, taxpayer-sponsored prevention research crossed a line when it took up morally repugnant topics.

The debates over HIV prevention also illustrate how the science-versus-politics topos can be used to limit the aims, methods, participants, and applications of science. Thus, another, related problem with the topos is that it can lead to a dangerous privileging of science and scientific discourse that excludes other participants, their "situated knowledges" (to borrow a term from Haraway, 1991), and their forms of knowledge making. Health officials did not see the need to invite community activists into the planning of its new science-based initiative, perhaps assuming that they already had all of the knowledge they needed. Earlier, public health officials, under pressure from politicians, removed and changed important information about condoms, partly in the name of science. As Condit (1996) argues in "How Bad Science Stays that Way," if we enable those speaking in the name of science to dismiss other, contradictory viewpoints, methods, interpretations, and applications as ideological and therefore nonscientific, we risk reinforcing the black box of science and privileging one set of partial knowledges over other, potentially enriching and beneficial knowledges.

The participation of a full range of stakeholders is especially important in debates about applications of science, such as HIV prevention policymaking. The purposes of such efforts extend beyond doing "science for science's sake," and the larger stakes of what is legitimated as scientific are more evident. People will be tested, exposed to certain prevention messages, and, if positive, face a range of needs that may or may not be met. Treichler (1999), Haraway (1991), and others have called for not only a broadening of the scientific but also a counterprivileging of those who have the most at stake, such as the targeted subjects of testing and prevention programs. Haraway reappropriates a scientific term in describing these alternative, usually dismissed, perspectives as examples of "embodied objectivity" (p. 188; see Treichler, 1999, p. 39).

In demarcating science from politics and ideology, the science-versus-politics topos makes a distinction that most science studies scholars and some scientists (e.g., Lewontin, 1991) would reject. Rhetoricians (e.g., Condit, 1996; Doyle, 1997; Lessl, 1988), sociologists and anthropologists (e.g., Latour & Woolgar, 1986; E. Martin, 1994), feminist critics (Fox Keller, 1985; Haraway, 1991; Spanier, 1995), and cultural critics (Terry, 1999; Treichler, 1999; Waldby, 1996) working in science studies have argued, to varying degrees, that scientific practice and knowledge are linguistically, socially, and culturally constructed and that, consequently, science is always contingent, partial, ideological (i.e., shaped by interpretive frameworks), and political (i.e., shaped out of power relations). Some of these scholars have shown, more specifically, how harmful, discriminatory ideologies such as sexism and homophobia can shape scientific practice and knowledge.[15] Some science studies critics, including Treichler and Donna Haraway, seem to reject any notion of a distinctly scientific realm, arguing instead for a notion of science as a fabric comprised of various cultural threads. Others, including Fox Keller and Condit, seem to recognize science as a somewhat distinct cultural domain, though not one free of politics and ideology and not one beyond external critique.

Many of the rhetors in the debate, too, likely view the relationship between science and politics or ideology in more complex, inter-related terms. Conservative lawmakers and activists, for example, clearly saw no conflict in shaping public health policy around their religious beliefs and political goals. HIV activists arguing against government policy have themselves argued that public health policy and research should be guided by moral as well as scientific criteria. Yet many of the rhetors cited earlier—especially those against recent shifts in prevention policy—have overdepended on arguments about the science behind their positions. It is tempting, no doubt, to build arguments around scientific evidence or the misappropriation thereof, as I did in my earlier critique of the knowledge

enthymeme, especially when one's adversaries present such easy targets. Upon close scrutiny, the arguments of those opposing the AHP
initiative and other policy shifts seem to have science on their side.
In addition, these opponents of government policy have, to a large
extent, been backed into a corner of arguing primarily from science,
as those in power have presented policy changes as science based and
pressured dissenters to prove the validity and efficacy of alternatives.
As prevention activists have pointed out, the positive effects of specific prevention efforts are difficult to "prove."

Basing arguments primarily on the science-versus-politics topos
has thus far been largely ineffective for those opposing policy shifts.
To be sure, this ineffectiveness can be explained by the power dynamics of the debate and the inartistic proofs of conservatives in power.
But it might also be explained by opponents' persistent (over)use of
the science-versus-politics topos, a framework that drastically limits
one's conceptual and rhetorical resources, that can be too-easily co-
opted to argue in the other direction, and that ultimately depends
on a distinction that just doesn't matter to some in the debate, even
though they might rhetorically deploy it. The debate over the federally sponsored prevention shift illustrates that arguments framed
by the science-versus-politics topos can be just as easily wielded to
argue for shortsighted or risky policy as against it, even when such
arguments do not stand up to scrutiny.

Given these problems with the science-versus-policy topos, we
would be wise to consider alternative rhetorical frameworks that
make possible other lines of arguments, evaluative and otherwise.
We could view science, as Treichler (1999) proposes, as just another
ideology, and not a wholly separate, complete, or coherent one. This
alternative might enable critics of shifts in HIV prevention policy to
more effectively articulate connections between scientific concerns
and other, more explicitly normative belief systems, as some conservatives have done. By recognizing the ideologic nature of their
own and others' arguments, critics might also be better positioned to
rearticulate and reappropriate these arguments as needed.

If taken too far, however, the position that science is just another ideology can abdicate the ethical evaluation of science and public health
policy, or at least makes such an evaluation more difficult. Furthermore, this position can be used to argue that distinguishing between
good and bad science or basing policy on science in the first place just
isn't that important. Conservative activists and lawmakers argued

against safer-sex programs and sex-based research less on the grounds that they were unscientific than on the grounds that they were morally offensive, sidestepping science in order to dismiss it. Haraway (1991) warns against such relativism as being the other side of totalization, explaining that both can fuel problematic fundamentalist positions, and that "both deny the stakes in location, embodiment, and partial perspective" (p. 191). In the debates over HIV prevention, the stakes are too high to abandon any critique of a policy characterized by a shortsighted and narrow focus on testing and management, limited prevention approaches, and questionable science. Science may be partial and limited, but that does not make its power any less potent, and sometimes this power works to neglect, oppress, or otherwise harm those whom it could serve.

Thus, these alternatives still leave us in a quandary about how to define and value science. Although I don't presume to have a solution, I think we need to recognize it as a quandary with which we, including those recognized as scientists as well as other stakeholders, must continuously grapple, and ideally not in an either–or way. Condit (1996) usefully explains that we can recognize the constructedness of science while also recognizing its "unique forms of contact with material realities" and also assess these forms of contact and the interpretations that they enable or disable (p. 101). Haraway (1991) offers a similar explanation of how to grapple with the disjunction between recognizing science's constructedness and partiality and recognizing its usefulness in interpreting the material world. In "Situated Knowledges," she proposes that we simultaneously juggle "an account of radical historical contingency for all knowledge claims and knowing subjects, a critical practice for recognizing our own 'semiotic technologies' for meaning-making, and a no-nonsense commitment to faithful accounts of a 'real' world" (p. 187). In this formulation, it is not enough to account for the constructedness and contingency of scientific knowledge, in part by tracing its conditions of possibility; we must also be inclusive of and responsive to the situated knowledges and embodied objectivities of the various stakeholders of this knowledge. We can assess these various knowledges, Haraway explains, according to their locatability, their effects, and their reflexivity (p. 191). It is important to note here that Haraway does not address motive, one of the main criteria for evaluating science in the HIV prevention debates. For Haraway, me, and, most likely, the millions of Americans affected by HIV prevention policy, the effects of this policy matter much more than its intent. In addition to recognizing both contingency and partial objectivity, Haraway adds the imperative to be self-reflexive about our rhetorical management of both in our interpretations and arguments.

Haraway's (1991) formulation gets away from the either–or logic of this topos and thereby opens up new questions and lines of arguments about HIV testing and prevention policy. Instead of determining whether prevention policy is based on science or politics, driven by scientific or ideological motives, we can start from the assumption that both sets of arguments are ideologically shaped and ask, "Who benefits and who loses from each ideology and its appropriations?" Instead of simply resigning ourselves to the idea that all scientific constructions are equally relative and useful, we can ask, "What locatable material 'actors' and practices do they reference, and how?" as well as "What are the effects of acting on these constructions in particular ways?" It is possible that even these questions, though more relevant, will not necessarily prompt more ethical policymaking, as policymaking and the science on which it depends are shaped not only by rhetors and their arguments but also by extrarhetorical actors and factors such as institutional arrangements, sociocultural movements (e.g., the shift toward privatization), economic conditions, and political climate. But such questions may move us in a more productive direction, especially if embedded in a wider range of arguments based on a broader, more imaginative network of beliefs, values, and desires (including "nonscientific" ones).

In the case of HIV prevention, the effects of government-sponsored policy shifts are mostly yet unknown, but we can hypothesize, based on good science, that the narrowing and standardization of prevention efforts will make prevention messages less accessible to and effective for more at-risk people, that the defunding of community-developed prevention programs will exacerbate risk within these communities, and that the simplification and expansion of testing will function more as a means of case identification than as an opportunity to provide prevention messages or link people to needed care.[16] In June 2005, the CDC announced its latest estimate of Americans living with HIV—an increase from around 900,000 to 1.18 million. The increase was not shocking, argued the head of the Community HIV/AIDS Mobilization Project, given the "potent mix ... of insufficient funding for science-based HIV prevention and an overdose of ideologically driven policy" (Community HIV/AIDS Mobilization

Project, 2005). Of course, others argued that the increase provided even more justification for the CDC's shifted prevention efforts, as their aim of testing and identification was apparently working. In the meantime, AIDS activists continue the struggle for more funding for comprehensive prevention efforts and for treatment and care, worried that policymakers won't be persuaded by the effects of inadequate HIV/AIDS efforts until they reach even more devastating proportions, if at all.

## Notes

1. In characterizing its proposed approaches this way, the CDC implied that existing approaches were relatively less proven and haphazard, a distinction that alludes to the long-standing accusation of "AIDS exceptionalism"—the claim that, because of the overpoliticization of AIDS, the public health response to the epidemic has been muted and has not treated it like other public health emergencies. This distinction of some prevention approaches as more proven and standardized than others also suggests a distinction between some approaches as more grounded in and verified by science.
2. According to a CDC study, approximately 30% of those who test positive do not return to learn their results, typically available 2 weeks after testing (CDC, 2003a, p. 330).
3. As the CDC (2003f) explained in one of its recommendations, one of the criteria for moving from selective testing to screening, or testing all persons in a defined population, is a test that is inexpensive and cost-effective.
4. In his *Washington Post* article "Testing Time," Matt McMillen (2003) describes his experience undergoing HIV testing with the OraQuick device at the Whitman Walker Clinic. Although this organization thoroughly trains its test counselors and takes counseling seriously, the pretest counseling session described by McMillen did little more than gloss over how HIV can be transmitted, without a discussion of the relative risks of transmission modes.
5. The CDC's relative de-emphasis on connecting those who test positive to prevention and other services is reflected in its primary performance indicators for funded HIV-testing programs: the number and percent of newly diagnosed HIV infections and HIV-positive test results returned to patients.
6. To its credit, the CDC does mention psychosocial factors that affect risk behaviors in its guidelines *Prevention Intervention with*

*Persons Living with HIV* (CDC, 2003e). This publication also discusses a wider range of prevention approaches.

7. The emphasis on the responsibility of HIV-positive individuals is even more blatantly reflected in the nationwide movement to criminalize HIV transmission. More than 20 states have passed laws against intentionally exposing someone to HIV, even through consensual sex (Russell, 2003).

8. None of Bush's appointees to PACHA were scientists specializing in HIV/AIDS, prompting one critic to call it a "freak show of fringe ideology, not science or sound judgment" (Salyer, 2003). Members included Patricia Ware, who had lobbied against including AIDS in the Americans for Disabilities Act, and, before he withdrew, Jerry Thacker, who had called AIDS a "gay plague."

9. In support of abstinence-based global programs, U.S. officials also argued that the promotion of abstinence led to lower rates of HIV in Uganda, prompting a Ugandan health official to respond that this argument was too simplistic and that Uganda's success was achieved through a "broad range of essential intervention" and prevention approaches (Serwadda, 2003). Later, supporters of the CDC's new initiative would argue that, in the United States, the epidemic was threatening to worsen precisely in the communities targeted by existing prevention efforts and funding (Weldon, 2003).

10. STOP AIDS was not awarded a grant in the next CDC funding cycle.

11. Pitts was the Congressman who amended the international AIDS bill to require that one third of the prevention money go to abstinence education.

12. In critiquing more recent conservative efforts to block FDA approval of a vaccine for the human papilloma virus, or HPV, renowned scientist and Nobel laureate David Baltimore similarly acknowledges the roles of politics and belief in science but drew the line at what he called "religious zealotry masked as politics" (Specter, 2006, p. 61).

13. Waxman's report foreshadowed some of the attacks on Bush during the 2004 presidential campaign. An October 2004 *USA Today* article titled "Science, Ideology Clash on AIDS Prevention" explained that the "tension between science and ideology has emerged as one of the central issues ... in the campaign" (Sternberg, 2004). The article cites John Kerry's claim that Bush "puts ideology ahead of science" as well as the Bush campaign's reiteration that previous prevention efforts were not effective. Even after the election, Bush opponents would continue to attack his policymaking through the

science-versus-politics framework, as illustrated by the book *The Republican War on Science* (Mooney, 2005).

14. The scientific advisory committees critiqued in *Politics and Science* (U.S. House, 2003) serve as clear examples.

15. Treichler (1999), for example, explains how homophobia shaped many early biomedical (mis)conceptions of AIDS that were taken as fact and that guided various cultural practices.

16. Determining the longer-term effects of the CDC's new prevention initiative on funding for community-based organizations is difficult. Much of the federal prevention funding shifted from one set of these organizations to another, many in the latter set offering testing and "science-based" rather than comprehensive and culturally contextualized prevention services. Although the federal funding for HIV prevention has remained stable over the last few years, the funding for testing and abstinence-only education has gone up (see, for example, AIDS Action, 2005).

## References

ACT UP. (2003, November). Activists march on White House: Bush lies on AIDS! Retrieved October 3, 2005, from http://www.actupny.org/reports/03WAD.html

AIDS Action. (2005). The federal HIV budget and advocacy (fact sheet). Retrieved January 8, 2006, from http://www.aidsaction.org/

Arnold, W. E., Harrington, M., & Baker, A. C. (2003, June 20). Letter to President George W. Bush. Retrieved December 9, 2004, from http://www.thebody.com/tag/oct03/bush_letter.html

Ayala, G. (2003). Changing how we think: HIV prevention in the U.S. AIDS Project Los Angeles. Retrieved September 1, 2005, from http://www.apla.org/apla/about/press/white_paper.pdf

Block, J. (2003, September 1). Science gets sacked. *The Nation*. Retrieved October 5, 2005, from http://www.thenation.com/doc/20030901/block

Centers for Disease Control and Prevention. (2001). Revised guidelines for HIV counseling, testing, and referral. *Morbidity and Mortality Weekly Report, 50* (RR-19), 1–58.

Centers for Disease Control and Prevention. (2002). *HIV counseling with rapid tests* [Fact sheet]. Retrieved March 1, 2003, from http://www.cdc.gov/hiv/pubs/rt-counseling.htm

Centers for Disease Control and Prevention. (2003a). Advancing HIV prevention: New strategies for a changing epidemic—United States, 2003. *Morbidity and Mortality Weekly Report, 52,* 329–332.

Centers for Disease Control and Prevention. (2003b). *CDC's new HIV initiative: Questions and answers.* Retrieved March 21, 2005, from http://cdc.gov/hiv/partners/question.htm

Centers for Disease Control and Prevention. (2003c). Incorporating HIV prevention into the medical care of persons living with HIV. *Morbidity and Mortality Weekly Report, 52,* 1–16.

Centers for Disease Control and Prevention. (2003d). *Prevention in medical care settings.* Retrieved March 21, 2005, from http://www.cdc.gov/hiv/partners/Interim/caresettings.htm

Centers for Disease Control and Prevention. (2003e). *Prevention interventions with persons living with HIV.* Retrieved March 21, 2005, from http://www.cdc.gov/hiv/partners/Interim/intervention.htm

Centers for Disease Control and Prevention. (2003f). *Routinely recommended HIV testing as part of regular medical care services.* Retrieved March 21, 2005, from http://www.cdec.gov/hiv/partners/Interim/routine.htm

Colfax, G. N., Buchbinder, S. P., Cornelisse, P. G., Vittinghoff, E., Mayer, K., & Celum, C. (2002). Sexual risk behaviors and implications for secondary HIV transmission during and after HIV seroconversion. *AIDS, 16,* 1529–1535.

Community HIV/AIDS Mobilization Project. (2005, June 13). *Number of Americans living with HIV exceeds 1 million, illustrating failure of federal government to implement prevention plan.* Retrieved October 5, 2005, from http://www.thebody.com/press/hiv_prevalence.html

Condit, C. (1996). How bad science stays that way: Brain sex, demarcation, and the status of truth in the rhetoric of science. *Rhetoric Society Quarterly, 26,* 83–109.

Connolly, C. (2003, June 14). U.S. warns AIDS group on funding; CDC cites S. F. programs that "appear to encourage" sex. *The Washington Post,* p. A14.

Crowley, S. (2006). *Toward a civil discourse: Rhetoric and fundamentalism.* Pittsburgh, PA: University of Pittsburgh Press.

Doyle, R. (1997). *On beyond living: Rhetorical transformations of the life sciences.* Stanford, CA: Stanford University Press.

Durbin, R. (2003, June 17). Letter to Tommy Thompson. Retrieved September 15, 2005, from http://www.aidschicago.org/pdf/durbin_letter_2.pdf

Fox Keller, E. (1985). *Reflections on gender and science.* New Haven, CT: Yale University Press.

Goode, E. (2003, April 18). Certain words can trip up AIDS grants, scientists say. *The New York Times,* p. A10.

Gorner, P. (2003, July 29). Ignorance hinders the AIDS fight, researchers say. *Chicago Tribune,* p. 13.

Haraway, D. J. (1991). Situated knowledges: The science question in feminism and the privilege of partial perspective. In D. J. Haraway (Ed.), *Simians, cyborgs, and women: The reinvention of nature* (pp. 183–201). New York: Routledge.

Higgins, D. L., Galavotti, C., O'Reilly, K. R., Schnell, D. J., Moore, M., Rugg, D. L., et al. (1991). Evidence for the effects of HIV antibody counseling and testing on risk behaviors. *Journal of the American Medical Association, 266,* 2430–2431.

HIV education up to doctors; Health groups urge detailed talks with infected patients. (2003, July 27). *Houston Chronicle,* p. A21.

HIV Prevention Defense Working Group. (2002). *HIV prevention saves lives.* Retrieved February 10, 2005, from http://www.gmhc.org/policy/prevention/prevention_defense.pdf

HIV/AIDS Federal Policy Year in Review. (2003). *Nov. 24 March on White House Coalition.* Retrieved September 1, 2005, from http://www.aidsinfonyc.org/yearinreview.pdf

Human Rights Watch. (2004). *The United States' "war on condoms."* Retrieved February 10, 2005, from http://www.hrw.org/backgrounder/hivaids/condoms1204/2.htm

Janssen, R. S., Holtgrave, D. R., Valdiserri, R. O., Shepherd, M., Gayle, H. D., & De Cock, K. M. (2001). The serostatus approach to fighting the HIV epidemic: Prevention strategies for infected individuals. *American Journal of Public Health, 91,* 1019–1024.

Kaufman, M. (2003, August 16). Sex-ed group faces new review. *The Washington Post,* p. A2.

Latour, B. (1987). *Science in action: How to follow scientists and engineers through society.* Cambridge, MA: Harvard University Press.

Latour, B., & Woolgar, S. (1986). *Laboratory life: The construction of scientific facts.* Princeton, NJ: Princeton University Press.

Lessl, T. M. (1988). Heresy, orthodoxy, and the politics of science. *Quarterly Journal of Speech, 74,* 18–34.

Lewontin, R. C. (1991). *Biology as ideology: The doctrine of DNA.* New York: HarperCollins.

Martin, E. (1994). *Flexible bodies: Tracking immunity in American culture from the days of polio to the age of AIDS.* Boston: Beacon Press.

Martin, M. A. (2003, June 16). *Letter to Secretary Tommy Thompson.* Retrieved October 3, 2005, from http://www.aidsaction.org/communications/letters/get_real.htm

McIlhaney, J. S. (2003, June 23). In the spotlight: AIDS a disease, not a political issue. *St. Paul Pioneer Press.*

McMillen, M. (2003, June 24). Testing time. *The Washington Post,* p. F1.

Meckler, L. (2002, Oct. 1). *HIV prevention groups say Bush administration is targeting their work.* Associated Press. Retrieved October 10, 2005, from http://www.aegis.com/news/ads/2002/AD021883.html

Medical Institute for Sexual Health. (2003). *Sex, condoms and STDs: What we know now.* Retrieved from http://64.49.226.96/ProductDetails. asp?ProductCode=1097

Mixed signals; Bush administration works at cross-purposes on AIDS research. (2003, May 4). *Buffalo News,* p. H2.

Mooney, C. (2005). *The Republican war on science.* New York: Basic Books.

Ornstein, C. (2003, April 18). Federal spending on HIV prevention to shift course. *Los Angeles Times,* p. A30.

Prelli, L. J. (1989). *A rhetoric of science: Inventing scientific discourse.* Columbia: University of South Carolina Press.

Roth, B. (2003, August 3). Bush's response to AIDS in U.S. draws skepticism. *Houston Chronicle,* p. A4.

Russell, S. (2003, September 21). Shift in AIDS prevention strategy: Emphasis now on accountability of those infected. *San Francisco Chronicle,* p. A3.

Russell, S. (2004, May 22). Priorities for AIDS funds shift; Federal grants focus on people with HIV. *San Francisco Chronicle,* p. B1.

Salyer, D. (2003). *Why the presidential advisory council on HIV and AIDS should be disbanded.* AIDS Survival Project. Retrieved October 5, 2005, from http://www.thebody.com/asp/mar03/lazarus.html

San Francisco AIDS Foundation. (2003, April 17). *SFAF supports efforts to expand HIV testing but expresses concerns about implementation of new CDC initiative.* Retrieved February 2, 2005, from http://www. sfaf.org/aboutsfaf/newsroom/cdc_testing.html

Scott, J. B. (2003). *Risky rhetoric: AIDS and the cultural practices of HIV testing.* Carbondale: Southern Illinois University Press.

Serwadda, D. (2003, May 16). Beyond abstinence. *The Washington Post,* p. A29.

Sherry, A. (2003, February 10). Rapid test for HIV lifts hope, worries. *Denver Post,* p. B1.

Spanier, B. (1995). *Impartial science: Gender ideology in molecular biology.* Bloomington: Indiana University Press.

Specter, M. (2006, March 13). Political science. *The New Yorker,* pp. 58–69.

Sternberg, S. (2003a, June 26). AIDS initiative targets those unaware they have the disease. *USA Today,* p. 9D.

Sternberg, S. (2003b, September 15). Top Democrats say Bush policy will weaken HIV prevention programs. *USA Today,* p. 7D.

Sternberg, S. (2004, October 28). Science, ideology clash on AIDS prevention. *USA Today,* p. 8D.

Terry, J. (1999). *An American obsession: Science, medicine, and homosexuality in modern society.* Chicago: University of Chicago Press.

Treichler, P. A. (1999). *How to have theory in an epidemic: Cultural chronicles of AIDS*. Durham, NC: Duke University Press.

U.S. Department of Health and Human Services. (2001, July 20). *Scientific review panel confirms condoms are effective against HIV/AIDS, but epidemiological studies are insufficient for other STDs*. Retrieved October 10, 2005, from http://www.hhs.gov/news/press/2001pres/20010720.html

U.S. House of Representatives Committee on Government Reform—Minority Staff. (2003). *Politics and science in the Bush administration*. Retrieved October 5, 2005, from http://www.democrats.reform.house.gov/features/politics_and_science/pdfs/pdf_politics_and_science_rep.pdf

Wahlberg, D. (2003, November 9). Conservatives accuse NIH of wasteful health research. *Atlanta Journal-Constitution*, p. A21.

Wahlberg, D. (2004, May 22). U.S. shifts strategy to curb HIV's spread. *Atlanta Journal-Constitution*, p. 5A.

Waldby, C. (1996). *AIDS and the body politic: Biomedicine and sexual difference*. New York: Routledge.

Weldon, D. (2003, September 23). Prevention programs don't curb AIDS. *USA Today*, p. 22A.

Weiss, R. (2003, October 30). NIH faces criticism on grants; Coalition assails "smarmy" projects. *The Washington Post*, p. A21.

Wolitski, R. J., MacGowan, R. J., Higgins, D. L., & Jorgensen, C. M. (1997). The effects of HIV counseling and testing on risk-related practices and help-seeking behavior. *AIDS Education and Prevention, 9* (Suppl. 3), 52–67.

Wyman, S. (2003, May 25). New policy changes HIV outreach. *South Florida Sun-Sentinel*, p. 1B.

# 12

# Health Literacy and AIDS Treatment and Prevention

*Seth C. Kalichman*
University of Connecticut

Literacy is generally defined as an individual's ability to read, write, compute, and solve problems at levels of proficiency necessary to function in society and achieve one's goals (National Literacy Act, 1991). As many as half of Americans have at least some difficulty reading and one in five adults demonstrate only rudimentary reading and writing skills. One in five high school graduates demonstrate poor literacy skills, with poorer literacy found in the southern United States than in other regions of the country. The U.S. National Literacy Survey showed that as many as 44 million Americans are functionally illiterate, with another 50 million having marginal literacy skills (Kirsh, Jungeblut, Jenkins, & Kolstad, 1993). As many as 90 million people in the United States lack adequate literacy for understanding health information (i.e., health literacy; Institute of Medicine, 2004). Even individuals with adequate literacy for familiar material can experience considerable difficulty understanding unfamiliar material, such as informed consent and health instructions (American Medical Association [AMA], 1999).

According to the Ad Hoc Committee on Health Literacy for the Council of Scientific Affairs of the AMA (1999), medical and health-related literacy poses significant threats to the public health because of poorer understanding of medical conditions and poorer treatment outcomes among persons with low literacy skills. Marginal and inadequate functional health literacy is prevalent among inner-city medical patients, with as many as 35% of English-speaking patients at public hospitals demonstrating inadequate functional health literacy (Williams et al., 1995). It has also been determined that inadequate health literacy is closely associated with poor health and negative treatment outcomes for people with diabetes, asthma, and other chronic illnesses (Dewalt, Berkman, Sheridan, Lohr, & Pignone, 2004). Baker, Parker, Williams, Clark, and Nurss (1997), for example, found that hospital patients who were unable to read commonplace medical instructions were significantly more likely to report poor health and a greater likelihood of having recently been hospitalized compared to persons with better literacy skills. One study of Medicare enrollees in managed care showed that one in five could not comprehend preparation instructions for an upper-gastrointestinal examination and 46% could not comprehend the rights and responsibilities section of a Medicaid application (Gazmararian et al., 1999). This same study showed that people who rated their health as fair or poor were twice as likely to have inadequate health literacy compared to those who viewed their health as good or excellent. In addition, individuals with chronic health conditions who demonstrate poor health literacy have limited knowledge and understanding of their illness. In a study of patients with hypertension and diabetes, for example, Williams, Baker, Parker, and Nurss (1998) found that poor health literacy was associated with less knowledge and less understanding of their chronic illness. Health literacy can particularly interfere with adherence to medical advice and treatment regimens.

In this chapter, I overview the area of health literacy in relation to HIV/AIDS treatment and prevention. After first defining health literacy, I review research concerning the role of health literacy in HIV treatment, focusing particularly on HIV treatment adherence. I then discuss interventions that may improve HIV treatment adherence among people with poor literacy skills. I then briefly discuss evidence that low literacy has important implications for HIV prevention.

Defining Health Literacy

Health literacy is a constellation of skills that include the ability to use printed, written, and verbal information for following medical and health care directions and improving health, such as reading and comprehending prescription bottles, dosage instructions, and appointment reminders (AMA, 1999). Although literacy can overlap with intellectual functioning and cognitive abilities, it should not be confused with these abilities. Also, literacy should not be mistaken with language-specific speaking and comprehension, such that individuals who can read in a language other than English should not be considered illiterate in English-dominant countries. Literacy is also not the same as education level; many individuals who have complete secondary education have poor literacy skills and many people with excellent literacy skills have few years of formal education.

Most research in health literacy operationally defines literacy by using scores on standardized tests. One common instrument for assessing health literacy is the Test of Functional Health Literacy for Adults (TOFHLA) (Parker, Baker, Williams, & Nurss, 1995; Williams et al., 1995). The TOFHLA uses a modified Cloze procedure, where individuals are asked to read a passage taken from actual medical instructions. Words are omitted throughout the passage and participants must select the correct word for each blank from four options, using a multiple-choice format. Three passages are completed within a 12-minute time limit. Researchers have used cut-scores below 75% to 85% correct on the TOFHLA to define lower health literacy.

Another common test for assessing health literacy is the Rapid Estimate of Adult Literacy in Medicine (REALM) (Davis et al., 1991). The REALM is a screening instrument used to determine a medical patient's ability to read and pronounce common medical terminology and lay terms for body parts and illnesses. The REALM was designed to guide the selection of health and medical educational materials and instructions, with the specific aim of identifying patients who read at levels below ninth grade. Scores on the REALM and TOFHLA correlate significantly with each other and both are considered excellent instruments for operationally defining health literacy in adults.

## Literacy Skills, Health Knowledge, and Health Care

The ability to read and comprehend medical instructions plays a particularly important role in health, health care, and treatment adherence, especially among low-income populations. Williams et al. (1995) showed that 42% of patients receiving care at public hospitals were unable to comprehend directions for taking medications on an empty stomach and 59% could not comprehend a standard medical informed consent form. Poor functional health literacy can also impede access to adequate health care. In addition to reading appointment cards and keeping a calendar, literacy skills are important in the interpretation and retention of information. Therefore, individuals with poor literacy skills are inclined to miss scheduled doctor's appointments, not follow examination preparation instructions, and often do not fully participate in treatment decisions. Research shows that patients with poor health literacy are less likely to understand and remember physician instructions for medications (Dewalt et al., 2004). Baker, Parker, and Williams (1996) found that health literacy was a stronger predictor of treatment adherence than was years of education. Persons with low literacy are more likely to take medications at the wrong dosage or frequency and are less likely to understand and monitor the adverse effects of medications.

Baker et al. (1997) described how poor literacy can affect treatment adherence across medical populations. First, low literacy can have direct effects on adherence by interfering with comprehension of dosing instructions. For example, 54% of patients with low literacy have been found unable to answer questions about when they should take a medicine with a label that read "Take this medicine on an empty stomach, 1 hour before or 2 hours after meals" (Gazmararian et al., 1999). An inability to read prescription labels requires patients to retain and recall verbal instructions given by physicians and pharmacists, therefore increasing the chances for memory errors. Second, Gazmararian et al. noted that low literacy precludes the use of written reminders and other verbal-based systems for enhancing adherence. Finally, patients with low literacy may not understand the repercussions of nonadherence, increasing the chance that they may intentionally miss doses of medications to relieve side effects, take a drug holiday, or cleanse their body of medications.

Several studies have now shown that poor health literacy is prevalent among people living with HIV/AIDS. Kalichman, Ramachandran, and Catz (1999) found that 14% of men and women living with HIV/AIDS experienced difficulty responding to a reading passage concerning preparation instructions for an upper-gastrointestinal series, and 36% experienced difficulty reading a Medicaid form. In a disease-tailored passage that presented a description of what to expect when having blood drawn for CD4 cell tests, 34% of participants had problems reading this information despite its likely familiarity to most participants. Similar difficulties were observed in terms of numerical health literacy—representing the ability to calculate and mathematically reason in health-related matters—with 17% of participants scoring between 75% and 89% correct, 50% scoring between 50% and 74% correct, and 9% scoring below 49% correct.

In another study that administered the three standardized passages from the TOFHLA reading comprehension scale, Kalichman, Catz, and Ramachandran (1999) once again found between 11% and 30% of people with HIV/AIDS demonstrated limited ability to read and comprehend medical information. The study found that 21% of the sample scored between 75% and 89% correct and 14% scored below 74% on the total reading comprehension scale of the TOFHLA. These studies documented rates of low health literacy in two samples of people living with HIV/AIDS that parallel those observed in other populations of persons receiving medical care from inner-city clinics (Baker et al., 1996; Parker et al., 1995; Williams et al., 1995). In addition, research has shown that functional health literacy is closely associated with but not synonymous to years of education. For example, 54% of HIV positive persons who score below 80% correct on the TOFHLA have obtained greater than 12 years of education (Kalichman, Benotsch, Suarez, Catz, & Miller, 2000).

There is now a substantial body of research that shows poor health literacy skills are closely related to knowledge and understanding of one's health, adherence to combination antiretroviral therapies, and health status in men and women living with HIV/AIDS (Van Servellen, Brown, Lombardi, & Herrera, 2003). In one study of HIV-positive men and women, it was clear that knowledge and understanding of HIV-related health status is impacted by health literacy skills (Kalichman et al., 2000). Using 79% correct on the TOFHLA Reading Comprehension scale as the cutoff for defining low literacy (Parker et al., 1995), the study identified 18% of people with HIV/AIDS as demonstrating poor health literacy. Individuals with lower literacy were nearly twice as likely not to know their CD4 count or their viral load. Among people who did know their CD4 cell count (the immune system cells that HIV specifically targets and kills), individuals with low literacy were three times more likely to state that they did not fully understand its meaning, and people with low literacy were almost four times as likely not to understand the meaning of their viral load. Knowing one's CD4 cell count and viral load are critical to understanding the progression of HIV disease and tracking one's progress on treatments. People with low literacy were also significantly more optimistic about HIV treatments and more likely to believe that it is safe to have unprotected sex when they have an undetectable viral load. Similarly, Kalichman and Rompa (2000) found that 49% of HIV-positive people with poorer health literacy incorrectly believed that the pulmonary infection Pneumocytis Carinii Pneumonia is a form of cancer, 72% believed that the first HIV medication AZT belongs to the newest class of medications protease inhibitors, and 32% believed that having an undetectable viral load means that HIV is completely eliminated from the body. Similar to studies with other medical populations, health literacy was associated with health-status knowledge among people with HIV/AIDS independent of education level. The relationships observed between health-related knowledge and health literacy can pose significant health risks when literacy interferes with HIV treatment adherence (Miller et al., 2003).

Wolf et al. (2004, 2005) provide further support for the association between HIV/AIDS disease knowledge and literacy skills among people with HIV. The study found that one in five people with HIV/AIDS studied in Chicago, Illinois, and Shreveport, Louisiana, had eighth-grade reading levels or lower. People with poorer literacy skills were less likely to accurately describe the meaning of the CD4 cell count and their viral load. Individuals with poorer reading skills were also less likely to correctly identify their antiretroviral medications, particularly when they were taking multiple medications. Persons with less than sixth-grade reading levels were significantly less likely to understand their CD4 count, viral load, and their medications compared to individuals with seventh- to eighth-grade reading levels who were in turn less likely to know about these aspects of their condition when compared to individuals with ninth-grade and higher reading levels.

Kalichman et al. (2000) reported that low-literacy skills are associated with several aspects of HIV-related quality of care. For example, individuals who have lower literacy scores are nearly three times less likely to report having an undetectable viral load, indicating a more rapidly progressing HIV disease process. Individuals with lower literacy more frequently visit their doctor, are significantly less likely to indicate that their doctors ask their opinions about their treatment, and are significantly less likely to state that they understand their doctor's explanation of their treatment. Individuals with lower literacy skills also report greater barriers to accessing HIV-related care, including being significantly more likely to feel they have been poorly treated by providers and more likely to distrust their doctors. Persons with lower literacy are also more likely to miss clinic appointments because they do not want to be seen receiving HIV-related care and because they have been intoxicated (Kalichman, Catz, & Ramachandran, 1999). Low literacy plays a critical role in the treatment of people living with HIV/AIDS, particularly with respect to treatment adherence.

## Health Literacy and HIV Treatment Adherence

Antiretroviral therapy represents the single most important advance in the treatment of HIV infection. Combination HIV treatments have had dramatic effects on reducing viral burden, improving health and quality of life of people living with HIV/AIDS, and contributing directly to significant declines in HIV-related mortality. When efficacy of treatment is assessed in clinical samples, viral load remains detectable and therapeutic effects are suboptimal in 30% to 70% of HIV infected patients. Although a number of factors contribute to HIV treatment failure, inconsistent adherence to therapeutic regimen is one of the most critical factors implicated in suboptimal response to therapy (Paterson et al., 2000). Adherence of 95% is now recognized as necessary for acceptable population-based viral suppression rates (Low-Beer, Yip, O'Shaughnessy, Hogg, & Montaner, 2000; Paterson et al., 2000). Clinical studies report that 26% to 35% of HIV-positive patients have difficulty maintaining even 80% adherence (e.g., Altice, Mostashari, & Friedland, 2001; Avants, Margolin, Warburton, Hawkins, & Shi, 2001).

There are known adverse health effects of poor treatment adherence in marginally literate people with HIV/AIDS, particularly with regard to measures of viral load, CD4 cell counts, and HIV-related symptoms. Specifically, individuals with poor literacy are less likely to have undetectable viral loads, have poorer immune function as indicated by lower CD4 cell counts, and have more HIV-related symptoms (Kalichman et al., 2000). Associations observed between health literacy and treatment adherence may indeed be a best-case scenario because persons with the poorest health literacy are often the least likely to be prescribed antiretroviral medications (Morse et al., 1991). The close association between AIDS and poverty suggests that the prevalence of illiteracy may even be higher in persons living with HIV/AIDS than that seen in general medical populations. Identifying low literacy as a factor in poor treatment adherence portends compelling opportunities for interventions to improve antiretroviral adherence. Unlike many of the other factors related to treatment nonadherence, such as adverse medication side effects, disease progression, substance abuse, and cognitive decline, low literacy can be directly addressed through patient education and behavioral interventions to improve antiretroviral adherence in people living with HIV/AIDS.

HIV treatment adherence is associated with literacy skills. In one study of 223 men and 93 women living with HIV/AIDS, Kalichman, Ramachandran, and Catz (1999) found that health literacy was significantly related to HIV treatment adherence, over and above other well-established adherence predictors, including social support and emotional distress. In fact, literacy skills predicted treatment adherence even after controlling for years of education. Kalichman et al. found that persons with literacy scores below 85% correct on the TOFHLA were four times more likely to have missed taking their antiretroviral medications in the previous 2 days. Among people with less than 12 years of education, 41% had missed at least one dose of their antiretroviral medications in the past 2 days. For persons with 12 or more years of education, adherence was associated with health literacy; 32% of people with low literacy had missed their HIV medications compared to 14% of people with higher literacy scores. Because literacy scores were associated with ethnic background in this study, the study also conducted subanalyses with African-American participants. The results showed that 40% of persons with lower literacy and less education had missed a dose of their anti-HIV medications in the past 2 days, a rate of nonadherence that was nearly twice that of persons with higher literacy and higher education levels. Individuals with lower literacy skills were significantly more likely to miss taking their antiretrovirals because they had been confused over dosing, because they were experiencing medication side effects, and because they wanted to cleanse their body of medications. The association between health literacy and antiretroviral adherence appears quite robust, with health literacy significantly predicting treatment adherence after controlling for social support, attitudes toward health care providers, HIV symptoms, income level, substance use, and even years of education.

Subsequent research has extended beyond treatment adherence and has demonstrated an association between health literacy and health status in people living with HIV/AIDS. In the most compelling study to date, Kalichman and Rompa (2000) found a significant association between health literacy and viral burden with individuals demonstrating higher health literacy as measured by the TOFHLA having significantly lower viral loads. Using indicators of health status abstracted from medical records, individuals with higher health literacy were more than six times as likely to have an undetectable viral load than were their lower literacy counterparts. Lower health literacy participants also had significantly lower CD4 cells counts and were significantly more likely to have CD4 cell counts below 300 cells/mm³ indicating clinically meaningful differences in health status. Individuals with higher health literacy were also significantly more likely to be currently receiving antiretroviral medications. This study also reported that there were no changes in the results for health-status markers after controlling for currently taking antiretrovirals. People with lower health literacy were significantly more likely to have been hospitalized three or more times for HIV-related conditions compared to people of higher health literacy. Lower health literacy was also related to individuals perceiving their health as poorer.

It is important to note that studies of health literacy in relation to HIV/AIDS treatment adherence have relied on cross-sectional study designs, so it is possible that the observed associations may be accounted for by other unmeasured confounding factors. Bolstering confidence in the findings from the cross-sectional research, however, is a prospective study reported by Golin, Liu, and Hays (2002). This study examined HIV treatment adherence over a 48-week period with assessments taken every 4 weeks. On average, study participants took 71% of prescribed doses and more than 95% of patients were less than 95% adherent. Several factors were independently associated with poorer adherence, including being African American, lower income and education, alcohol use, higher dose frequency, and using fewer adherence strategies such as pillboxes and timers. The study found that low literacy predicted nonadherence to antiretroviral therapies during the first 8 weeks of treatment but not thereafter. The study results therefore suggest that low literacy may be most problematic early in treatment with adjustments and individual strategies overriding the effects of low literacy at later time points.

## Interventions to Improve Adherence for People with Limited Literacy Skills

Complex treatment regimens require individuals to understand the importance of closely adhering to prescribed medications and the ability to follow dosing schedules. Interventions to increase and maintain combination antiretroviral adherence have relied on efforts to educate patients about the hazards of nonadherence, teach patients self-reminder skills, and instruct them in the use of timers, alarms, and other environmental cues to prompt doses (Rabkin & Chesney, 1999). Many techniques used to increase treatment adherence directly rely on reading comprehension skills, such as daily calendars, outlines of meal schedules, reminder notes, condensed schedules, and charts. Although devices used to prompt persons to take their medications do not necessarily rely directly on reading comprehension skills, individuals with low literacy skills frequently misinterpret medical instructions and experience difficulty translating medical instructions into actions, even when abstracting from simple concepts (Bernhardt & Cameron, 2003; Doak, Doak, & Root, 1996). In addition, memory cues only remind people when it is time to take medications without information about which medications to take, their dosing as well as dietary instructions. Low literacy can therefore interfere with the acquisition of information required to understand the importance of treatment adherence and the adoption of adherence strategies.

Previous research has shown that persons with low literacy are no more likely to be nonadherent due to memory lapses than are their higher literacy counterparts (Kalichman et al., 1999b). Rather, individuals with lower literacy are significantly more likely to miss taking a dose of their antiretrovirals because they become confused about dosing and because they believe that they should periodically cleanse their body of medications (Kalichman et al., 2000). These findings demonstrate that inadequate understanding of HIV treatments is associated with nonadherence, particularly among low-literacy people. Effective interventions for improving medication adherence in people with low literacy therefore require adaptation to match the individuals' reading comprehension and computational skills and abilities. For example, pictographs can assist in communicating concrete concepts that are required to increase adherence. In addition, adherence instructions can be translated to words and phrasing of characteristics optimal for comprehension by people with low literacy skills (Dowse & Ehlers, 2001). Color-coding medication schedules and dosage instructions can also simplify adherence to complex treatment regimens. Strategies to simplify instructions using minimal text, nonverbal descriptors, and behavioral cues have been effective in promoting health behaviors in low-literacy patients (e.g., Mayeux, Murphy, & Arnold, 1996). Jacobson et al. (1999), for example, demonstrated the efficacy of a one-page educational handout with pictographs and minimal text that did not exceed fifth-grade level to increase pneumococcal vaccination. Jolly, Scott, and Sanford (1995) also showed that simplifying emergency room discharge instructions significantly improved patient understanding and ability to carry out recommendations.

Failure to closely adhere to antiretroviral therapies seriously jeopardizes the potential benefits of HIV treatment advances. Because HIV builds rapid resistance and cross-resistance to antiretrovirals, providers may be reluctant to prescribe combination therapies to patients they believe will not be able to adhere, such as those patients who cannot demonstrate their understanding of dosage schedules. Drug resistance places serious limits on treatment efficacy and treatment options and nonadherence may pose risks to public health through the transmission of drug-resistant strains of HIV. Therefore, demonstrated prevalence of poor literacy in persons with HIV/AIDS suggests that limited reading comprehension and computational skills are a serious threat to personal and public health. To my knowledge, there has been only one attempt to design and examine an HIV treatment adherence intervention specifically for people with poor health literacy skills.

## HIV Treatment Adherence Counseling Intervention for People with Poor Health Literacy Skills

Following an extensive formative study period that included interviews, focus groups, and consultation from experts, Kalichman, Cherry, and Cain (2005) designed a treatment adherence intervention tailored for people with lower health literacy skills. The content of the intervention relied on pictographic information particularly relevant to an individual's medication regimen as well as his or her knowledge base, motivation to adhere to medications, and adherence skills. The intervention was designed to be similar to what may be delivered in clinical care settings, acknowledging the necessity of increasing intensity and duration to accommodate the needs of low-literacy people. The two–adherence improvement intervention session was followed by a single booster session, resulting in three sessions total, all delivered in individual counseling sessions by an HIV/AIDS specialist nurse. The intervention concentrated on delivering the most relevant information for treatment adherence including the importance of following prescribed instructions for each drug the person was taking. The sessions included motivational enhancement techniques, such as providing direct feedback on patient health status, and training in skills for self-monitoring changes in CD4 cell counts and viral load in relation to treatment adherence. For adherence skills building, the intervention tailored medication instructions to lower levels of reading literacy, including the use of memory cues and strategies for fitting medications into daily routines. Similar methods of simplifying treatment instructions have successfully improved patient comprehension of medical instructions (Jolly, Scott, Feied, & Sanford, 1993).

A primary aim of the intervention materials was to integrate intensive provider interactions with pictographic instructions (Houts et al., 1998). The intervention materials were developed with pictographs and minimal words, modeled after similar interventions that have been effective in other areas of health promotion (e.g., Houts et al., 1998; Jacobson et al., 1999). The intervention sessions were guided by a tabletop flipchart that moved the nurse and the patient through each intervention component together. In addition, a pocket-size pamphlet was developed with sticker-pictures of pills in actual sizes and colors representing an individual's medication regimen, as well as including the dosing times and administration instructions. A set of stickers was also used to place images on the pamphlet that were keyed to an individual's daily events, activities, and routines (home, car, work, food, TV, toothbrush, etc.). The nurse and the patient therefore created an individualized adherence plan within the context of two counseling sessions.

The adherence improvement intervention also relied on guidelines for developing medical education interventions for low-literacy patients. Doak et al. (1996) identified five principles for developing health education materials for individuals with poor literacy skills. Effective interventions and materials for low-literacy populations should set realistic objectives, focus on specific behaviors and relevant skill, create a context for new information before the new information is presented, partition complex instructions into smaller units, and use interactive techniques for instructing in new skills. The intervention embraced each of these important principles.

Consistent with behavioral theories and specific to instructing people with lower literacy, the intervention set realistic objectives targeted for persons taking antiretroviral therapies, such as taking medications at every dose and as instructed. To achieve this objective, skills were emphasized to establish medications as part of daily routines, adapt medication schedules to individual life circumstances, and receive feedback on CD4 counts and viral loads. Adherence instructions were presented in the context of the potential for successful treatment and all instructions were partitioned into meaningful units that avoided extraneous information. Finally, adherence instructions were presented in an interactive format and included skills-building exercises.

The counseling intervention was delivered in two sessions conducted 1 week apart with the third booster session convened 2 weeks after the second session for problem solving and to address maintenance issues. Each of the first two sessions was 90 minutes and the third booster session was 60 minutes; these sessions used elements of motivational interviewing to formulate the counseling experience (Miller & Heather, 1998; Miller, Zweben, DiClemente, & Rychtarik, 1992). The intervention was named "Stick to It!"—which became a theme in the counseling sessions as well as patient education materials. Following is a brief description of the intervention sessions.

### Session 1: Understanding HIV and HIV Medications

This first session focused on providing the patient with information about HIV disease processes, particularly with reference to changes in CD4 cell counts, viral loads, and opportunistic illness vulnerabilities. Through an interactive discussion guided by a tabletop flipchart, the nurse illustrated how HIV impacts the immune system and how antiretroviral medications slow the progression of HIV disease. Considerable emphasis was placed on interpreting the meaning of changes in CD4 counts and viral loads and how these changes are related to health and can be affected by medications. Thus, Session 1 was focused on providing accurate information about HIV disease and treatments, using an interactive and open exchange guided by pictographic and minimal verbal patient education materials.

## Session 2: HIV Medications and Your Health

The second session delivered the motivational and behavioral skills components of the intervention. Here, the patient was given his or her Personalized Feedback Report included in the patient pamphlet. Using motivational interviewing techniques (Miller et al., 1992), the nurse delivered feedback on the pattern of changes in CD4 counts and viral loads accessed via the patient's medical records and graphed on the pamphlet charts. The patient and nurse then discussed the patient's antiretroviral medications, one by one, identifying the medications by using sticker images and creating a profile of times and dosing on the pamphlet. The nurse engaged the patient in a discussion of his or her daily routines, integrating medications into their routines, and the barriers a patient may experience in taking his or her medications. The nurse and patient developed strategies for problem solving each barrier that the patient self-identified. Issues of side effects, drug allergies, and dosing instructions were included in discussing each medication.

Patients also discussed the last time they missed a dose of their medications and reenacted the situation with the nurse, role-playing the situation and generating strategies for how medications could have been taken on time in that situation, such as by using reminders, pillboxes, watch alarms, or enlisting a friend as a buddy to remind them to take their medications. Particular emphasis was placed on identifying people who can provide support and assistance in taking medications on schedule. At least two situations that challenged participants in taking their antiretroviral medications were role-played with the nurse offering constructive and corrective feedback. Participants worked through a series of practice exercises with the nurse where they used pillboxes and other strategies for improving organization and management of their medications. The medication management skills–building tasks were modeled after activities described by Albert et al. (1999). The session culminated with the nurse and the patient generating a personalized action plan for adhering to medications in difficult situations.

*Booster Session: Stick to It!: Maintenance*
*of Adherence Behaviors*

The third and final session was a booster session that focused on problem solving challenging situations that occurred since the previous session (2 weeks earlier). Situations in which medications may have been missed or not taken on schedule were re-created and role-played for problem solving with the aim of improving future adherence.

Outcomes of the Stick to It! Pilot Study.    The Stick to It! counseling intervention was examined for potential efficacy in a test of concept pilot study. The study enrolled 17 HIV positive men, 10 women, and 3 transgender persons who scored below 80% correct on the TOFHLA. All participants were currently taking a combination of at least two antiretroviral medications. Participants were counseled in the three-session Stick to It! intervention and were followed for 3 months after counseling (see Kalichman et al., 2005, for a complete report of the intervention outcomes). Results showed that knowledge of HIV disease processes as well as understanding of HIV-related health status improved significantly over the follow-up period. At baseline, 15% of participants understood the meaning of their viral load and 15% understood the meaning of their CD4 count compared to 46% of participants for understanding their viral load and CD4 counts at the follow-up. Scores on a standard HIV/AIDS disease-related knowledge test also improved from a mean of 57% correct at baseline to 80% correct 3 months later. Results also demonstrated significant increases in self-efficacy beliefs for being able to adhere to HIV medications. Most compelling were the results concerning medication adherence over time. These results are depicted in Figure 12.1. On average, participants missed 1.8 doses of antiretroviral medications in the 3 days before baseline compared to 0.5 doses at the 3-month follow-up. When divergence from scheduled dosing was included in the definition of nonadherence, participants went from a mean of 2.3 nonadherent doses to 0.6 three months later. The Stick to It! adherence-counseling intervention therefore demonstrated promising effects in the pilot study, suggesting that relatively brief and focused behavioral interventions can help improve HIV treatment adherence among persons with low literacy skills.

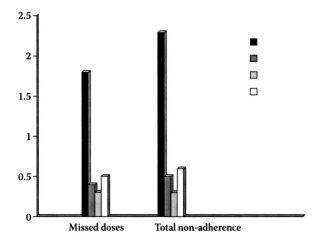

**FIGURE 12.1.** Adherence behavior outcomes for the Stick to It! pilot intervention trial. Note that missed dose = 3-day self-report total nonadherence defined as missing a dose or being off schedule by ± 2 hours.

*Lessons Learned.* The Stick to It! intervention was highly acceptable to our participants. We found patients eager to learn about their HIV medications and the proper use of these treatments. Our participants were also very motivated to better understand their health status and how it is affected by HIV treatments. Most patients did not understand the demands for high adherence to HIV medications because the connection between adherence, viral load, and viral resistance was not clear. Although the pictorial patient education materials we developed did assist in the delivery of this information, having adequate time with the nurse to ask and answer questions seemed most critical in improving patient understanding. In addition, the Stick to It! patient brochure, which provided a personalized adherence plan and grids for self-monitoring CD4 counts and viral load, also seemed key to assisting participants in improving their adherence.

There were also important limitations to the intervention that became apparent. Regardless of our efforts, it was not possible to develop patient education materials that were completely pictographic. The patient education flipchart and brochure included words, albeit as few as possible. The intervention required a considerable amount of time with a skilled nurse. Most HIV clinics are busy and it is likely infeasible with existing resources to deliver a three-session intervention to each patient, probably not even to each low-literacy patient. However, it is unlikely that the amount of time with the provider can be compromised with positive outcomes. It is also very unlikely that time with a provider can be replaced with a more cost-effective automated option, such as interactive computer programs or videotapes. Interventions for improving medication adherence in low-literacy populations will require an investment of time and resources if positive effects are expected.

## Health Literacy and HIV Prevention

There have been far fewer studies of health literacy as it may be related to HIV prevention compared to research on health literacy and HIV treatment adherence. However, the rationale for expecting such associations is the same: Individuals with poorer health literacy skills will likely experience less understanding of HIV prevention messages and will be more inclined to misunderstand risks and risk reduction. Although data are quite limited, there is support for this hypothesis. Fortenberry et al. (2001) for example, showed that 32% of individuals receiving treatment at sexually transmitted infections (STIs) clinics have reading levels below the ninth grade. The study showed that lower literacy patients perceive themselves to be at higher risk for STIs and yet are less likely to be screened for infection and are less likely to seek STI care.

Although people with lower literacy skills may be less likely to seek STI diagnostic and care services, they seem more likely to comply with providers in care settings. Barragan et al. (2005) found that clinic patients with poorer literacy skills are significantly more likely to comply with clinic procedures for HIV testing. In this case, the clinic used an opt-out procedure for HIV testing, where individuals have to actively opt out or they will be tested for HIV. Patients with poorer reading ability were more likely to comply with the testing request. Important to note, literacy was associated with complying with testing but education was not, once again illustrating the distinction between literacy skills and education.

In terms of HIV risks among people living with HIV infection, Kalichman et al. (2000) found that HIV-positive people with poor health literacy skills were more likely to endorse beliefs that HIV treatments reduce the risks for HIV transmission. For example, individuals with lower health literacy skills were six times more likely to believe that new HIV treatments make it easy to relax about unsafe sex and were six times more likely to agree that it is safe to have sex without a condom if their viral load was undetectable. These attitudes and beliefs have been associated with high-risk sexual practices across several studies (Crepaz, Hart, & Marks, 2004).

## Conclusions

The association between poor health literacy and HIV treatment adherence seems robust and reliable. Health literacy is related to knowledge and understanding of HIV disease and HIV treatment. Literacy skills are also related to HIV treatment adherence, perhaps most strongly in the initial weeks of starting therapy. Literacy is also related to detectable levels of virus in blood plasma, CD4 cell counts, hospitalizations for HIV, and subjective sense of well-being. Although there is less evidence supporting the association between literacy skills and HIV prevention activities, it appears that such associations do exist. Literacy skills must therefore be taken into account when designing HIV treatment and prevention programs.

Ultimately, the problems posed by poor literacy skills for health-related behaviors will best be overcome by improving the reading skills of medical patients. Literacy programs may very well be among the more important approaches to medical patient education. Brief and efficient patient educational counseling can also be effective in improving adherence to treatments among persons with low literacy skills. The need for HIV treatment and prevention interventions that are tailored for lower literacy populations is apparent in the United States, where growing numbers of people with HIV are of educationally disadvantaged backgrounds. The need is therefore even greater in developing countries where low literacy is far more wide-scale and HIV is far more prevalent. Research is needed to design and test adherence and prevention interventions for lower literacy adults across developed and developing countries.

## Acknowledgments

National Institute of Mental Health (NIMH) Grant R01MH071164 supported preparation of this chapter.

# References

Albert, S. M., Weber, C., Todak, G., Polanco, C., Clouse, R., McElhiney, M., et al. (1999). An observed performance test of medication management ability in HIV: Relation to neuropsychological status and medication adherence outcomes. *AIDS & Behavior, 3,* 121–128.

Altice, F. L., Mostashari, F., & Friedland, G. H. (2001). Trust and the acceptance of and adherence to antiretroviral therapy. *Journal of Acquired Immune Deficiency Syndromes, 28,* 47–58.

American Medical Association. (1999). Health literacy: Report of the council on scientific affairs. *Journal of the American Medical Association, 281,* 552–557.

Avants, S. K., Margolin, A., Warburton, L. A., Hawkins, K. A., & Shi, J. (2001). Predictors of nonadherence to HIV-related medication regimens during methadone stabilization. *The American Journal of Addictions, 10*(1), 69–78.

Baker, D. W., Parker, R., & Williams, M. (1996). The health care experience of patients with low-literacy. *Archives of Family Medicine, 5,* 329–334.

Baker, D. W., Parker, R. M., Williams, M. V., Clark, W. S., & Nurss, J. (1997). The relationship of patient reading ability to self-reported health and use of health services. *American Journal of Public Health, 87,* 1027–1030.

Barragan, M., Hicks, G., Williams, M., Franco-Paredes, C., Duffus, W., & del Rio, C. (2005). Low health literacy is associated with HIV test acceptance. *Journal of General Internal Medicine, 20,* 422–425.

Bernhardt, J., & Cameron, K. (2003). Accessing, understanding, and applying health communication messages: The challenge of health literacy. In T. Thompson, A. Dorsey, K. Miller, & R. Parrott (Eds.), *Handbook of health communication* (pp. 583–605). Mahwah, NJ: Lawrence Erlbaum Associates.

Crepaz, N., Hart, T., & Marks, M. (2004). Highly active antiretroviral therapy and sexual risk behavior: A meta-analytic review. *Journal of American Medical Association, 292,* 224–236.

Davis, T. C., Crouch, M. A., Long, S. W., Jackson, R. H., Bates, P., George, R. B., et al. (1991). Rapid assessment of literacy levels of adult primary care patients. *Family Medicine, 23,* 433–435

Dewalt, D. A., Berkman, N., Sheridan, S., Lohr, K., & Pignone, M. (2004). Literacy and health outcomes: A systematic review of the literature. *Journal of General Internal Medicine, 14,* 315–317.

Doak, C. C., Doak, L. G., & Root, J. (1996). *Teaching patients with low-literacy skills.* Philadelphia: Lippincott.

Dowse, R., & Ehlers, M. (2001). The evaluation of pharmaceutical pictograms in a low-literate South African population. *Patient Education and Counseling, 45,* 87–99.

Fortenberry, D., McFarlane, M., Hennessy, M., Bull, S. S., Grimley, D. M., St. Lawrence, J., et al. (2001). Relation of health literacy to gonorrhea related care. *Sexually Transmitted Infections, 77,* 206–211.

Gazmararian, J., Baker, D. W., Williams, M., Parker, R., Scott, T., Green, D., et al. (1999). Health literacy among Medicare enrollees in a managed care organization. *Journal of the American Medical Association, 281,* 545–551.

Golin, C., Liu, H., & Hays, R. D. (2002). A prospective study of predictors of adherence to combination antiretroviral medication. *Journal of General Internal Medicine, 17,* 756–765.

Houts, P. S., Bachrach, R., Witmer, J. T., Tringali, C. A., Bucher, J. A., & Localio, R. A. (1998). Using pictographs to enhance recall of spoken medical instructions. *Patient Education and Counseling, 35,* 83–88.

Institute of Medicine. (2004). *Health literacy: A prescription to end confusion.* Washington, DC: National Academy Press.

Jacobson, T. A., Thomas, D. M., Morton, F. J., Offutt, G., Shevlin, J., & Ray, S. (1999). Use of a low-literacy patient education tool to enhance pneumococcal vaccination rates. *Journal of the American Medical Association, 282,* 646–650.

Jolly, B. T., Scott, J. L., Feied, C. F., & Sanford, S. M. (1993). Functional illiteracy among emergency department patients: A preliminary study. *Annals of Emergency Medicine, 22,* 573–578.

Jolly, B. T., Scott, J. D., & Sanford, S. M. (1995). Simplification of emergency department discharge instructions improves patient comprehension. *Annals of Emergency Medicine, 26,* 443–446.

Kalichman, S. C., Benotsch, E., Suarez, T., Catz, S., & Miller, J. (2000). Health literacy and health-related knowledge among men and women living with HIV-AIDS. *American Journal of Preventive Medicine, 18,* 325–331.

Kalichman, S. C., Catz, S., & Ramachandran, B. (1999). Barriers to HIV-AIDS treatment and treatment adherence among African-American adults with disadvantaged education. *Journal of the National Medical Association, 91,* 439–446.

Kalichman, S. C., Cherry, J., & Cain, D. (2005). Nurse-delivered antiretroviral adherence counseling intervention for people living with HIV-AIDS who have poor reading literacy skills. *Journal of the Association of Nurses in AIDS Care, 16,* 3–15.

Kalichman, S. C., Ramachandran, B., & Catz, S. (1999b). Adherence to combination antiretroviral therapies in HIV seropositive men and women of health low literacy. *Journal of General Internal Medicine, 14,* 267–273.

Kalichman, S. C., & Rompa, D. (2000). Functional health literacy is associated with health status and health-related knowledge in persons living with HIV-AIDS. *Journal of Acquired Immune Deficiency Syndromes, 25,* 337–344.

Kirsh, I., Jungeblut, A., Jenkins, L., & Kolstad, A. (1993). *Adult literacy in America: A first look at the results of the National Adult Literacy Survey.* Washington, DC: National Center for Education Statistics, U.S. Department of Education.

Low-Beer, S., Yip, B., O'Shaughnessy, M., Hogg, R., & Montaner, J. (2000). Adherence to triple therapy and viral load response. *Journal of Acquired Immune Deficiency Syndrome, 23*(4), 360–361.

Mayeux, E. J., Murphy, P. W., & Arnold, C. (1996). Improving patient education for patients with low literacy. *American Family Physician, 53,* 205–211.

Miller, L., Liu, H., Hays, R., Golin, C., Ye, Z., & Beck, C. (2003). Knowledge of antiretroviral regimen dosing and adherence: A longitudinal study. *Clinical Infectious Disease, 36,* 514–518.

Miller, W., & Heather, N. (1998). *Treating addictive behaviors* (2nd ed). New York: Plenum.

Miller, W. R., Zweben, A., DiClemente, C., & Rychtarik, R. (1992). *Motivational enhancement therapy manual* (DHHS Publication No. ADM 92-1894). Washington, DC: U.S. Government Printing Office.

Morse, E. V., Simon, P. M., Coburn, M., Hyslop, N., Greenspan, D., & Balson, P. M. (1991). Determinants of subject compliance within an experimental anti-HIV drug protocol. *Social Science and Medicine, 32,* 1161–1167.

National Literacy Act. (1991). 20 USC 1201.

Parker, R. M., Baker, D. W., Williams, M. V., & Nurss, J. R. (1995). The test of functional health literacy in adults: A new instrument for measuring patients' literacy skills. *Journal of General Internal Medicine, 10,* 537–541.

Paterson, D. L., Swindells, S., Mohr, J., Brester, M., Vergis, E. N., & Squier, C. (2000). Adherence to protease inhibitor therapy and outcomes in patients with HIV infection. *Annals of Internal Medicine, 133*(1), 21–30.

Rabkin, J. G., & Chesney, M. (1999). Treatment adherence to HIV medications: The Achilles heel of the new therapeutics. In D. Ostrow & S. Kalichman (Eds.) *Behavioral and mental health impacts of new HIV therapies* (pp. 61–79). New York: Plenum.

van Servellen, G., Brown, J., Lombardi, E., & Herrera, G. (2003). Health literacy in low-income Latino men and women receiving antiretroviral therapy in community-based treatment centers. *AIDS Patient Care and STDs, 17,* 283–298.

Williams, M. V., Baker, D. W., Parker, R. M., & Nurss, J. R. (1998). Relationship of functional health literacy to patients' knowledge of their chronic disease: A study of patients with hypertension and diabetes. *Archives of Internal Medicine, 158,* 166–172.

Williams, M. V., Parker, R. M., Baker, D. W., Parikh, N. S., Pitkin, K., Coates, W. C., et al. (1995). Inadequate functional health literacy among patients at two public hospitals. *Journal of the American Medical Association, 274,* 1677–1682.

Wolf, M., Davis, T., Arozullah, A., Penn, R., Arnold, C., Sugar, M., et al. (2005). Relation between literacy and HIV treatment knowledge among patients on HAART regimens. *AIDS Care, 17,* 863–873.

Wolf, M., Davis, T., Cross, J., Marin, E., Green, K., & Bennett, C. (2004). Health literacy and patient knowledge in a southern U.S. HIV clinic. *International Journal of STD and AIDS, 15,* 747–752.

# 13

# Internet and Other Computer Technology-Based Interventions for STD/HIV Prevention

*Sheana Bull*

University of Colorado at Denver and Health Sciences Center

As of 2005, 68% of U.S. adults and 87% of youth aged 12 to 17 (Lenhart, Madden, & Hitlin, 2005; Lenhart et al., 2003) used the Internet. Estimates are that 81% of adults and 45% of youth own cell phones, and that whereas e-mail may be ubiquitous in the workplace and used widely among adults, youth appear to prefer instant messages for wireless text-based communication (Rheingold, 2002). Given the explosion in Internet, wireless, and computer-based technologies in the past 15 years, HIV/AIDS prevention and service providers are anxious to tap into opportunities to harness the potential of these powerful communication media to deliver effective HIV prevention interventions.

The promise of these communications is compelling—the Internet offers an unprecedented reach to populations at risk given the enormous number of persons who are online, and an ability to use technology to target that reach. Once we reach people over the Internet, computer and cell phone-based interventions can tailor communications about HIV/AIDS prevention to individual users, can offer interactive electronic forms of social support, and can be used adjunctively to tie in to or reinforce other face-to-face interventions.

Technology-based interventions—whether stand-alone efforts to promote HIV prevention or tied in to existing clinic-, school-, or community-based efforts—have been of particular interest in the past decade. Researchers have begun to demonstrate how we can use technology and communication to promote reductions in behavioral risk for chronic disease, improve quality of care and shared doctor–patient decision making, use Internet systems for home-based medical testing and access to the medical record, and use technology for improvements in surveillance.

The field of HIV prevention has been directly involved in the vanguard of Internet and other computer technology–based efforts to promote reduction in risk for acquisition and transmission. Investigations to date have focused on translating evidence-based community- and clinic-based interventions to technological versions of the same, and, though a solid evidence base of efficacy for specific interventions is still forming, we do have reason to consider Internet and other technology-based HIV/AIDS prevention interventions as highly promising.

As the use of technology in HIV prevention moves forward, it is important to consider some critical issues, particularly for researchers in communication and health. What is the potential of technology to realize a much faster and efficient system for rapid evaluation of interventions? What are the methodological limitations that should be kept in mind when considering both the efficacy and public health impact of a computer technology–based HIV prevention intervention? And to what extent do we consider the evolution of communication theories to address the ubiquitous role of computer-based technology as we embark on ever new and ever innovative approaches to prevent acquisition and transmission of HIV/AIDS?

In this chapter, we first examine what health professionals working outside HIV/AIDS have learned in using technology to address chronic illness and other infectious disease. Then we review current innovations in technology-based HIV/AIDS-related research. Readers are presented with considerations for anyone interested in using technology for HIV/AIDS-related research. Finally, we consider the implications of the current state of this field for the development of future dynamic theories of communication incorporating technology in American society.

## The State of the Art for Technology-Based
## Health Promotion Interventions

Researchers have been considering ways to incorporate Internet and other computer-based technologies into health promotion efforts for at least a decade—addressing everything from nutrition and weight loss to interventions for headache, tinnitus (ear ring-ing), chronic back pain, depression, and diabetes self manage-ment. Following are just a few examples of the growing literature from this field. Researchers implementing a randomized controlled trial (RCT) showed that using computer-based algorithms to pro-vide instant, tailored feedback to participants in an online nutrition intervention facilitated greater awareness of healthy nutrition habits and increased intentions to implement healthy nutrition behaviors (Oenema, Brug, & Lechner, 2001). An RCT of a weight loss program that utilized regular e-mail exchanges for communication between participants and counselors showed efficacy for achieving signifi-cantly greater weight loss for intervention versus control participants (Tate, Wing, & Winett, 2001). Investigators have shown an Internet-based intervention has promise for reducing headache symptoms and disability—and another for reducing distress, depression, and annoyance for persons with tinnitus—although these studies aren't conclusive given high attrition (50%–65%; Andersson, Bakhsh, Johansson, Kaldo, & Carlbring, 2005; Devineni & Blanchard, 2005; Strom, Pettersson, & Andersson, 2000). Diabetes self-management interventions online have demonstrated that recipients of tailored self-management messages online will improve self-management (Gottlieb, 2000). One of the better researched programs is a diabetes self-management program, called "Choosing Well," that focuses on these three key health risk behaviors, which are generally acknowl-edged to be the leading preventable causes of premature death and morbidity—physical activity, nutrition, and smoking. This program takes the user through a health risk assessment and provides tai-lored feedback regarding behavioral risk factors to the user through preprogrammed algorithms deployed during completion of the risk assessment survey. Following identification of risk factors, users are invited to set a goal for a behavioral change in one area—for exam-ple, increase physical activity, reduce fat intake, or quit smoking. An online role model—which can also be tailored to match the gender, age, and race/ethnicity of the user—can guide the user to identify possible barriers that exist for achieving their goal and strategies to overcome these barriers. The user can print out their goal, barriers, and strategies for later reference. The program has been found effec-tive for type 2 diabetes patients in group treatment settings, with older adults, when translated into a brief medical office–based inter-vention, and across multiple offices and interventionists (Glasgow,

2002; Glasgow & Toobert, 2000; Glasgow et al., 1997; Stevens, Glasgow, Toobert, Karanja, & Smith, 2003).

In addition to Internet and CD-ROM technologies for chronic illness interventions, investigators have explored the use of other technologies for health promotion as well. The use of interactive voice recognition (IVR) telephone communications for interventions has promise, and may be an ideal bridge for digital-divide concerns or to reach populations who might have access to the Internet and e-mail but simply prefer the telephone for most communication. IVR technology integrates computer and telephone technologies to create an automated system that can deliver brief behavioral assessments—which can also include tailored feedback—to an almost limitless number of participants over time. Studies have demonstrated that people perceive that recent IVR systems are similar to human telephone contact (Kaplan, Farzanfar, & Friedman, 2003). An example of IVR for chronic-illness prevention is a system used in the Veteran's Administration (VA) to improve diabetes self-management—researchers were able to show that persons with diabetes who regularly used the system, which incorporated preprogrammed algorithms to give feedback on specific diabetes self-management issues (e.g., getting foot checks, blood sugar levels and monitoring) significantly improved patient monitoring and glycemic control (Piette, 2000a, 2000b; Piette, Weinberger, & McPhee, 2000; Piette, Weinberger, McPhee, Mah, et al., 2000). Use of IVR systems tied to intervention or medical care rate highly on participant satisfaction. These systems have been tried and shown to be equally effective for Spanish speakers, who have higher system compliance and equally positive medical and self-management outcomes compared with other system users (Kaplan et al., 2003; Piette, McPhee, Weinberger, Mah, & Kraemer, 1999; Piette, 1999, 2000a, 2000b; Piette, Weinberger, & McPhee, 2000; Piette, Weinberger, McPhee, Mah, et al., 2000).

Recent reports from a pilot study using cell phones to deliver health-related interventions are also promising. Investigators using cell phones to send regular text messages to college students to assist them in achieving smoking cessation and reduction goals showed that 43% of participants had made at least one attempt to quit over a 24-hour period. Although these results are from pilot data, they point to options for considering communication beyond the Internet and computer and into the wireless-telephone environment (Ober-mayer, Riley, Asif, & Jean-Mary, 2004).

## Current Technology Innovations in HIV/AIDS-Related Research

### The Internet as a Risk Environment for Sexually Transmitted Diseases

HIV prevention using the Internet and other computer-based technologies differs in two important areas from the research described earlier. HIV prevention has an added dimension not seen in other areas. Not only are we challenged to use the potential of computer-based technology to prevent HIV, but we are also challenged to reduce the risk incurred by individuals who actively seek sex partners online, placing themselves at additional risk for sexually transmitted diseases (STDs). An early qualitative study in this area described the process whereby persons seek sex partners using chat rooms online (Bull & McFarlane, 2000). One of the first quantitative studies in this area showed that relative to STD patients not using the Internet to meet sexual partners, patients meeting sexual partners online reported more high-risk behaviors, including more past STDs, more sexual partners in the previous 12 months, more anal sex, and more exposure to partners known to be HIV-positive (McFarlane, Bull, & Rietmeijer, 2000). In a second study of the same clinic population, 7% of the sample had met a sexual partner over the Internet and 44% of the participants who found a sexual partner online did not use a condom the last time they had sex with an Internet partner (Rietmeijer, Bull, McFarlane, Patnaik, & Douglas, 2003). Data from a self-administered HIV STD behavioral risk assessment offered online—called Sex Quiz—revealed that among the 3,248 participants, 80% of men who have sex with men (MSM) and 32% of heterosexual men had sex with a partner initially met online (Bull, McFarlane, & Rietmeijer, 2001). The MSM reported an average of 9.0 Internet partners in the previous 12 months and 21.4 lifetime Internet partners. Heterosexual men reported an average of 4.2 Internet partners in the previous 12 months and 7.5 lifetime Internet partners. Fifty-five percent of heterosexual men and 29% of MSM indicated that they did not use a condom the last time they had vaginal or anal intercourse with a partner found online. Data analyses from this same study examining heterosexual risk behavior showed that among young heterosexual adults (aged 18–24) participants who had met a sexual partner via the Internet had nearly three times as many lifetime sexual partners (mean = 14.6) as participants not meeting a sexual partner online (mean = 5.8). Furthermore, 61% of participants who had met a partner online reported no condom use the last time they had vaginal or anal sex with an Internet partner (McFarlane, Bull, & Rietmeijer, 2002).

Studies with diverse populations have documented that using the Internet to seek a romantic or sexual partner is becoming a more and more common practice (Benotsch, Kalichman, & Cage, 2002; Bull, Lloyd, Rietmeijer, & McFarlane, 2004; Bull, McFarlane, & King, 2001; Bull, McFarlane, Lloyd, & Rietmeijer, 2004; Bull, McFarlane, & Rietmeijer, 2001; Cooper, McLoughlin, & Campbell, 2000; Elford, Bolding, & Sherr, 2001; Hospers, Harterink, Van Den Hoek, & Veenstra, 2002; Klausner, Wolf, Fischer-Ponce, Zolt, & Katz, 2000; Rietmeijer, Bull, et al., 2003; Rietmeijer, Patnaik, Judson, & Douglas, 2003). Meeting partners online has been shown across all of these studies to be a predictor of risk, even when controlling for demographics, attitudes regarding condoms, and substance use. A community-based study of MSM showed that more than one third (34%) of MSM attending a gay pride festival indicated that they had met a sexual partner online (Benotsch et al., 2002) and their HIV risks were high; that is, those with online partners had higher rates of unprotected sex and more sex partners. Individuals who find sexual partners online are also likely to continue to use the Internet as a source for new partners. A study of London MSM showed that most men (83%) who had sought partners online did so more than once (Elford et al., 2001).

In a study comparing risk behaviors for MSM recruited online and in gay bars, researchers documented higher HIV infection rates and greater frequency of STD history in the online sample compared to the gay-bar respondents. The online sample also had more sex partners in the past 30 days and less consistent condom use (Rhodes, DiClemente, Cecil, Hergenrather, & Yee, 2002). Researchers examining women's sexual risk behaviors among an online sample have shown that 30% of women engaged in sexual behavior the first time they met a partner they had initially contacted online, and 77% of women reported inconsistent or no condom use during vaginal intercourse (Padgett, 2003).

Most studies on Internet sexual risk behavior completed to date emphasize the digital divide in that they report findings from pri-

marily middle- to upper-income, well-educated, White populations. A notable exception is the work of Ross, Rosser, and Stanton
(2004), who have shown that Latino MSM have a similar risk profile to other MSM, but that it may require more perseverance to
recruit these men to participate in research online.

As mentioned previously, this early work included data from
largely well-educated, primarily White populations who had access
to health care through insurance. The evidence from these surveys
prompted researchers to consider whether and to what extent these
online populations would overlap with patients at publicly funded
STD clinics and HIV-testing sites. There was concern that online
partner seeking was occurring in a population not traditionally
reached with information and education about STD risk, and that
the newly documented information on linkages between online
partner seeking and STD risk was not widely disseminated among
people seeking sexual and romantic partners online.

The promise of the Internet was appealing—there was potential
to reach a wide number of people who may not otherwise be seen in
public clinics or community-based organizations where many HIV
prevention efforts occur. There was also consideration that communication about the links between online partner seeking and STD
risk would offer an important opportunity to raise awareness of risk
among online populations.

Researchers began to implement HIV and STD prevention interventions online largely by attempting to translate effective communication approaches from community- and clinic-based efforts to the
online environment. In an early HIV prevention intervention with
MSM online, researchers borrowed from the stage of change-based
role model story interventions used with success in the AIDS Community Demonstration Projects (Centers for Disease Control and
Prevention [CDC], 1999a), and capitalized on the unique capabilities
of the Internet to offer instant tailoring of materials to a participant.
Tailoring messages based on participant responses to a risk assessment already had substantial evidence of efficacy for developing
print materials, and researchers had shown that tailored materials
increased the relevance of information for readers, and were widely
preferred to nontailored materials for a wide variety of health promotion topics (Bental, Cawsey, & Jones, 1999; Campbell, Peterkin,
Abbott, & Rogers, 1997; Campbell et al., 1994; De Vries & Brug, 1999;
Kreuter & Strecher, 1995; Lipkus, Lyna, & Rimer, 1999; A. C. Marcus

et al., 1998; B. H. Marcus et al., 1998; B. H. Marcus, Owen, Forsyth, Cavill, & Fridinger, 1998; Rakowski et al., 1998; Rimer & Glassman, 1998; Rimer et al., 1999; Skinner, Siegfried, Kegler, & Strecher, 1993; Skinner, Strecher, & Hospers, 1994).

Participants in this early intervention study were recruited primarily via chat rooms to the study Web site, called Smart Sex Quest, and those who were eligible for the study (which focused on MSM) were invited to enroll, complete an informed consent process online, and take an HIV/STD behavioral risk assessment online. The computer randomly assigned men to an intervention or control group. Those in the intervention group received three online role model stories—one addressing condom use, one STD testing, and the third HIV testing. Photos of role models that matched their age and race/ ethnicity accompanied stories and each story was generated using a stage-of-change algorithm to match where participants were along the continuum of change for each behavior. This effort was plagued by high attrition of participants. Researchers successfully recruited more than 1,700 eligible participants to the Smart Sex Quest Web site, which was designed to test the efficacy of using messages tailored to participant stage of change and risk awareness for STD and HIV testing and condom use. Unfortunately, with only 20% participant retention, it was impossible for investigators to draw conclusions about study outcomes, although results did show a trend toward intervention efficacy for increasing HIV testing (Bull, Lloyd, McFarlane, & Rietmeijer, 2004).

There are multiple research studies currently under way examining the efficacy of the Internet for HIV prevention, but they are still in implementation stages and data on their efficacy are not yet available. The National Institute of Mental Health (NIMH) issued a request for applications (MH-01-003) called "Communications and HIV/STD Prevention" including requests for research proposals that examined the Internet environment and its relationship to HIV/STD risk. They funded several investigators to study Internet-related HIV/ STD risk and interventions. A study of rural MSM of an online education program to increase knowledge about HIV risk with a wait-list control showed efficacy for increasing knowledge over a 1-week follow-up period (G. C. Williams et al., 2005; M. Williams, 2005; M. L. Williams, Bowen, & Horvath, 2005). Currently under development or being investigated in randomized trials are Web sites that target (a) MSM seeking sex partners online with a highly interactive e-learning application designed to increase knowledge, awareness of HIV risk, and skills in reducing risk (Simon Rosser, principal investigator) and (b) a Web site testing the efficacy of tailored HIV prevention messages for youth (men and women, hetero and homosexual) aged 18 to 24 at risk for HIV (Sheana Bull, principal investigator).

Funded through other funding mechanisms are projects designed to test the efficacy of using the popular opinion leader (POL) model and an outreach model in an online environment. The POL model has been shown to have efficacy when used for face-to-face HIV risk reduction, and depends on training community members who are identified as leaders in their social circles (Kelly et al., 1991, 1992) to conduct peer-to-peer outreach. This is contrasted with an outreach model where a health department or community organization representative is doing education in community settings. Though both have been shown to have efficacy in community-based interventions, and though many community-based organizations are currently using the outreach model in chat rooms online, neither approach has been examined for feasibility or efficacy in the online environment. This recently funded research is under way, with results expected in 2007.

## Beyond Prevention—HIV-Related Technology-Based Interventions for HIV Positives and to Improve Care Provision

Computer-based technology interventions for HIV/AIDS prevention face the same perennial challenge that any HIV/AIDS prevention intervention must address: Whereas other interventions can focus on persons with a condition or disease who may be substantially motivated to make changes or obtain relief (e.g., from headache, back pain, diabetes), primary HIV/AIDS prevention must motivate individuals to make behavioral changes in advance of any infection or disease. Fortunately, there is promise as well for using technology in interventions that are aimed more toward persons infected with HIV. For example, in one study, investigators placed computers in the homes of people infected with HIV and provided them with Internet access and regular electronic communication with clinic staff. This increase in access to care showed both increased use of computers and self-disclosure of risk behaviors for patients with HIV for the intervention group (Gustafson, Hawkins, et al., 1999; Gustafson,

*dr knwmore about it so*
*screened more*

McTavish, et al., 1999; Gustafson, Robinson, Ansley, Adler, & Brennan, 1999c). Another study focused on providing both increased access to systems and social support to people with HIV showed that participants had greater satisfaction with HIV-related care, greater confidence in medical-related decision making, and decreased perception of social isolation (Flatley-Brennan, 1998).

Interventions to address HIV/AIDS can also happen at an organizational level, with activities such as physician training. Evidence from a recent study intervening to change physician behaviors is promising. The study compared the use of a multicomponent Internet-based continuing education intervention specific to Clamydia (CT) symptoms, complications, diagnosis, and treatment to a more generalized Internet-based continuing education program on women's health for physicians to increase CT screening. Physicians in the multicomponent Internet-based intervention had significantly higher CT screening than those completing the more general women's health module (Allison et al., 2005).

## Programmatic Efforts to Promote HIV/STD Risk Reduction

Other prevention efforts would be better categorized as programmatic rather than research based in that they aren't necessarily designed as research efforts or have yet to be formally evaluated. Nonetheless, these programmatic interventions are instructive in that they point to further areas for research of promising approaches online, including Web sites related to HIV prevention, partner notification online, and chat room–based and chat auditorium–style HIV prevention.

## STD/HIV Prevention-Related Web Sites

*taylor*

Several analyses have been conducted to document the extent of and type of HIV-related information available to persons on the Internet. As early as 1997, researchers were documenting the existence of HIV prevention resources online (Brettle, 1997) and offering suggestions on ways to make information relevant and appropriate for different risk groups. For example, Mallory (1997) documented the existence of a number of HIV prevention sites, but stressed that few were targeted toward women, and suggested that online communications should take into account gender differences that are important for HIV prevention and care.

Smith, Gertz, Alvarez, and Lurie (2000) completed a content analysis of sexuality-related Web sites to document the availability and quality of sex education online for adolescents. Using the Excite and Webcrawler search engines, they were able to identify 41 Web sites with sex education material. They concluded that some sites did provide relevant and accurate information and that it took about 4 minutes of searching to locate it. However, if people searching online are not aware of the specific keywords and navigation approaches needed to access this information, it could be challenging to find.

This early assessment of Web sites was limited primarily to reviewing the accuracy and relevancy of sex education information online. A subsequent review of Web sites used a similar methodology, but took the analyses beyond provision of information to consider the specific types of communication offered at the site, including whether sites offered detail on sexual behavior decision making and safer-sex negotiation as well as communication with partners (Keller, LaBelle, Karimi, & Gupta, 2002, 2004). Researchers identified 36 sites with sex education information and many that focused on partner communication in particular. Several also included tips on condom use and referrals for services.

The most recent assessment of sexual health information available online included more in-depth consideration of communication features online, including targeting, the use of behavior change theory, presence of interactivity, and presence of tailoring online. This assessment of 21 Web sites with relevant HIV prevention information showed that many do now target subgroups at risk for HIV, including heterosexuals, gay, lesbian, bisexual, and transgendered (GLBT) persons, and teens and young adults, but that more than half of the sites reviewed provided general rather than targeted information. Although there is strong evidence from meta-analyses regarding the consistent associations between specific theoretical constructs such as positive attitudes and norms, self-efficacy, and behavior change (Albarracin, Kumkale, & Johnson, 2004; Sheeran, Abraham, & Orbell, 1999), this analysis revealed that behavior change theory is rarely explicit on sexual health Web sites and when there are elements from which one could infer a theoretical framework they focus primarily on raising awareness or perceptions of susceptibility and severity of disease instead of attitudes and norms.

Some of the sites did include tips on condom negotiation and use, however, which could represent adherence to skills-building principles relevant for self-efficacy. The sites did include some interesting interactive components, such as quizzes, changing homepages, and message boards. It remains unclear to what extent these interactive features are important for facilitating behavior change. The authors indicated that bandwidth issues and other cost considerations may limit the ability of sites to include many interactive features (Noar, Clark, Cole, & Lustria, 2006).

### Partner Notification

The San Francisco Department of Public Health (SFDPH) has been an innovator in online HIV prevention since they first published their procedures for tracking a syphilis outbreak through cyberspace and conducting partner notification (PN) online (Klausner et al., 2000). SFDPH had syphilis-infected men with sex partners who were anonymous except for their e-mail address because they had solicited their partners via the Internet. SFDPH advises people implementing online PN to encourage the infected patient to be the first to notify their Internet sex partners of an infection, before the Health Department conducts any PN and to use the contact's Internet Service Provider (ISP) when possible to generate the Health Department online notification. They advise the use of credible agency logos and use of parsimonious subject lines regarding an urgent health matter, and underscore the importance of confidentiality by sending individual rather than group messages.

### Chat Room Outreach

Chat room outreach is the name given to the process whereby outreach workers from community-based HIV/AIDS service organizations go online to chat rooms that are oriented toward MSM, usually easy to identify because of the Web site hosting them (gay. com, manhunt.net, cruisingforsex.com) or because the room has a name that suggests it was established for MSM (sfmsm, menformen, bostonmfm, etc.; Bull & McFarlane, 2000). The outreach workers use the chat forum to share HIV prevention information. For

example, Howard Brown Health Center in Chicago conducts outreach in multiple venues (e.g., manhunt.net, gay.com, and America
OnLine [AOL]), logging in to the chat and then stating they are there
to answer HIV/STD-related questions. They have yet to complete
an evaluation of their program, but currently document the number of contacts made during various times of day, descriptions of
encounters, and number of referrals made. However, Chicago chat
rooms often include participants from other parts of Illinois, as well
as Wisconsin and Indiana, so determining if these referrals resulted
in clinic visits may not be feasible for this organization.

A similar project in Houston, Texas, at the Montrose Clinic is
called Project CORE (Cyber OutReach Education), and outreach
workers will, in addition to answering questions generated by chatters, post information or a question without waiting for a chatter to
approach them. They can use instant messaging (IM) or group chat
to connect to chatters. Project CORE is planning a qualitative analysis of all de-identified online conversations.

In Florida, United Foundation for AIDS (UFA) actively conducts
Internet-based outreach to MSM and has successfully used chat
room outreach to get 25 to 30 users of crystal methamphetamine
("crystal meth") to come to UFA for regular group risk reduction
workshops.

The SFDPH also conducts chat room outreach and has compiled
perhaps the most comprehensive evaluation of this type of intervention to date. Working with a consultant, Internet Sexuality Information Services, Inc. (ISIS), SFDPH spent 2 months doing chat room
outreach in three venues: AOL chat rooms specific to San Francisco,
Craigslist (San Francisco), and M4M4Sex. Outreach chatters covered topics such as STD symptoms, transmission and treatment, and
referrals to testing. Health professionals responded to questions and
provided syphilis fact sheets and online coupons for syphilis testing
at the public STD clinic.

Study staff spent 57 hours conducting outreach in the three online
venues, and documented 212 interactions (67 on M4M4Sex; 21 on
Craigslist; 124 on AOL). The rate of coupon redemption for clinic-
based testing was 16% (35 coupons redeemed).

In another form of online outreach, SFDPH again collaborated
with ISIS to establish seven auditorium-style chats with online visitors
to gay.com. Auditorium-style chats are also known as "moderated" or
"scheduled" chats, where there is a scheduled time for the chat and

people can see ahead of time who will be moderating the session or in the role of "guest speaker" or "expert." Chatters pose questions to the moderator or guest speaker, who posts a response in real time that can be viewed by all participating in the session. In these seven 1-hour sessions, there was an average of 120 people per session attending and between 10 and 50 people in the session at any one time, with an average of 15 questions each hour.

*Banner Advertisements*

Banner advertising online is similar to the use of billboards in the physical environment. They are of varying size and shape, but generally consist of small boxes of information that are posted on high traffic areas of the Internet, with the intent of attracting an Internet user to click on the advertisement. This will lead an individual to the advertiser's Web page. For HIV prevention, this can mean linking the individual to a Web site with HIV prevention content. Banner ads can be targeted to a particular page on a site, and can be geo-targeted for placement on Web pages for a specific city, ZIP code, or census tract. They can also be geo-targeted for pages that attract certain demographics, for example, men, people aged 18 to 25, African Americans, and so forth. In this way, banner ads can offer much more of a "narrowcasting" than broadcasting approach, while stopping short of tailoring, but still taking advantage of technology to segment ads for more specific audiences. The evaluation of the reach of banner ads is fairly straightforward. Web sites can count the number of people who click on the banner; in fact, some advertisers pay for the number of click-throughs, rather than the number of impressions (the number of times a banner ad is shown online). Once a user has clicked on the banner, however, it can be difficult to document the effect the information on the linked Web page has on behavior. One Web site, manhunt.net, an online sex-seeking venue, has established links from banner ads on their site to local syphilis-testing opportunities, in an effort to promote awareness of STD among MSM. Manhunt and their various health department partners have not yet documented the efficacy or effectiveness of this approach (S. Adelson, personal communication).

## Considerations for Those Interested in Using Technology for HIV/AIDS-Related Research

The proliferation of use of the Internet and other computer technologies suggests these modalities are becoming normative in the United States and their use for research is likely to continue and evolve. Given this assumption, it is worth considering some important limitations specific to HIV prevention when relying on technology either for assessment of risk or to deliver HIV-related interventions. Researchers in this area have identified specific sampling, recruitment and retention of study participants, verification of study participants, and data security among other issues as key methodological considerations for technology-based HIV-related research.

### Sampling

Investigators have shown time and again that Internet-based recruitment can yield much larger samples than those obtained through more traditional methods (e.g., face-to-face, telephone, and mail; Bull, McFarlane, & Rietmeijer, 2001; Rhodes, DiClemente, Yee, & Hergenrather, 2001). However, for HIV-related research in particular, we need to be concerned about targeting people who are at risk and being able to recruit the most appropriate individuals to participate in research. Higher reach alone will not likely yield a sample of persons at increased risk for HIV—indeed, having a substantial reach may reduce our ability to sample people at elevated risk for HIV. We should consider specific tools to improve sampling of populations at risk. For example, we can identify ZIP codes or census tracts with higher than average rates of STD or HIV infection and with residents representing groups at greater risk. We can then geo-target banner advertisements to people in these ZIP codes. We can also use this information to search for chat rooms from specific areas (e.g. "East-LAM4M") and include those chat rooms in a sampling frame.

### Recruitment, Retention, and Security of Study Participants

In addition to concerns regarding sampling, investigators have already documented multiple challenges to recruitment and retention of online samples (Andersson et al., 2005; Bull, 2005; Bull, McFarlane, et al., 2004; Devineni & Blanchard, 2005; Glasgow, Boles, McKay, Feil, & Barrera, 2003; Strom et al., 2000). Of particular relevance for HIV prevention initiatives online is the need for research credibility to enhance motivation for participation. Given the easy access to sexually explicit Web sites online, as well as the frequent media attention to such issues as online pedophilia, investigators conducting any research that involves collection of data related to sexual risk behavior should take extra care in establishing themselves as credible. Ways to do this include offering links to university Web sites with detailed information on investigators (including telephone and e-mail contact information) and links to funding agencies sponsoring the research. Investigators can also offer more detailed information in the "Frequently Asked Questions" (FAQ) sections on Web pages that offer specific information on why questions are being asked and what is likely to be done with the data.

Retention of study participants may be enhanced by having mechanisms that can facilitate personal contact, such as telephone reminders to return to the Web site, or e-mail contact with study staff. These techniques have yet to be proven efficacious for retention of study participants online and are potentially relevant for all Internet research, not only HIV-related research online. However, it is possible that people providing regular data on sexual behavior may benefit from human contact as a way to address any concerns that the data are being used, stored, or shared inappropriately.

Security of data for HIV prevention research online is of particular importance. Institutional review boards, university information technology (IT) departments, researchers, and participants have justifiable concerns regarding ways that data are stored and transferred online. We need to take extra care that sexual risk behavior data cannot be accessed beyond study staff and that researchers adhere to the strictest security protocols possible. At the University of Colorado at Denver and Health Sciences Center, for example, the IT Department, Colorado Multiple Institutional Review Board, and Burser's Office have all established protocols for computer-based data security, in part to be in compliance with the Health Insurance Portability and Protection Act (HIPPA) and in part to avoid incentive fraud. Protocols include data encryption online, standardization of secure-socket-layer (SSL) protection procedures for every Web site, and data storage behind computer server firewalls.

## Conclusions and Future Considerations

In this chapter, we have considered the current state of the art of Internet and other computer-based technological interventions as they related to HIV and other chronic illness, both research based and program based, and we have offered some cautions related to the evaluation of technology-based interventions. Given this review, what is the future of technology-based HIV/AIDS-related research?

### What Is the Potential of Technology to Realize a Much Faster and Efficient System for Rapid Evaluation of Interventions?

It is interesting to note that the majority of publications on technology-based HIV/AIDS and other interventions discussed here are from the year 2000 or later. The rapid change in the field in the past decade showcases this area as a new frontier for research. One very promising consideration for the field, assuming methodological challenges can be addressed, is the development of rapid, "real-time" systems of evaluation that can substantially speed up the turn around for intervention evaluation. With increased reach afforded by technology, and possibilities for methods such as random sampling online, it is within reason to consider we may soon be prepared to develop technology-based interventions and quickly assemble a large study population and assess intervention efficacy in a matter of months rather than years. This may, in turn, position us more effectively to conduct much needed assessments of external validity—for example, intervention effectiveness for diverse populations or subgroups within a sample; intervention adoption and diffusion, and intervention maintenance over time.

### How Will We Overcome Limitations and Maximize Both the Efficacy and Public Health Impact of a Computer Technology-Based HIV/AIDS-Related Intervention?

It is not completely clear how the methods for technology-based HIV/AIDS research will evolve. There is, however, an interesting opportunity for us to consider the development of methodologies and protocols that are specific for HIV-related technology applications. Work in the area of sampling for online populations to ensure inclusion of high-risk individuals is needed. Taking steps to ensure study credibility and state-of-the-art data security is critical. We can experiment with novel and innovative approaches beyond the traditional RCT because the evolution of these media is such that the traditional time lines to implement such trials are so long as to potentially render any efficacy observed through rigorously controlled research obsolete in the face of fast-paced new technological innovation. Consider, for example, recent advances that allow wireless access to streaming video through the telephone, and ability to check e-mail, weather, stocks, and so forth on a mobile device. How long will it be before we have regular streaming video of counselors reminding HIV-positive patients to take medication? When will we experience text messaging of young adults on Friday nights to buy condoms before going out as normative? If we plan for new standards in technology-based research methodologies, we can be poised to make this a reality much more quickly.

## To What Extent Do We Consider the Evolution of Communication and Technology Theories in HIV/AIDS-Related Research?

We have a substantial body of research elucidating the importance of theory to guide behavioral and other intervention development and evaluation, including multiple meta-analyses and reports regarding the practical use of theory and evidence that theory-based interventions for HIV appear to have greater efficacy than those that are not theory based (Galavotti, Saltzman, Sauter, & Sumartojo, 1997). To date, the majority of these theories focus on behavioral changes at the individual level and/or how change is operationalized at the individual level. Development of theory that more fully explores issues of technology for health promotion is needed. For example, as the digital divide persists, it is of value to consider how different groups acculturate or assimilate to the dominant cultural norms regarding technology. As multimedia forms of communication become more prevalent, theories about learning and behavior change within a multimedia and multimodal communication context would be highly instructive.

## The Future of Technology-Based or Technology-Assisted HIV Prevention

It is clear that the Internet, telephone, and cell phone technologies are or are soon to be endemic in most parts of the world. We have made important strides in HIV prevention in the past decade, and now have a substantial evidence base of effective interventions that work in face-to-face circumstances (CDC, 1999b). We may be entering a new period of HIV prevention that can take this evidence base and translate it for applications online or via telephone or other handheld devices. We can also consider the possibilities for new and unique interventions that are technology specific. We can also consider approaches that might blend existing effective interventions with new technology-based interventions to facilitate achievement of the combined promise of technology for substantially increasing reach while simultaneously making interventions personalized and relevant (Cassell, Jackson, & Cheuvront, 1998).

Our efforts to date to use the Internet for HIV prevention have been concentrated on translation of "what works" in face-to-face environments to the Internet and testing for efficacy. In the short term, one can expect that we will develop technology-specific methodological protocols that can facilitate the rapid assessment and dissemination of interventions, overcoming the current challenges related to recruitment, retention, and security online. Given the currently funded research on technology-based HIV prevention initiatives, we are only a couple of years from learning about the efficacy of using theoretically framed, tailored risk reduction messages online to promote condom use, and of using highly interactive approaches such as simulations and games to reduce HIV risk for MSM.

Somewhat further in the future are answers to questions regarding the use of more complex HIV prevention counseling and prevention training online and the use of other technologies—for example, cell phones and IVR systems to promote HIV prevention.

As is true with the introduction of any new technology, we need to consider the importance of using these new technologies as both adjunctive as well as stand-alone mechanisms to promote behavior change. There may be little reason to consider developing an Internet-based intervention as a stand-alone counseling tool, for example, when it may have higher efficacy when used in conjunction with prevention services available in clinic settings. However, as we recognize the limitations clinicians have in reaching all persons at risk for HIV, it is important to turn to technological innovations to increase reach.

Technologies such as the Internet and telephone can offer substantial reach while delivering a consistent and standard message. At the same time, the message can be tailored as needed to increase the relevance for the receiver. Future interventions are likely to capitalize on this hybrid feature—it is not far off to conceptualize programs where individuals share a few select details about their risk behavior and are instantly offered a personalized risk reduction message online or via e-mail or telephone.

Interactive features are becoming commonplace both online and via telephone. It is likely that bandwidth issues will be less constraining in the future and that messages will be much more interactive than passive, allowing for branching, deeper tailoring, and higher engagement with the communication process by participants.

With an ever-changing technology environment, we face myriad exciting opportunities to harness the potential of the Internet, computer, and wireless systems for HIV/AIDS-related research and programs. It is primarily with excitement for the promise of these media that we can look forward to the possibility of making significant impacts on HIV in years to come.

## References

Albarracin, D., Kumkale, G. T., & Johnson, B. T. (2004). Influences of social power and normative support on condom use decisions: A research synthesis. *AIDS Care, 16,* 700–723.

Allison, J. J., Kiefe, C. I., Wall, T., Casebeer, L., Ray, M. N., Spettell, C. M., et al. (2005). Multicomponent Internet continuing medical education to promote chlamydia screening. *American Journal of Preventive Medicine, 28,* 285–290.

Andersson, G., Bakhsh, R., Johansson, L., Kaldo, V., & Carlbring, P. (2005). Stroop facilitation in tinnitus patients: An experiment conducted via the world wide web. *Cyberpsychology and Behavior, 8,* 32–38.

Benotsch, E. G., Kalichman, S., & Cage, M. (2002). Men who have met sex partners via the internet: Prevalence, predictors, and implications for HIV prevention. *Archives of Sexual Behavior, 31,* 177–183.

Bental, D. S., Cawsey, A., & Jones R. (1999). Patient information systems that tailor to the individual. *Patient Education and Counseling, 2,* 171–180.

Brettle, R. P. (1997). The Internet and medicine: related sites including HIV/AIDS. *International Journal of STDs and AIDS, 8,* 71–77.

Bull, S. (2005, July). *Methodological considerations for sampling and recruitment of online populations.* Paper presented at the 2005 International Society for Sexually Transmitted Disease Research Conference, Amsterdam.

Bull, S., Lloyd, L., McFarlane, M., & Rietmeijer, K. (2004). *Men who have sex with men and women (MSM/W): Their use of Internet and related HIV/STD risk.* Unpublished manuscript.

Bull, S. S., Lloyd, L., Rietmeijer, C., & McFarlane, M. (2004). Recruitment and retention of an online sample for an HIV prevention intervention targeting men who have sex with men: The Smart Sex Quest Project. *AIDS Care, 16,* 931–943.

Bull, S. S., & McFarlane, M. (2000). Soliciting sex on the Internet: What are the risks for sexually transmitted diseases and HIV? *Sexually Transmitted Diseases, 27,* 545–550.

Bull, S. S., McFarlane, M., & King, D. (2001). Barriers to STD/HIV prevention on the Internet. *Health Education Research, 16,* 661–670.

Bull, S. S., McFarlane, M., Lloyd, L., & Rietmeijer, C. (2004). The process of seeking sex partners online and implications for STD/HIV prevention. *AIDS Care, 16,* 1012–1020.

Bull, S. S., McFarlane, M., & Rietmeijer, C. (2001). HIV and sexually transmitted infection risk behaviors among men seeking sex with men online. *American Journal of Public Health, 91,* 988–989.

Campbell, E., Peterkin, D., Abbott, R., & Rogers, J. (1997). Encouraging underscreened women to have cervical cancer screening: The effectiveness of a computer strategy. *Preventive Medicine, 26,* 801–807.

Campbell, M. K., DeVellis, B. M., Strecher, V. J., Ammerman, A. S., DeVellis, R. F., & Sandler, R. S. (1994). Improving dietary behavior: The effectiveness of tailored messages in primary care settings. *American Journal of Public Health, 84,* 783–787.

Cassell, M. M., Jackson, C., & Cheuvront, B. (1998). Health communication on the Internet: An effective channel for health behavior change? *Journal of Health Communication, 3,* 71–79.

Centers for Disease Control and Prevention. (1999a). Community-level HIV intervention in five cities: Final outcome data from the CDC AIDS Community Demonstration Projects. *American Journal of Public Health, 89,* 336–345.

Centers for Disease Control and Prevention. (1999b). *Compendium of HIV prevention interventions with evidence of effectiveness.* Atlanta: Author.

Cooper, A., McLoughlin, I. P., & Campbell, K. M. (2000). Sexuality in cyberspace: Update for the 21st century. *Cyberpsychology & Behavior, 3,* 521–536.

De Vries, H., & Brug, J. (1999). Computer-tailored interventions motivating people to adopt health promoting behaviors: Introduction to a new approach. *Patient Education and Counseling, 36,* 99–105.

Devineni, T., & Blanchard, E. B. (2005). A randomized controlled trial of an Internet-based treatment for chronic headache. *Behaviour Research and Therapy, 43,* 277–292.

Elford, J., Bolding, G., & Sherr, L. (2001). Seeking sex on the Internet and sexual risk behaviour among gay men using London gyms [comment]. *AIDS, 15,* 1409–1415.

Flatley-Brennan, P. (1998). Computer network home care demonstration: A randomized trial in persons living with AIDS. *Computers in Biology & Medicine, 28,* 489–508.

Galavotti, C., Saltzman, L. E., Sauter, S. L., & Sumartojo, E. (1997). Behavioral science activities at the Centers for Disease Control and Prevention. A selected overview of exemplary programs. *American Psychology, 52,* 154–166.

Glasgow, R. E. (2002). Evaluation models for theory-based interventions. In K. Glanz, B. Rimer, & F. Lewis (Eds.), *Health behavior and health education* (3rd ed., pp. 530–544). San Francisco: Jossey-Bass.

Glasgow, R. E., Boles, S. M., McKay, H. G., Feil, E. G., & Barrera, M. (2003). The D-Net diabetes self-management program: Long-term implementation, outcomes, and generalization results. *Preventive Medicine, 36,* 410–419.

Glasgow, R. E., La Chance, P. A., Toobert, D. J., Brown, J., Hampson, S. E., & Riddle, M. C. (1997). Long-term effects and costs of brief behavioural dietary intervention for patients with diabetes delivered from the medical office. *Patient Education Counseling, 32,* 175–184.

Glasgow, R. E., & Toobert, D. J. (2000). Brief, computer-assisted diabetes dietary self-management counseling: Effects on behavior, physiologic outcomes, and quality of life. *Medical Care, 38,* 1062–1073.

Gottlieb, S. (2000). Study explores Internet as a tool for care of diabetic patients. *British Medical Journal, 320,* 892.

Gustafson, D. H., Hawkins, R., Boberg, E., Pingree, S., Serlin, R. E., Graziano, F., et al. (1999). Impact of a patient-centered, computer-based health information/support system. *American Journal of Preventive Medicine, 16,* 1–9.

Gustafson, D. H., McTavish, F. M., Boberg, E., Owens, B. H., Sherbeck, C., Wise, M., et al. (1999). Empowering patients using computer based health support systems. *Quality Health Care, 8,* 49–56.

Gustafson, D. H., Robinson, T. N., Ansley, D., Adler, L., & Brennan, P. F. (1999). Consumers and evaluation of interactive health communication applications. The Science Panel on Interactive Communication and Health. *American Journal of Preventive Medicine, 16,* 23–29.

Hospers, H. J., Harterink, P., van Den Hoek, K., & Veenstra, J. (2002). Chatters on the Internet: A special target group for HIV prevention. *AIDS Care, 14,* 539–544.

Kaplan, B., Farzanfar, R., & Friedman, R. H. (2003). Personal relationships with an intelligent interactive telephone health behavior advisor system: A multimethod study using surveys and ethnographic interviews. *International Journal of Medical Information, 71,* 33–41.

Keller, S. N., LaBelle, H., Karimi, N., & Gupta, S. (2002). STD/HIV prevention for teenagers: A look at the Internet universe. *Journal of Health Communication, 7,* 341–353.

Keller, S. N., LaBelle, H., Karimi, N., & Gupta, S. (2004). Talking about STD/HIV prevention: A look at communication online. *AIDS Care, 16,* 977–992.

Kelly, J. A., St. Lawrence, J. S., Diaz, Y. E., Stevenson, L. Y., Hauth, A. C., Brasfield, T. L., et al. (1991). HIV risk behavior reduction following intervention with key opinion leaders of population: An experimental analysis. *American Journal of Public Health, 81,* 168–171.

Kelly, J. A., St. Lawrence, J. S., Stevenson, L. Y., Hauth, A. C., Kalichman, S. C., Diaz, Y. E., et al. (1992). Community AIDS/HIV risk reduction: The effects of endorsements by popular people in three cities. *American Journal of Public Health, 82,* 1483–1489.

Klausner, J. D., Wolf, W., Fischer-Ponce, L., Zolt, I., & Katz, M. H. (2000). Tracing a syphilis outbreak through cyberspace. *Journal of the American Medical Association, 284,* 447–449.

Kreuter, M. W., & Strecher, V. J. (1995). Changing inaccurate perceptions of health risk: Results from a randomized trial. *Health Psychology, 14,* 56–63.

Lenhart, A., Horrigan, J., Rainie, L., Allen, K., Boyce, A., Madden, M., et al. (2003). The ever-shifting Internet population: A new look at Internet access and the digital divide. Retrieved from http://www.pewinternet.org/PPF/r/88/report_display.asp

Lenhart, A., Madden, M., & Hitlin, P. (2005). Teens and technology: Youth are leading the transition to a fully wired and mobile nation. Retrieved from http://www.pewinternet.org/PPF/r/162/report_display.asp

Lipkus, I. M., Lyna, P. R., & Rimer, B. K. (1999). Using tailored interventions to enhance smoking cessation among African-Americans at a community health center. *Nicotine & Tobacco Research, 1,* 77–85.

Mallory, C. (1997). What's on the Internet? Services for women affected by HIV and AIDS. *Health Care for Women International, 18,* 315–322.

Marcus, A. C., Heimendinger, J., Wolfe, P., Rimer, B. K., Morra, M., Cox, D., et al. (1998). Increasing fruit and vegetable consumption among callers to the CIS: Results from a randomized trial. *Preventive Medicine, 27,* 16–28.

Marcus, B. H., Emmons, K. M., Simkin-Silverman, L. R., Linnan, L. A., Taylor, E. R., Bock, B. C., et al. (1998). Evaluation of motivationally tailored vs. standard self-help physical activity interventions at the workplace. *American Journal of Health Promotion, 12,* 246–253.

Marcus, B. H., Owen, N., Forsyth, L. H., Cavill, N. A., & Fridinger, F. (1998). Physical activity interventions using mass media, print media, and information technology. *American Journal of Preventive Medicine, 15,* 362–278.

McFarlane, M., Bull, S. S., & Rietmeijer, C. A. (2000). The Internet as a newly emerging risk environment for sexually transmitted diseases [comment]. *Journal of the American Medical Association, 284,* 443–446.

McFarlane, M., Bull, S. S., & Rietmeijer, C. A. (2002). Young adults on the Internet: Risk behaviors for sexually transmitted diseases and HIV(1). *Journal of Adolescent Health, 31,* 11–16.

Noar, S. M., Clark, A., Cole, C., & Lustria, M. (2006). Review of interactive safer sex websites: Practice and potential. *Health Communication, 20*(3), 233–241.

Obermayer, J. L., Riley, W. T., Asif, O., & Jean-Mary, J. (2004). College smoking-cessation using cell phone text messaging. *Journal of American College Health, 53,* 71–78.

Oenema, A., Brug, J., & Lechner, L. (2001). Web-based tailored nutrition education: Results of a randomized controlled trial. *Health Education Research, 16,* 647–660.

Padgett, P. (2003, August). *The effects of the Internet on women's sexual health and sexuality.* Paper presented at the STD/HIV Prevention and the Internet Conference, Washington, DC.

Piette, J. D. (1999). Patient education via automated calls: A study of English and Spanish speakers with diabetes. *American Journal of Preventive Medicine, 17,* 138–141.

Piette, J. D. (2000a). Interactive voice response systems in the diagnosis and management of chronic disease. *American Journal of Managed Care, 6,* 817–827.

Piette, J. D. (2000b). Satisfaction with automated telephone disease management calls and its relationship to their use. *Diabetes Education, 26,* 1003–1010.

Piette, J. D., McPhee, S. J., Weinberger, M., Mah, C. A., & Kraemer, F. B. (1999). Use of automated telephone disease management calls in an ethnically diverse sample of low-income patients with diabetes. *Diabetes Care, 22,* 1302–1309.

Piette, J. D., Weinberger, M., & McPhee, S. J. (2000). The effect of automated calls with telephone nurse follow-up on patient-centered outcomes of diabetes care: A randomized, controlled trial. *Medical Care, 38,* 218–230.

Piette, J. D., Weinberger, M., McPhee, S. J., Mah, C. A., Kraemer, F. B., & Crapo, L. M. (2000). Do automated calls with nurse follow-up improve self-care and glycemic control among vulnerable patients with diabetes? *American Journal of Medicine, 108,* 20–27.

Rakowski, W., Ehrich, B., Goldstein, M. G., Rimer, B. K., Pearlman, D. N., Clark, M. A., et al. (1998). Increasing mammography among women aged 40-74 by use of a stage-matched, tailored intervention. *American Journal of Preventive Medicine, 27,* 748–756.

Rheingold, H. (2002). *Smart mobs: The next social revolution.* New York: Basic Books.

Rhodes, S. D., DiClemente, R. J., Cecil, H., Hergenrather, K. C., & Yee, L. J. (2002). Risk among men who have sex with men in the United States: A comparison of an Internet sample and a conventional outreach sample. *AIDS Education and Prevention, 14,* 41–50.

Rhodes, S. D., DiClemente, R. J., Yee, L. J., & Hergenrather, K. C. (2001). Correlates of hepatitis B vaccination in a high-risk population: An Internet sample. *American Journal of Medicine, 110,* 628–632.

Rietmeijer, C. A., Bull, S. S., McFarlane, M., Patnaik, J. L., & Douglas, J. M. (2003). Risks and benefits of the internet for populations at risk for sexually transmitted infections (STIs): Results of an STI clinic survey. *Sexually Transmitted Diseases, 30,* 15–19.

Rietmeijer, C. A., Patnaik, J. L., Judson, F. N., & Douglas, J. M. (2003). Increases in gonorrhea and sexual risk behaviors among men who have sex with men: A 12-year trend analysis at the Denver Metro Health Clinic. *Sexually Transmitted Diseases, 30,* 562–567.

Rimer, B. K., Conway, M., Lyna, P., Glassman, B., Yarnall, S. H., Lipkus, I., et al. (1999). The impact of tailored interventions on a community health center population. *Patient Education and Counseling, 37,* 125–140.

Rimer, B. K., & Glassman, B. (1998). Tailored communication for primary care settings. *Methods of Information in Medicine, 37,* 171–178.

Ross, M. W., Rosser, B. R., & Stanton, J. (2004). Beliefs about cybersex and Internet-mediated sex of Latino men who have Internet sex with men: Relationships with sexual practices in cybersex and in real life. *AIDS Care, 16,* 1002–1011.

Sheeran, P., Abraham, C., & Orbell, S. (1999). Psychosocial correlates of heterosexual condom use: A meta-analysis. *Psychological Bulletin, 125,* 90–132.

Skinner, C. S., Siegfried, J. C., Kegler, M. C., & Strecher, V. J. (1993). The potential of computers in patient education. *Patient Education and Counseling, 22,* 27–34.

Skinner, C. S., Strecher, V. J., & Hospers, H. (1994). Physician recommendation for mammography: Do tailored messages make a difference? *American Journal of Public Health, 84,* 43–49.

Smith, M., Gertz, E., Alvarez, S., & Lurie, P. (2000). The content and accessibility of sex education information on the Internet. *Health Education and Behavior, 27,* 684–694.

Stevens, V. J., Glasgow, R. E., Toobert, D. J., Karanja, N., & Smith, K. S. (2003). One-year results from a brief, computer-assisted intervention to decrease consumption of fat and increase consumption of fruits and vegetables. *Preventive Medicine, 36,* 594–600.

Strom, L., Pettersson, R., & Andersson, G. (2000). A controlled trial of self-help treatment of recurrent headache conducted via the Internet. *Journal of Consulting and Clinical Psychology, 68,* 722–727.

Tate, D. F., Wing, R. R., & Winett, R. A. (2001). Using Internet technology to deliver a behavioral weight loss program. *Journal of the American Medical Association, 285,* 1172–1177.

Williams, G. C., McGregor, H., Zeldman, A., Freedman, Z. R., Deci, E. L., & Elder, D. (2005). Promoting glycemic control through diabetes self-management: Evaluating a patient activation intervention. *Patient Education and Counseling, 56,* 28–34.

Williams, M. (2005, July). *Sexual health and Internet.* Paper presented at the International Society of Sexually Transmitted Disease Research Conference, Internet Symposium, Amsterdam, the Netherlands.

Williams, M. L., Bowen, A. M., & Horvath, K. J. (2005). The social/sexual environment of gay men residing in a rural frontier state: Implications for the development of HIV prevention programs. *Journal of Rural Health, 21,* 48–55.

# II

*Intervention Exemplar Chapters*

# 14

# Reducing Risky Sex Through the Use of Interactive Video Technology

*Paul Robert Appleby*

*Carlos Godoy*

*Lynn Carol Miller*

*Stephen J. Read*
University of Southern California

The goal of the current project was to produce three HIV prevention interactive videos (IAVs), one for each of the highest risk ethnic groups (African American, White, and Latino) of young men who have sex with men (MSM), to reduce HIV risk taking. The overall structure and content of each of the videos was identical except that each of the videos was designed to be appropriate for each group. Pilot research and community advisory boards (CABS), which represented each of the ethnic groups, informed the culturally specific elements for each script (i.e., slang for sexual terms and drugs, proxemics, etc.) These IAVs use a DVD platform, which allowed for greater interactivity (i.e., more choice points), more content, and higher quality content than had our prototype CD-ROM reported in Read et al. (2006).

## Description of IAVs

Each IAV is played on a DVD with a standard television and remote control. When played, two guide characters begin by explaining the objectives of the video and setting the story up for the user. Men who use the video are asked to identify with the main character and are given the opportunity to make choices, seek advice, and guide their character's actions (using their remote control). The user is then taken on a virtual date where he can make choices about where he meets his partner (club or Internet), whether he accepts drugs or alcohol, and finally the type of sex he wants to have, ranging from safe (mutual masturbation) to very risky (unprotected anal sex) or somewhere in between (e.g., oral sex, protected anal sex). The guide characters are always available to give advice about what choice to make. They also reinforce safer choices and gently rebuff the user if his choices are risky. At the end of the video, recaps of the user's choices and the implications of each choice are reviewed by the guides and a condom demonstration is played.

## Theory and Development

In developing the content for the IAVs, a review of the literature was conducted and key psychosocial variables were identified. Our previous research indicated that feelings of trust are often barriers to using condoms (Appleby, Miller, & Rothspan, 1999) and that eliciting consideration of future consequences might reduce risk taking (Appleby et al., 2005). We therefore integrated a discussion of consequences (e.g., "even though there are treatments for HIV, they don't work for everyone and the side effects are no picnic") and addressed feelings of trust by introducing the possibility that some partners, no matter how attractive and healthy they appear, may lie, or not know, about their HIV-positive status. We were also influenced by Bandura's cognitive social learning theory and worked hard to create realistic social situations that would simulate the circumstances under which different types of negotiation might occur. Our goal was to create the *when, where,* and *how* of risk-reducing safe-sex negotiations. Using research on implemental intentions (Gollwitzer, 1990; Gollwitzer & Moskowitz, 1996), we sought to *activate* a series of narrative linkages for viewers according to those specific circumstances they would most likely encounter in real life. Drawing on work by Miller and Read (1991) and Read and Miller (1995), we constructed narratives that served as a self-regulatory "glue" with the intention of increasing safer sex behavior in a variety of future contexts (Miller & Read, 2005; Read et al., 2006). By allowing viewers to create their own context-specific narratives, we sought to build concrete intentions that would likely be processed heuristically under future similar circumstances. One strength of the video is that it can be sexually arousing, increasing the similarity between the intervention and a typical sexual encounter. Instruction that occurs under psychological and emotional states similar to those under which the behavior will be enacted should improve transfer to the subsequent situation. Because our IAV incorporates safer sex education into a semirealistic context (including sexual arousal), this should greatly enhance the recall and application of critical cognitive and behavioral skills, such as self-control strategies and sexual-negotiation techniques.

Through the use of guide characters, whose role was to provide feedback on *a real-time* basis, we were able to incorporate frame specific messages according to the type of behaviors selected. For example, prior research has shown that gain frames work best for prevention (i.e., giving praise for *successfully* negotiating safer sex) whereas loss frames work better in more risky situations (i.e., emphasizing the dangers of deciding *not* to use a condom). The guides also, in conjunction with the overall narrative structure, provided countermessages, or resistance strategies potential partners might use to avoid practicing safe sex in order to inoculate and teach viewers how to negotiate around these potential pitfalls.

Pilot research was conducted to identify typical sexual scripts including both verbal and nonverbal communication modalities involved in sexual negotiation and intimate encounters. Pilot questions also focused on specific elements that were intended to be part of the storyline so that the narrative would be authentic for the audience. For example, our pilot data informed us that young MSM are typically connecting for casual sex at bars or clubs and over the Internet. Finally, after preliminary scripts were developed, CABS were used to help modify and strengthen our preliminary scripts.

## Production

The production process is complex and demands collaboration with cinema experts. There are two lessons we learned when undertaking production. First, actors, directors, cinematographers, and production designers often want to impose their own creative vision on the production. There are times when such creativity is appropriate and times when it is not. It is therefore necessary to have a social science representative from the project on site during filming. Sometimes improvisation is inconsequential; sometimes it has great consequence if it changes your message. The director must be taken aside by the on-set researcher and told immediately if there is a problem, so that the scene can be reshot with the appropriate dialogue in the appropriate manner. If this is not done, much of what you need from a research/educational perspective may not get filmed. Second, half of your production budget should be slated for postproduction. In this media form, postproduction is much greater than just editing, color correction, and music. The programming aspect of interactive technology—which allows the viewers to experience their choices in the order of their choosing—is elaborate. Programming is thus labor intensive, and there are few programmers who have learned to push the limits of DVD technology to our level of interactive sophistication. This increases postproduction costs.

Preliminary Evaluation

We are early in the evaluation process of the IAVs, but preliminary results are promising. Participants (ages 18–30) were recruited from Los Angeles County through venue-based sampling and advertising (Internet and print) and must have engaged in unprotected anal sex with either a primary or nonprimary partner in the past 3 months. Participants who viewed the IAV reported significantly higher levels of sexual arousal than those who did not view the IAV (control group). This is important because sexual arousal is a key part of our hypotheses with respect to the recall and application of information contained in the IAV to real-life experiences. Furthermore, behavioral intentions to practice safer sex and self-efficacy (i.e., confidence about one's abilities to negotiate safer sex) were significantly greater for the IAV group than for the control group.

Those who have viewed the IAVs have generally evaluated them positively. On scales ranging from (1) *not at all* to (10) *very much,* median scores were 8 or above on the following key variables: believability of guide characters, cultural and age appropriateness of information, and relevance of the information.

## Conclusion

Behavioral data from our prototype study and preliminary data from our current study support the efficacy and salience of IAV as an HIV intervention for young MSM. This relatively new paradigm for health intervention provides a rich integrative theoretical and methodological framework for reaching, tailoring to, and connecting with at-risk individuals who have "tuned out" traditional approaches to behavior change.

## Acknowledgments

The project described was supported by Grant R01 AI052756 from the National Institute of Allergy and Infectious Diseases (NIAID). Its contents are solely the responsibility of the authors and do not necessarily represent the official views of the NIAID.

## References

Appleby, P. R., Marks, G., Ayala, A., Miller, L. C., Murphy, S., & Mansergh, G. (2005). Consideration of future consequences and unprotected anal intercourse among men who have sex with men. *Journal of Homosexuality, 50*(1), 119–133.

Appleby, P. R., Miller, L. C., & Rothspan, S. (1999). The paradox of trust for male couples: When risking is a part of loving. *Personal Relationships, 6*, 81–93.

Gollwitzer, P. M. (1990). Action phases and mind-sets. In E. T. Higgins & R. M. Sorrentino (Eds.), *Handbook of motivation and cognition: Foundations of social behavior* (Vol. 2, pp. 53–92). New York: Guilford.

Gollwitzer, P. M., & Moskowitz, G. B. (1996). Goal effects on action and cognition. In E. T. Higgins & A. W. Kruglanski (Eds.), *Social psychology: Handbook of basic principles* (pp. 361–399). New York: Guilford.

Miller, L. C., & Read, S. J. (1991). On the coherence of mental models of persons and relationships: A knowledge structure approach. In G. J. O. Fletcher & F. D. Fincham (Eds.), *Cognition in close relationships* (pp. 69–99). Hillsdale, NJ: Lawrence Erlbaum Associates.

Miller, L. C., & Read, S. J. (2005). Virtual sex: Creating environments for reducing risky sex. In S. Cohen, K. Portnoy, D. Rehberger, & C. Thorsen (Eds.), *Virtual decisions: Digital simulations for teaching reasoning in the social sciences and humanities* (pp. 137–159). Mahwah, NJ: Lawrence Erlbaum Associates.

Read, S. J., & Miller, L. C. (1995). Stories are fundamental to meaning and memory: For social creatures, could it be otherwise? In R. S. Wyer, Jr. (Ed.), *Advances in social cognition: Vol. 8. Knowledge and memory: The real story* (pp. 139–152). Hillsdale, NJ: Lawrence Erlbaum Associates.

Read, S. J., Miller, L. C., Appleby, P. R., Nwosu, M. E., Reynaldo, S., Lauren, A., et al. (2006). Socially optimized learning in a virtual environment: Reducing risky sexual behavior among men who have sex with men. *Human Communication Research, 32*, 1–34.

# 15

# The Internet
## Accessible and Affordable HIV Prevention for Rural MSM

*Sara Clayton*

*Candice M. Daniel*

*Anne Bowen*
University of Wyoming

HIV/AIDS cases in rural areas are predominantly among men who have sex with men (MSM; Wyoming Department of Health [WDH], 2005). Rural MSM are often socially isolated (Cody & Welch, 1997), hiding their sexual preference because of the conservative nature of rural areas. In the last 10 years, rural MSM have increasingly utilized the Internet as a mechanism for communication with other MSM. The Internet's availability, affordability, and anonymity (Cooper, 1998) have provided rural men with a vehicle for learning about gay lifestyles, coming out, finding sex partners, and unfortunately increased incidence of sexually transmitted diseases (STDs) and possibly HIV. The high frequency of Internet use along with the ability of the men to remain anonymous also makes the Internet a potentially ideal mechanism for contacting and recruiting rural MSM and providing them with prevention materials.

The Wyoming Rural AIDS Prevention Project (WRAPP) began in 2001 with an overall goal of developing an Internet-delivered HIV prevention program to rural MSM. To this end, we developed three Internet prevention modules (Project HOPE) based on Internet survey data collected in the first 2 years of the project. Social cognitive theory (Bandura, 1986) was used as a foundation for both the survey and the interventions. The three interventions of Project HOPE include knowledge, contexts of risk, and sexual partners. Each intervention includes two 20-minute modules and the men may participate in all three interventions.

The knowledge intervention focuses on (a) understanding HIV infection, including medications, side effects, and testing, and (b) prevention behaviors including correct condom use. There are many interactive activities within the knowledge intervention, such as the Wheel of Risk, the Condom Slot Machine, a Handful of Pills, and the Body. In the Wheel of Risk, participants can click on a different section of the wheel to see how things like STDs, Feelings, the Internet, Alcohol and Drugs, Anal Sex, and Oral Sex can contribute to HIV risk. The Condom Slot Machine gives you two credits to start. Each time the participant "spins," he gets some mixture of a condom, a condom with a slash through it, or a picture of a virus. If the participant spins three condoms, he wins a credit. For any combination of no condom or virus, the participant loses credits. The Handful of Pills shows a hand holding all the different HIV medications. The participant can roll over each pill to learn more about it, as well as the daily and yearly cost of each medication. Finally, the Body allows participants to roll over different parts of the body to see how HIV medications affect the body's functioning.

The sexual partners intervention modules discuss issues specific to new and casual partners. The new partners module has the participant identify a life goal and then procedes through an interactive dialogue that examines how that goal would be affected if the participant became infected with HIV. Participants may repeat the "conversation" with a different goal or pick different responses as often they like. The module ends with participants choosing a personal approach to introducing condoms with a new partner. The casual partner module begins with an interactive conversation about renegotiating safer sex with a casual partner and then in high-risk contexts such as when the participant is lonely or drunk. Each participant's personalized feedback sheet summarizes his life goals and how they may be affected by HIV, communication skills for negotiating condom use that he would be comfortable using, and personal excuses that may hinder him from using condoms.

The short-term acceptability and efficacy of the knowledge intervention has been tested in a pilot randomized control trial with a wait-list control (Bowen, Horvath, & Williams, 2006). Group 1 received the intervention immediately with a pretest, posttest, and 1-week follow-up. Group 2 took the pretest, waited 1 week and retook the pretest, then entered the intervention and took the posttest. Outcome measures included retention, acceptability, knowledge, self-efficacy, and outcome expectancies. Ninety men were recruited, with 80% retention, and data were analyzed using an intent-to-treat model. The men rated the intervention as highly acceptable with a slightly lower rating by men who had slower access to the Internet. The men's knowledge, self-efficacy, and outcome expectancies increased significantly, contingent on participation in the intervention, and no changes were seen as a result of assessment only.

The recruiting phase of the WRAPP project is complete and we are currently collecting follow-up data. The primary goal of the study is to assess the acceptability and short-term efficacy of three interventions. Currently, data are available from 202 men, who have completed the three intervention modules and their associated posttests. Qualitative feedback has been generally positive and preliminary data analyses indicate that there are positive and significant changes in knowledge, self-efficacy, and outcome expectancies. The data also indicate that order of participation in the intervention modules may be important. It appears that participation in the knowledge intervention, either first or alone, causes negative outcome expectancies for condom use to become more negative. On the other hand, participation in either the context or partner intervention first, with knowledge as the last intervention, results in significant reductions in negative outcome expectancies. Though changes in cognitive predictors of risk behavior are positive, behavioral outcomes are not yet available.

## References

Bandura, A. (1986). *Social foundations of thought and action: A social cognitive theory.* Englewood Cliffs, NJ: Prentice-Hall.

Bowen, A., Horvath, K., & Williams, M. (2006). Randomized control trial of an Internet delivered HIV knowledge intervention with MSM. *Health Education and Research, 22*(1), 120–127.

Cody, P. J., & Welch, P. L. (1997). Rural gay men in northern New England: Life experiences and coping styles. *Journal of Homosexuality, 33,* 51–67.

Cooper, A. (1998). Sexuality and the Internet: Surfing into the new millennium. *Cyber Psychology & Behavior, 1,* 187–193.

Wyoming Department of Health. (2005). *Wyoming HIV/AIDS surveillance report*. Retrieved April 18, 2006, from http://wdh.state.wy.us/HIV-Surveillance/statpage.asp

# 16

# Using Communication Strategies in an HIV Prevention Curriculum to Enhance African-American Adolescents' Adoption of HIV-Preventive Behaviors

*Ralph J. DiClemente*

*Nikia D. Braxton*

*Jessica McDermott Sales*

*Gina M. Wingood*
Emory University

Unprotected sexual activity increases the risk of young people acquiring sexually transmitted diseases (STDs), including HIV. Indeed, nearly one half of all newly diagnosed STDs occur among adolescents ages 15 to 24 (Cates, Herndon, Schulz, & Darroch, 2004). The adverse health and social consequences of STD/HIV are not uniform across adolescents. African-American women and girls have been identified at particularly high risk for acquiring STD/HIV, thereby making STD/HIV interventions specifically tailored for this subgroup a public health priority.

Although a number of factors have been suggested to influence adolescent sexual risk taking (DiClemente, Salazar, Crosby, & Rosenthal, 2005), one factor that has been consistently associated with increased safer sex is sexual communication (DiClemente & Crosby, 2003). Sexual communication is particularly critical for young women who may be the "gatekeepers" in their relationships, as they decide where, when, or if sex should occur, and must negotiate this with their male partners.

Refusal skills are also especially important among young girls who may experience substantial pressure for unwanted sex. Furthermore, sexual communication with regard to condom use is uniquely important for women and girls; because they cannot use condoms independently, they must negotiate their use with male partners. Thus, it is imperative that interventions designed to impact the adoption and maintenance of safer-sex behavior prominently emphasize enhancing adolescents' communication and negotiation skills.

To address the aforementioned health disparity, our research team recently developed and evaluated a theory-guided, culturally appropriate, and gender-tailored sexual risk reduction program, with an emphasis on sexual communication skills, for African-American female adolescents, called SiHLE (*Sistas Informing, Healing, Living and Empowering*). SiHLE was conceptualized by Drs. DiClemente and Wingood and is a modified version of an established and efficacious HIV intervention for African-American women 18 to 29 years of age that has been adopted by the Centers for Disease Control and Prevention (CDC) in their *Compendium of HIV Prevention Programs with Demonstrated Evidence of Effectiveness* (DiClemente & Wingood, 1995).

## Study Participants and Procedures

The study included 522 African-American adolescent females, 14 to 18 years of age, who reported being sexually active in the preceding 6 months. The study design was a randomized controlled trial. Participants were randomly assigned to either the SiHLE HIV intervention or a time-equivalent general health promotion (GHP) comparison condition. The SiHLE intervention and GHP comparison condition each consisted of four, 4-hour interactive group sessions, implemented over consecutive Saturdays. Each session averaged 10 to 12 participants, and was implemented by a trained African-American female health educator and was cofacilitated by two African-American female peer educators.

## HIV Intervention Condition

The aim of SiHLE was to reduce the risk of HIV and STDs among sexually active African-American adolescent females (DiClemente et al., 2004). Social cognitive theory (Bandura, 1994) and the theory of gender and power (Wingood & DiClemente, 2000) were complementary theoretical frameworks guiding the design and implementation of the SiHLE. Social cognitive theory addresses both the psychosocial dynamics facilitating health behavior and the methods of promoting behavior change (i.e., modeling). Applying the gender-relevant theoretical framework of the theory of gender and power was critical as it highlighted HIV-related social processes prevalent in the lives of African-American female adolescents such as having older male sex partners and lack of communication skills relevant for enhancing safer sex. Ultimately, by creating an intervention for adolescent females grounded in both social cognitive theory and the theory of gender and power, both of which highlight, to varying degrees, the importance of effective communication, we hoped to more fully address the processes impeding women's adoption of health-promoting behaviors while teaching multidimensional strategies, including communication skills, to reduce STD/HIV-associated risk behaviors.

## Communication Is Key

Young women must feel confident and competent to assertively convey their sexual intentions and possess effective communication skills to negotiate safer sex. Many of the SiHLE intervention activities addressed the multiple dimensions of effective communication skills. Specifically, SIHLE provides training in both verbal and nonverbal communication. In addition, SiHLE differentiates and provides training in different communication styles, such as passive, assertive, and aggressive communication styles. Furthermore, SiHLE uses a gradient of emotion-laden topics to rehearse resisting partner pressures to engage in unsafe sex, using both refusal skills and condom negotiation skills. Role-playing scenarios were initially used to model assertive communication in nonsexual scenarios and, once proficient, in more emotionally laden sexual situations (e.g., demanding that their male sex partner use condoms). Adolescents' participation in these guided role-playing scenarios enhanced their proficiency in communication skills and, as a consequence, increased their sense of communication self-efficacy. Additionally, facilitators provided positive reinforcing feedback for role plays that used assertive communication and appropriate skills and corrective feedback for role plays that did not apply assertive communication and skills.

## Efficacy of the SiHLE Intervention

To assess the efficacy of the SiHLE intervention, data collection occurred at baseline (i.e., before participating in the intervention), as well as 6 and 12 months after participating in the intervention. Relative to participants in the GHP condition, participants in the SiHLE HIV intervention condition were more likely to report using condoms consistently in the 30 days preceding the 6-month assessment (Intervention = 75.3% vs. Comparison = 58.2%), and at the 12-month assessment (Intervention = 73.3% vs. Comparison = 56.5%). Likewise, participants in the HIV intervention were more likely to report using condoms consistently during the 6 months prior to the 6-month assessment (Intervention = 61.3% vs. Comparison = 42.6%), and at the 12-month assessment (Intervention = 58.1% vs. Comparison = 45.3%). Additionally, participants in the HIV intervention were more likely to report using a condom at last vaginal sexual intercourse, less likely to self-report a pregnancy, and less likely to report having a new vaginal sex partner in the 30 days prior to assessments. Important to note, the SiHLE intervention was also effective at reducing the incidence of chlamydia infections and pregnancy over the entire 12-month follow-up period.

The SiHLE intervention also had marked effects on empirically and theoretically derived psychosocial mediators of STD/HIV-preventive behaviors. Participants in the SiHLE intervention reported fewer perceived partner-related barriers to condom use, more favorable attitudes toward using condoms, more frequent discussions with male sex partners about HIV prevention (one measure of communication), higher condom use self-efficacy scores, and higher HIV prevention knowledge scores, and demonstrated greater proficiency in using condoms at the 6- and the 12-month assessments and over the entire 12-month period.

## Lessons Learned

SiHLE is the first HIV/STD intervention to not only enhance theoretically important mediators of safer-sex behavior and reduce risk behaviors associated with disease acquisition, but also to decrease adverse biological sequelae, such as STDs and unintended pregnancy, among a vulnerable adolescent subgroup. Though effective, there is always the opportunity to learn from our research and optimize future interventions. One important lesson learned was that communication skills are central to the behavior change process, particularly for young adolescent females, many of whom are in power imbalanced relationships. Indeed, although highly effective, future studies may consider engaging young men in role-playing scenarios with participants to increase the "realism" of the training.

## Dissemination of SiHLE

Ultimately, controlling the HIV/STD epidemic among youth is dependent not only on the development of effective behavioral interventions, like SiHLE, but perhaps more importantly, on how effectively these interventions can be disseminated and integrated into sustainable community, school, and clinic programs. With respect to SiHLE, the CDC DEBI program has adopted SiHLE for national dissemination through training institutes held across the United States. We are currently developing a training curriculum to assist the CDC in these efforts. In addition, though SiHLE was tailored for African-American female adolescents, there is growing interest in developing comparable programs tailored to other ethnic/racial populations (i.e., Latinas, White, Asian) as well as programs designed to be gender and culturally appropriate for male adolescents, in particular, African-American male adolescents. Currently, we are collaborating with CDC on developing a systematic protocol for the adaptation of SiHLE for other at-risk adolescent populations.

## Implications

In an era when adolescents are one of the fastest-growing groups acquiring STD/HIV, it is crucial that effective sexual-risk reduction interventions are created and implemented in an attempt to curtail this physically, emotionally, and financially devastating epidemic. Although a multitude of factors undoubtedly influence adolescents' adoption of safer sexual practices, this study suggests that focusing on improving sexual communication and negotiation skills in young women is a key ingredient for reducing risky sexual practices in this at-risk population. Future interventions for adolescents, especially female adolescents, need to further enhance their emphasis on communication and negotiation skills as a critical factor for promoting the adoption and maintenance of STD/HIV preventive practices.

## References

Bandura, A. (1994). Social cognitive theory and exercise of control over HIV infections. In R. J. DiClemente & J. L. Peterson (Ed.), *Preventing AIDS: Theories and methods of behavioral interventions* (pp. 25–29). New York: Plenum.

Cates, J. R., Herndon, N. L., Schulz, S. L., & Darroch, J. E. (2004). *Our voices, our lives, our futures: Youth and sexually transmitted diseases.* Chapel Hill: School of Journalism and Mass Communication, University of North Carolina at Chapel Hill.

DiClemente, R. J., & Crosby, R. A. (2003). Sexually transmitted diseases among adolescents: Risk factors, antecedents, and prevention strategies. In G. R. Adams & M. Berzonsky (Eds.), *The Blackwell handbook of adolescence* (pp. 573–605). Oxford, England: Blackwell.

DiClemente, R. J., Salazar, L. F., Crosby, R. A., & Rosenthal, S. L. (2005). Prevention and control of sexually transmitted infections among adolescents: The importance of a socio-ecological perspective: A commentary. *Public Health, 119,* 825–836.

DiClemente, R. J., & Wingood, G. M. (1995). A randomized controlled trial of an HIV sexual risk-reduction intervention for young adult African-American women. *Journal of the American Medical Association, 274,* 1271–1276.

DiClemente, R. J., Wingood, G. M., Harrington, K. F., Lang, D. F., Davies, S. L., Hook, E. W., III, et al. (2004). Efficacy of an HIV prevention intervention for African American adolescent girls: A randomized controlled trial. *Journal of the American Medical Association, 292,* 171–179.

Wingood, G. M., & DiClemente, R. J. (2000). Application of the theory of gender and power to reexamine HIV related exposures, risk factors and effective interventions for women. *Health Education and Behavior, 27,* 313–347.

# 17

# Social and Sexual Networks at STOP AIDS Project

## A New Strategy for Diffusing Messages

*Jennifer Hecht*
STOP AIDS Project

STOP AIDS Project, an HIV prevention organization run by and for gay men in San Francisco, has remained at the cutting edge of prevention for more than 20 years by maintaining a close relationship with community members and HIV prevention researchers. Our work focuses on behavioral interventions designed to reduce men's risk for HIV and other sexually transmitted diseases (STDs). A major tactic in achieving this goal is the creation of prevention messages and targeted campaigns that help gay men make conscious and informed decisions about their sexual behavior. Recently, we have augmented our HIV prevention strategies with an innovative approach focused on social and sexual network interventions. Our goal is to modify sexual network research for use in on-the-ground HIV prevention strategies.

A sexual network is a group of individuals who are connected through common sex partners. From this perspective, HIV and other STDs move through a population like electricity on a transmission grid. By modifying the grid (or sexual network), we can affect how quickly transmission occurs. In this way, targeted interventions with a select group of individuals or venues can reduce HIV and STD transmission for entire groups of men. Examples of sexual network intervention goals are: (a) changing network structure directly by affecting partner selection patterns, (b) targeting men who are influential in network structure (men who "bridge" one sexual network to another or those who are highly sexually active and centrally positioned in a given network), and (c) targeting venues that bridge one sexual network to another. Through this network paradigm we aim for outcomes such as: increasing disclosure of HIV status, decreasing sexual partnerships between high and low-risk MSM, increasing the frequency of HIV and STD testing, and facilitating sero-sorting (choosing a partner based on his sero-status) (Truong & McFarland, 2004).

Sexual networks and social networks often overlap. Our model uses a two-pronged approach: (a) structural interventions to modify sexual networks, which are in turn supported by (b) social network interventions that affect social norms. Our social network interventions employ the popular opinion leader (POL) model to diffuse messages (Kelly et al., 1991). The POL model relies on diffusion of innovations theory, which is a process for spreading new ideas throughout a population (Rogers, 2003). POLs are defined as people within a network who are most well-connected and influential, allowing for messages to be diffused and adopted more quickly by others in the network.

Our programming is designed around six groups, aimed to exemplify sexual networks, which consist of high-risk individuals and/or places where men meet other men for sex: bars/clubs, Internet, gyms, sex clubs and outdoor cruising spots, African American gay venues, and leathermen. Each network was chosen because it represents a group or place that men at high risk meet sex partners; decisions were based on epidemiologic data and anecdotal evidence from outreach in the community. Each network has an intervention coordinator responsible for organizing a team of volunteers, conducting outreach shifts in appropriate locations, staffing a community advisory board (CAB), and keeping a pulse on that network.

Prevention messages are developed and targeted for each network based on information collected formally through input of CAB members and network member interviews as well as informally through hundreds of one-on-one conversations during outreach shifts. Based on both qualitative and quantitative data collected within each network, messages are targeted to the HIV risks that are most relevant to that network. Messages are further tailored to individuals during one-on-one outreach conversations.

## Sample Messaging: Leather

In our leather network, we are attempting to increase the safety of sex that occurs between older and younger men. Older men are more likely to be HIV-positive than younger men and intergenerational sexual relationships are common in the leather network. To develop a campaign targeted toward this pattern of partner selection we took the mantra "safe, sane, and consensual," used by leathermen to guide negotiations of play scenes, and applied it to safer sex. With this underlying value of taking care of one another, we developed a campaign titled, "Protect your Daddy, Protect your Boy," which will encourage HIV disclosure and negotiation of safer sex.

The leather network has high social and sexual network overlap. By maintaining a presence at leather bars and play parties, recruiting POLs from within the leather community, and holding workshops, leather network members receive targeted messages from multiple sources to change the norms in the leather community.

## Sample Diffusion Methods: Bars/Clubs

The bars/clubs network is spreading messages using light-emitting diode (LED) belt buckles, allowing for a programmable sign like those seen on billboards to appear on their belts. A few of their messages said, "Thanks for playing safe!" "Stop Staring and Take my Condoms," and "Keep it Safe, Ho." POLs recruited from each of the clubs will diffuse these messages by wearing the belt buckles when they go out.

## Sample Diffusion Methods: Internet

An entirely different approach has been necessary for the Internet network. The medium of the Internet does not lend itself readily to the POL model, as POLs can be neither identified nor recognized by other Internet users. Our strategy for the Internet capitalizes on the strengths of that medium, namely guerilla marketing. We have developed a new symbol, much like existing emoticons (i.e., the smiley face that sometimes appears in e-mails) that depicts a preference for safer sex. The image is a condom unrolled to look like an exclamation point. The user attaches the emoticon to his profile in a posting for a sex encounter or while hooking up in a chat room. The emoticon is diffused via popular networking Web sites, using an Internet-adapted version of POLs, for example, men on myspace.com, friendster.com, and tribe.com with many "friends." These men are encouraged to post the new emoticon in their profiles to help create an online norm supporting negotiation about safer sex. When clicked, the emoticon reveals a safer-sex pledge and STOP AIDS Project's Web site URL.

## Outcomes

Tracking any network is an imperfect science. Where does the leather network end and another network begin? Researchers of sexual networks have traditionally asked study participants identifying information (such as names) to map networks, a feat that seems both impractical and unacceptable at the community level. We recognize that conducting network interventions in a community setting requires us to find alternative means of measuring networks. We ask men where they meet their sex partners; those who identify leather bars as places where they meet sex partners are included in leather network analyses for program planning and evaluation.

Our goal is to reach 20% to 30% of each network population, as suggested by the diffusion of innovations model. It is not yet feasible for us to determine whether we have achieved this goal. We do not have the resources to randomly sample these networks for evaluative purposes, nor do we know the size of each network. We are investigating new strategies for measuring networks that are within our financial means. We intend to measure changes in perception about safer sex, HIV-testing frequency, sero-sorting, sexual partnerships between high- and low-risk MSM, and rates of disclosure of HIV status within each network by conducting follow-up evaluations of men who attend our workshops.

## Challenges to the Model

Translating research into practice is not without challenges. We have applied sexual network characteristics from a research model to HIV prevention practice using sample sexual networks. Each network differs in its level of social/sexual network overlap, making some networks more appropriate for the POL model and diffusion of targeted messages. In addition, as we gain a better understanding of each network, our messaging and prevention strategies evolve to better reflect our target audience. Many questions remain after our first year of implementation: Have we chosen the right networks? What are the appropriate structural and social norms interventions for each network? How will we document changes by network?

## Conclusion

STOP AIDS Project's new effort, focused on using social networks to support sexual network interventions, is a hybrid model designed to capitalize on the strengths of each prevention model as well as the strengths of our agency and staff. Using the creative energy and localized knowledge of our teams of outreach workers, we are able to diffuse creative, tailored messages that are relevant to each network.

## References

Kelly, J. A., St. Lawrence, J. S., Diaz, Y. E., Stevenson, L. Y., Hauth, A. C., Brasfield, T. L., et al. (1991). HIV risk behavior reduction following intervention with key opinion leaders of population: An experimental analysis. *American Journal of Public Health, 81,* 168–171.

Rogers, E. M. (2003). *Diffusion of innovations* (5th ed.). New York: The Free Press.

Truong, H. M., & McFarland, W. (2004, February). *Increases in "serosorting" may prevent further expansion of the HIV epidemic among MSM in San Francisco.* Paper presented at the 11th Conference on Retroviruses and Opportunistic Infections, San Francisco.

# 18

## Leveraging Entertainment Media to Communicate About AIDS
### The Kaiser Family Foundation Media Partnership Model

*Tina Hoff*

*Julia Davis*

*Matt James*
The Henry J. Kaiser Family Foundation

When there were three broadcast networks that everyone watched, getting out public service messages was pretty straightforward. But, today, in an age where there is a cable or satellite channel for every possible interest, the one-size-fits-all approach no longer works. Americans consume more media today than ever before. From digital video recorders that offer more control over when and how we view our favorite television shows to the array of devices for sending and receiving information, from instant messaging and streaming content on computers to text messaging on cell phones, to downloading music, news, and video on palm-size MP3 players, how we use media is rapidly changing and with it traditional approaches to advertising are being challenged. In this new media environment, public service advertising needed to become more sophisticated or risk being lost in the crowd.

In the mid-1990s, the Kaiser Family Foundation, a nonprofit independent health information and research organization, began exploring different approaches to getting out public health information through entertainment media. Central to our strategy was an idea that we could more effectively reach our target populations if we partnered with media companies popular with those audiences, and if we secured donated airtime upfront for our campaigns. Our first such "entertainment media partnership" with a television network was with Music Television (MTV) in 1997, followed shortly thereafter by one with Black Entertainment Television (BET) in 1998, and a number of others in the years to come, including UPN, CBS, Nickelodeon, Fox, and Univision. Prior to that, the Foundation had teamed up with popular women's and teen's magazines, such as *Glamour*, *Self*, *seventeen*, and *YM*, employing a new editorial partnership model, to reach readers with critical reproductive health information.

In 2003, the Foundation forged a ground-breaking public education partnership with Viacom, Inc. and CBS Corporation, the corporate parents of the publisher Simon & Schuster, broadcasters CBS and the CW, Paramount Pictures, King World, CBS Radio and Outdoor, and an array of cable properties including Vh1, Comedy Central, Country Music Television, and Showtime, among others. This new effort—called *KNOW HIV/AIDS*—signified an unprecedented commitment by a media company to address HIV/AIDS (let alone any single public health issue) in a cross-platform manner more commonly used for commercial ventures but never before for social causes. In the most recent year of the campaign, 2005, Viacom estimated the value of ad space devoted to the campaign exceeded $200 million. Particularly notable, however, was the way the partnership leveraged Viacom's content with the Foundation's substantive expertise to incorporate the campaign issues and messages into top-rated television programming from *Girlfriends* to *Judging Amy* to *Jeopardy!*

## A New Approach

In working with the media, our approach is flexible, strategic, and opportunistic. We seek partners our target audiences already value and consume and then look to utilize the full array of their assets and brand appeal to advance a particular social issue. For example, when we wanted to reach African Americans—one of the most impacted racial/ethnic groups—with information about HIV/AIDS, BET was a logical partner to work with to develop a public education partnership. As the nation's only dedicated television network for African Americans, BET is available in 8 million homes in the

United States, Canada, and the Carribean, and BET.com is the number one Internet portal for African Americans. Similary, when we looked for outlets that resonated with people under 25, MTV was one of the first partners we approached about developing a targeted sexual health campaign. This type of partnered approach to public education campaigns represented a significant departure from traditional social marketing strategies that tended to invent new messaging "products," like public service announcements (PSAs), which then effectively had to be "sold" as something of value to the target. Our campaigns built on the established credibility of brands that already had appeal with the populations we were trying to reach.

We found we were not only better able to target messages to specific audiences, but also secure up-front commitments of media space to ensure those messages were seen. By working directly with channels like MTV or BET, we could create programming that we knew would reach our target groups of youth and African Americans because those are the viewers who watch these networks. Rather than sending the same message out to all channels and hope for placement during times when our targets may be watching, we could develop advertising and other types of content specifically tailored to our primary targets, who are the majority of audiences that MTV and BET reach. Our messages—all of which offer a clear call to action, be it "get tested," "get more information," or "talk with..."—are developed to appeal to our target audiences, reflecting their unique information needs and circumstances. Also critical to our approach was to diversify the means we used to get out messages, and not rely solely on PSAs, but rather to use the full assets available from our media partners. We work with our partners both to seamlessly insert information into the storylines of television shows that are popular with our target audiences, as well as to coproduce original long-form programming, including public affairs, news, documentary, and entertainment shows. We have also employed "product placements" for campaign messages, for example, in the back of books and in inserts in CDs and DVDs with related themes produced by Viacom, as well as sought alliances with other complementary corporate brands to extend the reach of a campaign. Our media partners' Web sites—themselves popular online destinations for our target audiences—offer yet another platform extending the reach of our messages.

All of our campaigns offer free resources and referral services. In a 10- or 30-second television PSA, the scope of information that can be conveyed is limited, so our goal is to capture a viewer's attention and communicate a simple message (e.g., get tested for HIV, protect yourself, or talk with your health care provider) and direct them to other sources—a toll-free hotline or Web site—to find out more. Additionally, we seek to link our on-air and online campaigns with organizations serving our target groups on the ground, like health departments, schools, and youth-serving organizations.

## A Coordinated Strategy with Broad Reach

Collectively, the Foundation's ongoing U.S. public education campaigns—with BET, MTV, Univision, and Viacom—represent the largest coordinated media efforts in this country today addressing HIV/AIDS and related issues. Though each campaign is tailored to the audience and assets of the particular media partner, our involvement ensures that the efforts complement and reinforce one another for a greater overall impact.

In response, more than 2.5 million young people to date have called one of our dedicated hotlines to get free information or be connected to the Centers for Disease Control and Prevention's (CDC's) national HIV/STD counseling and referral service, and even more have gone online to get information from one of our Web sites. Approximately 1.3 million copies of one of our free informational guides have been distributed. Hundreds of millions of young people across the United States and in other parts of the world have seen the programming we produce with partners like MTV or BET.

A nationally representative telephone survey of younger African Americans conducted in 2004 confirmed that our information—primarily on BET, but also including some targeted messages in our campaign with Viacom—was reaching them. Fully 9 out of 10 (92%) of those aged 18 to 24 were familiar with the BET campaign brand (*Rap It Up*). Most reported having seen a recent PSA or longer-form show we produced, and the majority of those definite viewers report that they had learned something or taken action as a result of what they saw (Kaiser Family Foundation, 2003).

Eight in 10 (82%) learned something about how HIV/AIDS affects the African-American community; and a majority (57%) learned how prejudice may affect the fight against AIDS. Forty-five percent learned how to talk to a sexual partner about the issue. Half (52%)

reported that they were moved to do this by the ads or shows they saw. More than one in three viewers in this age group (37%) reported that they either visited a doctor or got tested for HIV because of the programming they saw (Kaiser Family Foundation, 2004).

An assessment of our campaign with MTV in 2003 found similar results. A nationally representative survey of 1,100 adolescents and young adults ages 16 to 24 found that three in five knew of *Fight For Rights: Protect Yourself,* the name of our campaign with MTV. Nearly three fourths (73%) of those who had seen our content on MTV reported being likely to take their sexual relationships "more seriously" as a result. Those who were already sexually active said they were more likely to use condoms (73%) and get tested for HIV or other STDs (65%) in response (Kaiser Family Foundation, 2003).

Our findings are corroborated by the research of others. In May of 2003, researchers from the CDC conducted an innovative study measuring the impact of a series of HIV-themed storylines on the UPN program *Girlfriends*—part of our *KNOW HIV/AIDS* campaign. The study found that viewers of the storylines produced as part of our campaign had developed more sympathetic attitudes toward people living with HIV/AIDS and were more likely to consider getting tested themselves after watching the show (Kennedy et al., 2007).

We do not expect our campaigns to single-handedly change the face of HIV/AIDS and sexual health in the United States; rather, we see the possibility of media to add a powerful dimension to efforts under way by many others, including federal, state, and local governments, national AIDS service organizations, and grassroots groups. We also believe that by engaging the media as allies on HIV/AIDS, the partnership models we are creating today will have long-term benefits for an array of social issues that will outlive any single campaign we could create.

## References

Kaiser Family Foundation. (2003). *Reaching the MTV generation: Recent research on the impact of the Kaiser Family Foundation/MTV public education campaign on sexual health.* Menlo Park, CA: Author.

Kaiser Family Foundation. (2004). *Assessing public education programming on HIV/AIDS: A national survey of African-Americans.* Menlo Park, CA: Author.

Kennedy, M. G., O'Leary, A., Wright-Fofanah, S., Dean, E., Chen, Y., & Baxter, R. (2007). *Effects on HIV stigma of viewing an HIV-relevant storyline in a television situation comedy.* Manuscript submitted for publication.

# 19

## "For People Like Us"
### Mobilizing Communities for HIV/AIDS Prevention, Treatment, Care, and Support

*John Howson*
International HIV/AIDS Alliance

*Kim Witte*
Michigan State University

In early 2003, the Health Communication Partnership[1] (HCP) in Namibia was challenged[2] with developing health communication interventions to: reduce the incidence of HIV infections, increase access to HIV counseling and testing and prevention of mother-to-child transmission services, help coordinate and harmonize communication interventions, and design, plan, and undertake a strategic information system to give program implementers the information they needed to plan interventions, as well as track behavioral changes over time.

HIV prevalence in Namibia was 22% (UNAIDS, 2004), with significant regional variations. Communication efforts were largely focused on mass media approaches to condom promotion and stigma reduction. Community-based responses were limited and organized largely by the churches.

Through our discussions with civic and community leaders, community members, and program implementers, we found that although awareness of HIV was almost universal there was little appreciation of the ways that the behavior of individuals and community norms might fuel the epidemic, and community members had little confidence that they could effect change. This passive response appeared to be caused by feelings of hopelessness about being able to do anything about HIV/AIDS, and was complicated by an expectation that solutions to the problem would come from outside of the communities.

This is a classic situation encountered by health communication specialists. The communities appeared to be engaged in a "fear control" process, where they felt personally threatened by a serious disease, in this case HIV, yet they believed there was nothing they themselves could do to avert the threat, and even if there was something, it probably wouldn't work anyway.[3]

HCP decided that the initial goal of communication efforts should be to help stimulate a collective sense of understanding and ownership of the problem, and move away from passive fatalism through increased community participation and increased individual and collective self-efficacy. The team also wanted to gain a better appreciation of how the different sections of the communities understood and conceptualized HIV so as to better contextualize communication messages to fit the reality of people's everyday lives. The challenge was how to do this at scale in an incredibly diverse country.

In dialogue with the funders, HCP decided that our initial response to the first two challenges was to facilitate participatory, reflective processes about HIV/AIDS in representative communities of the target population, as this would be the best hope of reducing individual and community paralysis in response to HIV. Through a process of community dialogue, communities could articulate their problems and identify collective solutions resulting in action toward necessary social change. One of the most eloquent and influential theorists for this type of approach is the Brazilian educator, Paulo Friere (1984). Friere emphasized that through dialogue and reflection the most marginalized in society would be better able to comprehend and analyze their situation, find their voice, and effect necessary, contextually appropriate and sustainable social change.

Central to this approach is the principle that those infected and affected by the epidemic must participate in the analysis of their own problems. As opposed to top-down approaches, participatory community mobilization helps communities and implementers better understand how they see and understand their problems and helps them identify their untapped community assets; therefore, the process acts as an intervention in and of itself. It is a process that fosters hope by helping community members appreciate that they have the power and tools at their disposal to create real and lasting change.

The participatory community mobilization program was developed using Participatory Learning and Action (PLA)-type approaches, modified and designed with a view to rapid scale-up. Following is a description of the participatory communication intervention, which HCP is now implementing in more than 10, soon to be 13, sites across Namibia.

1. *Community meetings.* As part of the preparation for this activity, community leaders were informed that the process they were about to undertake would necessarily stimulate discussion about issues that most people find uncomfortable discussing in public—for example, issues related to sexual behavior, gender relations, alcohol and substance misuse, partner abuse, and their relationship with the church. In particular, sexual behavior would be explored in some depth: Without the community having a collective understanding of how HIV had become such a problem, it would be unlikely that a collective response could be successfully agreed upon and developed.

2. *Trained peer facilitators.* Peer facilitators were trained during a weeklong workshop on how to facilitate community dialogue among their own peers using a participatory assessment tool, called "For People Like Us" (HCP-Namibia, 2005).[4] The aim of the training was to help the facilitators understand and practice dispassionate observation, gain skills in encouraging dialogue and reflection, and learn the skills necessary to guide and support the participants through the PLA exercises.

3. *Peer facilitator–led sessions.* The peer facilitators then led four sessions with approximately 15 members of six peer groups: young women/young men aged 16 to 25, women/men aged 25 to 45, older women/older men aged 46+. The participants were chosen by the community leaders because as individuals they were seen by their peers as being representative of that peer group. All the exercises were done using symbols so as not to exclude those in the community who might be illiterate. As we were interested in understanding the collective perception and behavior of the distinct peer groups, we asked the peer representatives to answer all the questions asked by thinking about it "for people like you." Although this approach has its limitations, it did allow for more candid discussion of sensitive issues and also helped the community and the program understand better the varying needs and perspectives of the different peer groups.

4. *Plenary community meeting held.* Following completion of the peer sessions, a community meeting was held where each of the

peer groups fed back to the larger community their own responses to the questions asked. This format proved essential to the process of helping the communities explore, for instance, collective taboos about sexual behavior, sexual partner preferences, and collective perceptions of "blame" and "innocence" that were associated with stigmatizing behaviors. Following the presentation of results, there was much community dialogue and debate about the findings. This led to the community members collectively developing a vision of what changes they would like to see in their community in 3 years' time and how they might achieve that vision.

5. *Develop community action forums.* To sustain the process, each community developed a community action forum, which acted as the community coordinating body for the various interventions implemented by community members. These action forums work in close cooperation with provincial HIV/AIDS coordinating mechanisms as well as all local actors—hospitals, clinics, nongovernmental organizations (NGOs), community-based organizations, and faith-based organizations—working in the area of HIV and community development. To help build the capacity of these forums and nurture incipient initiatives, some communities had the on-site support of Peace Corps volunteers and all have regular contact and support from HCP staff and other local NGOs.

This holistic and dynamic approach helped each peer group, and the community as a whole, gain a better understanding of how the attitudes, beliefs, and behaviors of each of the peer groups influenced both individual and collective risk of HIV. It also helped the communities identify those most vulnerable to infection and discrimination and those most in need of protection. This approach also helped identify factors that enabled or inhibited access to health care and other services. What emerged so powerfully in all the groups was the collective recognition that they needed to find ways of addressing the underlying factors that increase vulnerability to HIV infection: stigma, alcohol and drug use, gender and sexual norms, violence, and fear of change.

Through the community action forums, the communities are implementing their own interventions based on their own analysis, with the support of, and in collaboration with, HCP and other local actors.[5] A second round of household and social network analysis data is currently being collected to try to quantify changes in risk perception, individual and collective efficacy, as well as knowledge, access, and use of services.

## Notes

1. Health Communication Partnership is a 5-year global health program funded by USAID. It is led by the Johns Hopkins Bloomberg School of Public Health Center for Communication Programs in partnership with the Agency for Education and Development, Save the Children (United States), the International HIV/AIDS Alliance, and Tulane University.
2. This program is funded by the President's Emergency Plan for AIDS Relief (PEPFAR) through USAID.
3. The theoretical grounding for this perspective is from the extended parallel process model (EPPM), where fear motivates people to either control the danger (if they feel able to engage in an effective response to combat the threat) or control their fear (if people feel unable to effectively address the threat). See Witte, Meyer, and Martell (2001) for complete description of the theory.
4. Available on request from the first author at jhowson@jhuccp.org.
5. Given that the nature of this intervention is participatory and the intervention aims to build collective self-efficacy and social change, much of the impact evaluation has been at the level of community-reported changes following the intervention. Most notably this has included the development of community alcohol misuse programs to address what the communities themselves perceive to be the greatest challenges they confront in terms of sexual risk taking and gender-based violence. Although the information we have collected at the community level is very informative, we acknowledge that the data primarily are anecdotal in nature.

## References

Freire, P. (1984). *Pedagogy of the oppressed* (translated from the original 1968 Portuguese manuscript by Myra Bergman Ramos). New York: Continuum.

HCP-Namibia. (2005). *For people like us.* Windhoek, Namibia: Johns Hopkins University Center for Communication Programs.

UNAIDS. (2004). 2004 Report on the global AIDS epidemic. Geneva, Switzerland: WHO/UNAIDS.

Witte, K., Meyer, G., & Martell, D. (2001). *Effective health risk messages: A step-by-step guide.* Newbury Park, CA: Sage.

# 20

# A Network-Oriented HIV Prevention Intervention
## The SHIELD Study

*Carl A. Latkin*

*Amy R. Knowlton*
Johns Hopkins University Bloomberg School of Public Health

The SHIELD (Self-Help in Eliminating Lethal Disease) project, initiated in 1996, was a theory-based, culturally tailored, experimental behavioral HIV prevention intervention targeting injection drug users and their social network members. The goal of the program was to train high-risk former and current drug users to promote HIV-preventive practices among their social network members, a critical strategy for health education of hard-to-reach drug-using populations. The targeted behavioral outcomes were reduction in injection drug risk practices, risky sexual practices, and injection drug use. The project utilized small-group, multisession training in peer health education skills, and a harm reduction perspective. Participants were encouraged to disseminate risk reduction messages to their drug and sex risk networks, that is, drug-sharing ties and sex partners. Participants were recruited in high-risk neighborhoods of Baltimore, Maryland. A randomized controlled study design was used, with an equal-attention control arm, and pre- and posttest evaluation. Both quantitative and qualitative methods were used for study evaluation.

## Theoretical Framework

The study's theoretical framework drew from theories of social identity, diffusion of innovations, social networks, active learning, and cognitive dissonance. It was theorized that promoting a social identity of peer educator would motivate participation in the group sessions and participants' HIV prevention education of network members in natural settings. Based on prior research, it was theorized that risk network members comprise proximal influences on HIV risk behaviors, and that participants would be most influential to risk behaviors among risk network members as compared to strangers or mere acquaintances. Active learning and cognitive dissonance principles were employed with the anticipation that the peer educators' promoting risk reduction among network members would lead to a reduction of their own risk behaviors as a result of any ambiguity between their risk reduction messages and their own behavior. It was also anticipated that performance of a peer educator role would generate social rewards within this marginalized population's larger community, which would lead to more sustained behavior change as compared with traditional individual-focused intervention approaches.

## Social Network Orientation

The intervention used a social network approach to motivate and reinforce risk reduction. Accordingly, the intervention emphasized the importance of participants' interpersonal relationships in influencing their HIV infection or transmission risk, and emphasized risk reduction as a means of protecting one's family and friends. Participants' network members were a key focus of the intervention. Participants were trained in social influence techniques for promoting risk reduction among their network members. Training sessions emphasized group problem solving for improved, culturally tailored, audience-specific communication of prevention messages. It was theorized that a network approach would facilitate diffusion of prevention messages and behavior change through the participants' social networks, potentially altering network norms of risk behaviors and establishing new norms of safer injection practices and sexual behaviors.

## Participants

Study participants were recruited through street outreach in areas of Baltimore identified through ethnography and geographic mapping as areas of high prevalence of drug use. Eligibility criteria included at least weekly contact with current drug users, willingness to talk with friends about HIV prevention, and being willing to recruit to the clinic for assessment at least one at-risk network member. Therefore, though not a requirement of study eligibility, 99% of those recruited reported to be current or former illicit-drug users. There were 250 individuals who enrolled in the intervention, with a random assignment of 2:1 to the experimental group. The control group received equal-attention sessions and the attrition was similar in both groups. The 6-month follow-up rate was 92%.

## Communications

Communication skills building was the focus of the training sessions. Our prior studies suggested that individuals in drug-using communities infrequently discussed HIV prevention, and that HIV discussions often focused on gossip about individuals who were infected. Seldom were everyday conversations about strategies for preventing HIV infection (Smith, Lucas, & Latkin, 1999).

The highly scripted 10-session training curriculum focused on motivating participants to communicate HIV prevention messages and on methods of effective communication with peers. Extensive role playing, modeling, practice in community settings, and other skills-building exercises were utilized to enhance communication skills. Intervention topics included how to evaluate a situation and to determine appropriate situations for bringing up the topic of HIV prevention, how to model injection risk reduction behaviors, how to initiate a conversation about HIV prevention, how to enhance and maintain credibility as a peer health educator, how to understand and cope with negative verbal and nonverbal feedback, and how to provide positive verbal and nonverbal feedback to others.

After basic communications training, intervention facilitators accompanied participants in the community to practice performing the communication skills. In each of the sessions, the group facilitators would model effective communications techniques. In some sessions, the facilitators would role-play ineffective communications and encourage the participants to critique them and to role-play more effective methods. In sessions, participants discussed prior homework assignments that involved communicating with a network member or others in the community about HIV prevention and their involvement in the SHIELD program. During this feedback, the facilitators identified and socially rewarded examples of applying effective communication. The feedback sessions were guided to facilitate group members' collective problem solving in order to refine communications techniques to their cultural norms, and to model effective communication skills for each other.

Outcomes

The 6-month posttest evaluation revealed that individuals in the experimental condition, as compared to those in the control condition, reported statistically significantly reduced frequencies of sharing needles and cookers, injection drug use, and unprotected sex with casual partners (Latkin, Sherman, & Knowlton, 2003). The vast majority of participants reported that their family members and friends were proud of their training to be peer educators, and they also appeared to value the role of outreach "worker," one of the few prosocial, formal economy roles available to them (Dickson-Gomez, Knowlton, & Latkin, 2004). Results also indicated that former drug users as compared to current drug users tended to engage in more frequent peer education. However, current drug users were more likely than former drug users to talk to active injectors about reducing their HIV risk behaviors (Latkin, Hua, & Davey, 2004).

Lessons Learned

One of the major lessons learned from this intervention was to keep simple the communication skills training. Similarly, we found it useful to have only a few program goals, which were repeated and built upon throughout the sessions, and to emphasize the practice of communication skills. Intervention components that did not appear to enhance communication skills or motivation were omitted from the training. For example, we found that many drug users in this community are highly knowledgeable about modes of HIV infection and that increasing knowledge was not an efficient use of time. Even essential informational materials were easily integrated into communication skills training. We also found that often participants enter programs for extrinsic rewards such as food and money. One of the major program goals was to alter the participants' motivation for engagement in priority risk reduction activities so that they became intrinsic and, hence, sustainable. We found that providing informational materials other than HIV prevention, such as resources for HIV care, drug treatment, and soup kitchens and shelters, enhanced participants' motivation to attend and their credibility as peer outreach workers. Relevance was also enhanced by having the program meet participants' other basic needs. The SHIELD program was design to enhance participants' respect in the community and enhance their communication skills so that they could communicate more effectively with family, friends, and social service agencies.

Interventions should allow sufficient training time for improving communication skills. One of the most common sources of miscommunication of peer educators is that they tend to be preachy, telling others what to do. Training peer educators to be more affirming and positive and to engage others in discussion can significantly alter their style and effectiveness in interpersonal communication, with potential implications to HIV prevention.

## References

Dickson-Gomez, J. B., Knowlton, A., & Latkin, C. (2004). Values and identity: The meaning of work for injection drug users involved in volunteer HIV prevention outreach. *Substance Use and Misuse, 39,* 1259–1286.

Latkin, C. A., Hua, W., & Davey, M. (2004). Factors associated with peer HIV prevention advocacy in drug using communities. *AIDS Education and Prevention, 16,* 499–508.

Latkin, C. A., Sherman, S., & Knowlton, A. R. (2003). HIV prevention among drug users: Outcome of a network-oriented peer outreach intervention. *Health Psychology, 22,* 332–339.

Smith, L. C., Lucas, K. J., & Latkin, C. (1999). Rumor and gossip: Social discourse on HIV and AIDS. *Anthropology and Medicine, 6,* 121–131.

# 21

# Faith and the ABCs of HIV
## *The Approach of "I Choose Life-Africa"*

*Ann Neville Miller*
Daystar University

HIV/AIDS-related governmental and nongovernmental organizations (NGOs) have long used the shorthand of ABC to describe the foundation of comprehensive prevention programs. "A" stands for abstaining if one is single, "B" for being faithful to one HIV-negative partner if one is either married or unable to abstain, and "C" represents condom use for individuals who either choose to have multiple sexual partners or have a partner who is HIV-positive. Many faith-based organizations (FBOs) and denominations, most notably the Catholic church worldwide, have concluded that to promote both the "A" and the "C" components of the well-known AIDS alphabetical is to offer contradictory messages. They argue that if they are preaching the ideal of abstinence until marriage, encouraging condom use will dilute their focus, and even promote the behavioral patterns they are trying to discourage.

I Choose Life-Africa (ICL), the largest HIV/AIDS intervention targeting university students in Kenya, is based in a Christian worldview, and is distinctive among NGOs in its apparently equal emphasis on all three components of the ABC prevention model. Operating at five of the six Kenyan public universities and one private university, its stated purpose is to prevent HIV transmission through facilitating "caring communities that make possible responsible decisions regarding life and HIV/AIDS through peer education training." In congruence with the collective nature of Kenyan culture, it aims at developing a university environment where students can feel affirmed and even proud to make responsible choices.

This community-oriented intervention task is addressed through a multilayered process. After baseline analysis, intervention on campus begins with a search for leaders in various subsets of the student body. Sports figures, student government officials, and other students who are certifiably "cool" by campus standards are invited to participate in a high-energy 3-month HIV/AIDS training program from which they graduate at a highly publicized ceremony.

During training students pair up to initiate "behavior change communication groups" (BCCGs) that are developed around common interests of participants—anything from Salsa dancing to financial management—but all additionally committed to building an environment conducive to support and sustain changes in risky behavior. Communication within the training modules and BCCGs is comprised of a range of interactive techniques including brainstorming, panel discussions, case studies, quizzes on sexuality, role plays, games, movie clips, debates, and assignments. The organization runs an on-campus resource center to provide peer educators with a range of information, education, and communication (IEC) materials including videos, brochures, pamphlets, posters, magazines, handouts, and other current HIV-related publications.

Following graduation, peer educators may enroll in a 3-week life skills course designed to empower them toward effective decision making. The course covers topics like managing emotions, values, interpersonal negotiation skills, and self-esteem. At the next level, participants gather in large groups for monthly themed activities that may involve visiting homes of people living with HIV/AIDS, volunteering at AIDS orphanages, assisting in HIV-related research, or other consciousness-raising experiences. Once per quarter these large-group gatherings culminate in a giant high-profile campuswide event.

In conjunction with this progression of community building, ICL also organizes multiple mobile voluntary counseling and testing (VCT) clinics for student participants and the campus at large. Posttest clubs supplement that emphasis. At one university a "Mr. and Miss Status" contest is run as part of an annual HIV-testing day, with contestants allowed to compete only if they have been tested for HIV.

Although ICL emerges from a faith-based orientation, it does not identify itself as a strictly religious organization in its campus work. Thus, Bible verses are incorporated into certain units of the training, but many other perspectives are also brought to bear on each topic.

In all activities, approximately equal weight is given to presenting abstinence, being faithful, and condom use as prevention strategies. That balance, however, represents a shift from the organization's initial approach when the strongest component of the message was that of abstaining. T-shirts proclaimed "for the infected and affected: Abstinence" and a push was made for participants to sign pledge cards committing to secondary abstinence. More recently, although the secondary abstinence pledges are still a feature of the ICL message, t-shirts advocate general sexual responsibility and small- and large-group messages on "B" and "C" are alternated with calls to save sex until marriage.

Staff members are firmly convinced that the current approach is appropriate for two reasons. First, they suggest that the motivations for abstinence and condom use are different. People who sign private abstinence pledges frequently do so from cultural, moral, or religious convictions; for them health concerns are a secondary consideration. People who commit to condom use are centrally motivated by health concerns for themselves and/or their partners. The introduction of information about condom use is, therefore, believed not to dissuade individuals already inclined toward abstinence.

Second, ICL asserts that by the time youth reach university age they are capable of grasping the fact that trainers can present multiple options for responsible sexual behavior, even when they personally consider one option to be preferable to others. Students can, for instance, understand why one especially enthusiastic staff member can be a committed Christian determined to live abstinence in his own life, and at the same time facilitate excellent informational sessions on condom purchase and use. As an educated population, students are able to hold these facts in paradoxical tension and make their own decisions.

Since its inception in 2002, ICL has trained a total of 45 staff trainers and 2,901 peer educators. The peer educators have reached approximately 40,091 students across six campuses. Forty-two BCCGs have been formed, mobile VCTs at six campuses have recorded 3,235 student HIV-testing visits, and more than 61,000 pieces of related IEC material have been distributed.

The first impact assessment of the program, at Kenyatta University, revealed a number of positive trends. ICL evidenced a strong impact on HIV testing, with the proportion of students reporting ever having been tested increasing from one fourth to more than half between 2004 and 2006. Much of the testing occurred at ICL events. Levels of HIV/AIDS-related knowledge and training increased significantly and ICL was mentioned as the most influential source of HIV/AIDS information among on-campus NGOs. Condom use across the student body as a whole also showed a modest but significant increase, and the first-year "gold rush"—the term used to describe the practice of upper-level male students targeting naïve female first-years—showed signs of declining.

At the same time, the mean number of reported sexual partners and the proportion of students who said they had never had sex did not change. Whether decreasing sexual contact is simply a much more difficult goal to achieve than other behavioral objectives, or whether an abstinence-only focus would have produced greater shifts among students toward abstinence and secondary abstinence was not possible to demonstrate without a comparison group.

Thus, the jury is still out on the effect of the ICL model on abstinence uptake. In any case, not all religiously based interventions will or should consider the ICL multi-option message. Churches may see their role in prevention as stressing abstinence and leave other entities to advance other safer-sex messages; FBOs working with high school–age youth may evaluate their audience as unready for a contingent moral reasoning that at once states its ideals while at the same time offering health-based alternatives to people who choose not to commit to those ideals. Nevertheless, the experience of ICL offers the possibility of integrating faith- and health-oriented perspectives in one program, and may serve as a useful resource to assist churches and other religiously based organizations in making informed decisions about potential interventions aimed at the same sort of population.

# 22

# A TTM-Tailored Condom Use Intervention for At-Risk Women and Men

*Colleen A. Redding*

*Patricia J. Morokoff*

*Joseph S. Rossi*

*Kathryn S. Meier*
University of Rhode Island

Effective models and methods for reaching those at risk for HIV are needed, especially for those from diverse urban, poor areas where rates of HIV are highest. In the United States, high-risk heterosexual contact is the largest risk category for women of color and the second largest for men of color for HIV/AIDS (Prejean, Satcher, Durant, Hu, & Lee, 2006), and internationally, heterosexual sex is a primary exposure category for HIV/AIDS. Consistent condom use offers the best hope of reducing rates of infection. Public health and behavioral research communities are seeking effective interventions to increase condom use that can be delivered at low cost to large segments of the at-risk population. This study, Rhode Island Project RESPECT, developed and evaluated a theoretically and empirically tailored expert system (ES) intervention based on the transtheoretical model (TTM) to increase condom use in at-risk heterosexually active women and men. This intervention combines the reach of large-scale public health efforts with the efficacy of more traditional clinical interventions, potentially enhancing public health impact. This TTM-tailored intervention was designed to intervene with participants at all stages of condom use and was delivered via a multimedia computer-based ES that has the potential to be both cost-effective and widely disseminated.

The theoretical basis for this study was the TTM, which includes the following constructs: stages of change, decisional balance, self-efficacy, and processes of change (Prochaska, Redding, & Evers, 1997). TTM research has found both that people progress toward health behavior change in a series of stages of change and that different intervention messages and content are effective for participants at different stages of change. These ideas are the foundation for tailoring. The empirical foundation for this study was based on TTM-tailored ES outcomes across various samples and behaviors. Among adults, a series of three TTM-tailored text-based ES feedback reports (Prochaska et al., 1997; Velicer, Prochaska, & Redding, 2006) outperformed both stage-targeted manuals and a generic smoking cessation manual, demonstrating efficacy for smoking cessation. Subsequent studies have both replicated this finding in larger samples and extended it to additional single health risk behaviors, as well as to multiple risk behaviors (Prochaska et al., 1997; Velicer et al., 2006).

Multimedia interactive computer feedback is more immediate, novel, and accessible than text-based feedback reports. Multimedia ES programs to increase both smoking cessation and condom use were developed for urban adolescent girls in family-planning clinics (Prochaska et al., 1997; Redding et al., 1999; Redding, Prochaska, et al., 2002). Both ES feedback and counseling in the treatment group were tailored for female adolescents at all stages of readiness to change both smoking and condom use. This randomized trial of a TTM-tailored intervention package increased condom use in sexually active female teens (14–17 years old), as well as increased cessation among smokers, compared to a usual care comparison group (Redding, Prochaska, et al., 2002).

The next project adapted existing adolescent multimedia programs for a new adult male and female at-risk population. The ES incorporated pictures, background music, brief movies, and voice feedback through earphones, which enhanced our ability to reach and interact with a range of individuals, including those with limited literacy skills. A pilot study of 100 women evaluated one session using the adolescent system (Brown-Peterside, Redding, Ren, & Koblin, 2000) and found that most women rated the system and its feedback very interesting and useful, as well as clear and user-friendly. Many women appreciated its confidentiality and all said that they felt able to answer questions honestly. The enthusiasm and positive feedback expressed by these women supported this system's feasibility, laying the foundation for further adaptation for adults.

This ES was adapted in several ways: Feedback was rewritten for adults using communication and TTM intervention principles (Redding et al., 1999). The ES provided feedback on all TTM constructs, specifically stage of readiness to use condoms consistently, pros and cons of condom use, confidence, and processes of change. Processes of change include 16 specific ways people can progress toward using condoms more consistently, including: learn more about it (consciousness raising), realize their risk (dramatic relief), adjust their self-image (self-reevaluation), talk to their partner about condoms (communication), be clear and firm about using condoms (condom assertiveness), make using condoms more enjoyable (eroticize condom use), reward themselves for using condoms (reinforcement management), keep and carry condoms (stimulus control), date people who support condom use (interpersonal systems control), use healthier alternatives instead of unprotected sex if, for example, condoms aren't available (counterconditioning), and notice how the social environment and norms increasingly support safer sex (environmental reevaluation) (Noar, Morokoff & Redding, 2001; Redding, Morokoff, et al., 2002) . Participants enjoy reading feedback that is tailored to their own responses because it is more personal and engaging than more generic information/advice. For each stage of readiness, both a simple reflection of the participant's readiness, a reinforcement of any positive behaviors or progress, and a suggestion to take the next step forward were provided. For example, for a Precontemplator (not considering using condoms every time in the next 6 months), the stage feedback would be along these lines:

> You are not thinking about using condoms more often right now. Every time you have sex without condoms, you could catch a sexual disease that you probably don't want to deal with. You probably want to make the best choices for yourself and your future. Read on for some ideas that could help you make your best choices.

Stage-tailored feedback for a participant in Preparation (using condoms almost every time) or Action (using condoms every time) would also reflect where they were and then would also reinforce safer behaviors with a statement like, "Great job. You are taking steps to reduce your sexual risks by using condoms every time you have sex." All participants received feedback that was tailored to their stage of condom use across all constructs, and in addition, feedback for the Pros and Cons, Confidence, and Processes of change was also compared to a normative cutoff at both baseline and follow-up timepoints (normative feedback). At follow-up timepoints, an individual's feedback also referred back to her previous scores on the same construct (ipsative feedback), allowing even relatively small changes over time to be reinforced. For example, "Good work. You are keeping and carrying condoms more often than before. This will help you stay on track." Feedback on readiness to use condoms with both main and other partners was integrated into the ES. Male voice recordings to complement on-screen feedback were added to a parallel ES for men. Pilot testing of the TTM measures and normative cutoffs demonstrated that their psychometric structures were sound and that they accounted for important variance in condom use among both at-risk men and women (Redding et al., 2001; Redding, Morokoff, et al., 2002). Although the ES could accommodate gender-specific normative cutoffs, subsequent data demonstrated that this was unnecessary.

This randomized community-based trial included clinics and substance abuse treatment settings where at-risk populations could be recruited near Providence, Rhode Island, as well as in the Bronx, New York. Potential participants were approached and screened for eligibility by one of several trained health educators. Once eligible and enrolled, participants were randomly assigned to either a TTM-tailored, individualized ES intervention, or to a generic information and advice comparison group. The computer delivered all intervention feedback, except group-specific manuals. After baseline, two more intervention sessions took place at 2 months and 4 months. The TTM-tailored group received individualized, TTM-tailored feedback and stage-tailored manuals, whereas the generic information comparison group received nontailored HIV information/advice and a generic condom information manual.

Baseline demographic and sexual risk variables were analyzed to reveal both that the two randomized groups were comparable and that the sample was diverse and sexually at risk. Analysis of 6-month outcomes revealed that the TTM intervention group used condoms more often and progressed further in the stages of condom use than did the comparison group (Redding et al., 2004).

## Conclusion

This chapter described the development and evaluation of an effective computer-delivered TTM-tailored ES intervention to increase condom use and readiness to use condoms in diverse at-risk adult heterosexual men and women recruited from a range of urban settings. Some may find interacting with a computer more acceptable than attending a clinic-based HIV prevention intervention. Alternatively, a computer-based intervention could enable reaching a wide audience and then a clinic-based intervention could be utilized only for those who need it most, in a stepped-care model. This computer-delivered intervention has the potential for adaptation and dissemination to a wide variety of settings including health care clinics, schools, worksites, prisons, and the Internet. The main strengths of this intervention are: tailoring that targets adults at all stages of readiness to use condoms; and both theoretical and empirical tailoring on the TTM variables that have demonstrated strong relationships to condom use and readiness to use condoms across many at-risk samples. These innovative features have the potential to increase both population reach and effectiveness for HIV prevention, thereby increasing their public health impact.

## Acknowledgments

This research was supported by Grant AI/MH 41323 from the National Institute of Allergy and Infectious Disease. Various aspects of this project have been presented at the annual meetings of the Society of Behavioral Medicine.

## References

Brown-Peterside, P., Redding, C. A., Ren, L., & Koblin, B. A. (2000). Acceptability of a stage-matched expert system intervention to increase condom use among women at high risk of HIV infection in New York City. *AIDS Education and Prevention, 12,* 171–181.

Noar, S. M., Morokoff, P. J., & Redding, C. A. (2001). An examination of transtheoretical predictors of condom use in late-adolescent heterosexual men. *Journal of Applied Biobehavioral Research, 6,* 1–26.

Prejean, J., Satcher, A. J., Durant, T., Hu, X., & Lee, L. M. (2006). Racial/ethnic disparities in diagnoses of HIV/AIDS—33 States, 2001–2004. *Morbidity and Mortality Weekly Report, 55*(5), 121–125.

Prochaska, J. O., Redding, C. A., & Evers, K. (1997). The transtheoretical model and stages of change. In K. Glanz, F. M. Lewis, & B. K. Rimer (Eds.), *Health behavior and health education: Theory, research, and practice* (2nd ed., pp. 60–84). San Francisco: Jossey-Bass.

Redding, C. A., Meier, K. S., Noar, S. M., White, S. L., Rossi, J. S., Doherty-Iddings, P., et al. (2001). The transtheoretical model for condom use in a community sample of at-risk men and women. *Annals of Behavioral Medicine, 23*, S135 (Abstract).

Redding, C. A., Morokoff, P. J., Noar, S. M., Meier, K. S., Rossi, J. S., Koblin, B., et al. (2002). Evaluating transtheoretical model-based predictors of condom use in at-risk men and women. *Annals of Behavioral Medicine, 24*, S021 (Abstract).

Redding, C. A., Morokoff, P. J., Rossi, J. S., Meier, K. S., Hoeppner, B. B., Mayer, K., et al. (2004). Effectiveness of a computer-delivered TTM-tailored intervention at increasing condom use in at-risk heterosexual adults: RI Project Respect. *Annals of Behavioral Medicine, 27*, S113 (Abstract).

Redding, C. A., Prochaska, J. O., Pallonen, U. E., Rossi, J. S., Velicer, W. F., Rossi, S. R., et al. (1999). Transtheoretical individualized multimedia expert systems targeting adolescents' health behaviors. *Cognitive & Behavioral Practice, 6*, 144-153.

Redding, C. A., Prochaska, J. O., Rossi, J. S., Armstrong, K., Coviello, D., Pallonen, U., et al. (2002). Effectiveness of a randomized clinical trial of stage-matched interventions targeting condom use and smoking in young urban females. *Annals of Behavioral Medicine, 24*, S061 (Abstract).

Velicer, W. F., Prochaska, J. O., & Redding, C. A. (2006). Tailored communications for smoking cessation: Past successes and future directions. *Drug and Alcohol Review, 25*, 49–57.

# 23

# Partnership for Health Program Development
*A Brief Safer-Sex Intervention for HIV Outpatient Clinics*

## Jean L. Richardson

## Joel Milam

## Lilia Espinoza
University of Southern California

Rationale for Importance of Area and Intervention

The Centers for Disease Control and Prevention (CDC) estimates that approximately 900,000 persons are living with HIV in the United States. Until recently, most prevention programs have been developed for HIV-negative persons to provide them with information and skills to avoid HIV. Few prevention programs address behaviors of people living with HIV/AIDS (PLWHA) even though many studies have documented that approximately one third of those diagnosed and in care engage in unsafe sexual behavior that may lead to new infections (Richardson, Milam, Stoyanoff, et al., 2004).

The Partnership for Health (PfH) Study was a controlled intervention trial that tested brief provider-delivered safer-sex counseling with PLWHA during routine clinic visits. The safer-sex counseling was provided in two different communication styles: gain (or advantages) frame at two clinics and loss (or consequences) frame at two clinics, and each was compared to two control clinics that received medication adherence counseling (Richardson, Milam, McCutchan, et al., 2004).

## Theoretical Framework

Three compatible behavioral theories were incorporated into the PfH model. *Message framing* was formally tested and was supported by the *mutual participation* and the *stages of change* models.

Message framing links a behavior with an outcome. Information that instills recognition of risk and motivation to reduce risk can be conveyed to patients in a way that emphasizes the positive consequences of performing a healthful behavior (gain frame) or the negative consequences of not performing a healthful behavior (loss frame) (Rothman & Salovey, 1997). Different presentations of factually equivalent information encoded as relative gains or relative losses will be perceived and acted on differently.

Examples of advantages (gain) and consequences (loss) frame messages include:

*Advantages:* "If you and your partner use latex condoms while having sex, you protect yourself from other sexually transmitted diseases."
*Consequences:* "If you and your partner don't use latex condoms while having sex, you may expose yourself to other sexually transmitted diseases."

Both gain and loss frame messages can be delivered in a supportive manner and need not be fear appeals. Framing effects may be moderated by a number of factors including the patient's psychological status, beliefs in personal efficacy to enact the behavior, and perceptions of proximal or distal effects. Prior studies of message framing have not, for the most part, been conducted in diseased people who may be particularly receptive to messages about potential health risks.

The mutual participation model of provider–patient relations (Szasz & Hollender, 1956) suggests the patient and provider(s) work together as a team to formulate goals, expectations, responsibilities, and commitments regarding health care. Provider–patient interactions improve patient understanding of their disease and its treatment, satisfaction with health care, adherence to medical treatment regimens, and compliance with prescribed health promotion activities. Health care providers can be effective agents of behavior change because they are respected sources of prevention messages and can assess and counsel patients repeatedly during routine visits to address risky sexual behaviors. However, during medical exams most HIV clinicians do not inquire about condom use and the patient's number of sexual partners (Marks et al., 2002).

The transtheoretical model of behavior change (TTM) is well known for describing how people change health behaviors in the natural environment. This description includes five *stages of change: precontemplation, contemplation, preparation, action,* and *maintenance* (Prochaska, Redding, Harlow, Rossi, & Velicer, 1994). In PfH, *catalysts* that help to create the motivation for behavior change include a caring provider, strategically placed posters, appropriate referrals, encouraging responses, repetition, expectations for gradual movement from smaller to larger goals, and framed messages.

The TTM was used as a concept to explain different stages of patient thinking and behavior, the breadth of responses the patient may express, and the progression of goals that might be appropriate including:

1. All people can be inconsistent in their behavior, can be highly risky in one situation and highly protective in another, and can make little changes or dramatic changes.
2. Patients will not progress step-by-step through these levels of behavior change.
3. Small steps forward are successes.
4. Slip-ups are expected.
5. Some people will not change specific risky behaviors and alternative ways to increase protection need to be discussed.

## Intervention

In order to fully integrate the intervention into the clinic, *all* clinic staff persons were trained in the conduct of the intervention. The intervention is supported by materials developed for patients, providers, and staff. Materials included brochures, posters, flyers, counseling pocket guides for providers, and medical-chart stickers. The 4-hour training program was delivered to the staff at each clinic and included modules on communicating gain or loss frame messages to patients, conducting a brief counseling session, responding to patients' questions, and role plays. The training was supplemented with a booster session 6 weeks later.

The intervention emphasizes the importance of a patient–provider team approach to help patients stay as healthy as possible and also help protect others from getting infected. During each clinic visit, the provider refers to the partnership theme and engages the patient in a brief (3–5 minute) interaction. The patient and provider touch on one or all of the three core messages: self-protection, partner protection, and disclosure of HIV status. All PfH materials support the patient–provider partnership theme. The provider is able to tailor safer-sex messages that promote the adoption of safer behaviors and explore possibilities for disclosure. All of the primary care providers (nurse practitioners, physician assistants, physicians) in each clinic participated in the intervention. The only aspect that systematically differed between clinics was the framing (gain or loss) of the prevention messages delivered to patients. Thus in the gain frame clinics, exam room posters, brochures for patients, and provider counseling were all framed with gain frame messages; in the loss frame clinic, each of these were framed with loss frame messages.

## Results

The PfH study was the first study to test prevention message framing among people infected with HIV. People in the loss frame intervention arm who had two or more partners at baseline reduced high-risk sexual behavior (unprotected anal or vaginal [UAV] sex) by 38% over the course of the study. The likelihood of UAV at follow-up was significantly lower in the loss frame arm compared with the control arm (OR = .34; 95% CI = .24–.49, $p$ = .0001), after adjusting for baseline differences in UAV, demographic, and HIV-medical variables. No change was found for participants in the gain frame arm or for those who had one main partner (Richardson, Milam, McCutchan et al., 2004), perhaps because UAV was already lower among those with one partner. Behavior change with steady partners may require discussion between the partners and mutual agreement to reduce unsafe sex.

## Discussion/Interpretation

Why are loss frame messages more effective with higher risk patients with HIV disease than gain frame messages? Loss frame messages address the potential serious consequences of the high-risk patient's *current* behavior; thus, patients may easily recognize their own risk and the risk they pose to others. Few patients actually want to infect another person. Loss frame messages may be consistent with the patient's own perceptions and values and more likely to evoke the serious concern that another person actually could become infected. Patients with a serious illness may find that emphasizing actions that may cause the disease to worsen may be particularly salient, creating greater motivation for self-protection as well. Finally, loss frame messages may appear to be more to the point and serious and when delivered by a highly credible health care provider, may be the expected norm in the health care setting, and may tap into the patient's heightened concerns and increase the extent the message is cognitively and emotionally processed and acted on.

The PfH program offers great potential to prevent new HIV infections and to protect the health of people already infected. The message-framing techniques are easily learned and yield impressive prevention results when put in the hands of health care providers.

## Acknowledgments

This work was supported by the California Universitywide AIDS Research Program (Grant ID04-USC-042) and the National Institute of Mental Health (Grant RO1MH57208).

## References

Marks, G., Richardson, J. L., Crepaz, N., Stoyanoff, S., Milam, J., Kemper, C., et al. (2002). Are HIV care providers talking with patients about safer sex and disclosure?: A multi-clinic assessment. *AIDS, 16,* 1953–1957.

Prochaska, J. O., Redding, C. A., Harlow, L. L., Rossi, J. S., & Velicer, W. F. (1994). The transtheoretical model of change and HIV prevention: A review. *Health Education Quarterly, 21,* 471–486.

Richardson, J. L., Milam, J., McCutchan, A., Stoyanoff, S., Bolan, R., Weiss, J. M., et al. (2004). Effect of brief safer-sex counseling of HIV-1 seropositive patients: A multi-clinic assessment. *AIDS, 18,* 1179-1186.

Richardson, J. L., Milam, J., Stoyanoff, S., Kemper, C., Bolan, R., Larsen, R. A., et al. (2004). Using patient risk indicators to plan prevention strategies in the clinical care setting. *Journal of AIDS, 37,* S88-S94.

Rothman, A. J., & Salovey, P. (1997). Shaping perceptions to motivate healthy behavior: The role of message framing. *Psychological Bulletin, 121,* 3-19.

Szasz, T., & Hollender, M. (1956). A contribution to the philosophy of medicine: The basic models of the doctor–patient relationship. *Archives of Internal Medicine, 97,* 585-592.

# 24

# Using Technology to Prevent Teen Pregnancy, STDs, and HIV

*Anthony J. Roberto*

*Kellie E. Carlyle*
The Ohio State University

"Welcome to A Date with Destiny. In this activity, you will be making decisions about alcohol, dating, and sex. Please click 'Continue' to begin." So began the Choose Your Own Adventure CD-ROM, which was one part of the six-lesson computer- and Internet-based pregnancy, sexually transmitted disease (STD), and HIV prevention intervention that is discussed in this chapter. Imagine being a high school sophomore going on a "virtual date" where you have to make a variety of important choices that ultimately influence how the adventure will end. Will you buy condoms? Will you go to a party? If you go to the party, will you drink alcohol or go to a room to be alone with your date? And if so, will you give in to the pressure to have unprotected sex? If you do have sex, what happens next? Nothing? Do you or your partner get pregnant? HIV? Some other STD? And then what would you do? "This ends the activity. Would you like to start again and see what might happen if you made different choices?"

The use of computers and the Internet in HIV prevention interventions has a number of important strengths. For example, such technologies are available on demand, provide a cost-effective means to segment a large number of users, allow for individually tailored messages, can be regularly updated, and provide researchers and practitioners with a high level of control over implementation and monitoring. In spite of these advantages, research regarding the effectiveness of such interventions is still limited, particularly in the area of pregnancy, STD, and HIV prevention. The balance of this chapter provides a brief overview of one such intervention. The target audience was adolescents in rural Kentucky, though we believe the information presented here is generalizable to other adolescents as well. The goal of this project was to determine how technology might help change, shape, and reinforce a number of theoretically important variables that should ultimately lead to a delay in the initiation of sexual activity and to increased condom use among those who are sexually active.

## Formative Evaluation and Program Design

For this project, formative evaluation consisted of four focus groups and more than 1,700 surveys with rural adolescents. Survey data revealed that nearly 96% of the target audience had access to the Internet and a CD-ROM drive. Thus, using a computer- and Internet-based intervention with this target audience seemed feasible. Focus group participants indicated that they would be unlikely to participate in activities not required by school without incentives of some sort. Therefore, the intervention included a few minor monetary incentives to encourage participation in the weekly activities. Finally, survey and focus group data clearly suggested that perceived susceptibility and self-efficacy needed to be increased. As these variables are directly related to the extended parallel process model (Witte, Meyer, & Martel, 2001), it was selected to inform the development of the intervention.

## Program Implementation and Process Evaluation

The 7-week intervention included 6 computer-based activities. One activity was put online for each of the first 6 weeks, and all six activities were put online during Week 7 (dubbed "Make-Up Week"). This time frame allowed students more time to process information and encouraged students to complete an activity more than once. It also provided time to promote each of the activities, and allowed participants to think about the larger issue for a longer period of time. Most activities took about 15 minutes to complete. Though facilitated through schools, all activities were designed to be completed outside of class time. Some of the activities were developed specifically for this intervention, whereas others were adapted from Barth's (1996) *Reducing the Risk* curriculum. Whenever possible, materials were also adapted for rural adolescents based on feedback received during the formative evaluation. A brief overview of each of the six computer- or Internet-based activities follows.

Two of the activities asked students to fill out the sensation-seeking and impulsive-decision-making scales. Individuals received tailored information about these personality traits, how they relate to their risk-taking behavior, and things they might do to reduce their risk. Two of the activities asked students to identify whether various statements were "truth" or "myth," or whether various behaviors were "very risky," "a little risky," or "not risky." Individuals received tailored feedback to each answer and also regarding their final score. The refusal skill/delaying tactic activity asked students to imagine they were in a situation where their date wanted to have sex and they did not, and to submit their best refusal or delaying response. Finally, there was the Choose Your Own Adventure CD-ROM, which was introduced in the opening paragraph of this chapter.

Process evaluation results indicate that although participation tended to decrease as the intervention progressed, nearly 90% of students completed at least one of the six activities ($M = 3.5$ for those doing at least one activity). Furthermore, students' opinions were generally very favorable toward the intervention as a whole, and toward each individual activity. Though seemingly simple, these were important steps as they ensured the intervention was implemented as intended, and therefore provided greater confidence in the outcome evaluation results presented next.

## Outcome Evaluation

Two different studies were conducted to determine the effects of the intervention. First, we conducted a small-scale study at two high schools using a pretest–posttest control-group design (Roberto, Zimmerman, Carlyle, & Abner, 2007). More than 85% of eligible students completed the survey at both points in time ($N = 326$). Results show that individuals in both the treatment and control groups were nearly identical on all variables at the pretest. However, by the posttest, the treatment group demonstrated significantly greater knowledge, more positive attitudes toward waiting to have sex, and greater condom negotiation and situational self-efficacy, and was also significantly less likely to initiate sexual activity than individuals in the control group ($ps < .05$).

In a second study (Roberto, Zimmerman, Carlyle, Abner, Cupp, et al., 2007), we implemented and evaluated the intervention on a larger scale at nine high schools using a pretest–posttest "institutional cycle design" (Campbell & Stanley, 1963). This design entailed collecting data for the control group during one institutional cycle (or school year), and data from the treatment group during the following school year. Nearly 62% of eligible students completed the survey at both points in time ($N = 887$). The treatment and control groups were again found to be nearly identical at the pretest. By the posttest, however, the treatment group had significantly greater knowledge, more positive attitudes toward waiting to have sex, greater perceived condom self-efficacy, and greater perceived susceptibility to HIV ($ps < .05$).

## Conclusion and Recommendations

This investigation provides evidence that even modest computer-based interventions can influence several theoretically important variables, and even short-term behavior. These findings are particularly notable because participation in the intervention was optional, not required; took place outside of class/school, rather than during class/school; and contained only six short (15-minute) activities, rather than a larger number of longer (full class period) activities. Though results were promising, we have a few recommendations for those interested in undertaking a similar endeavor. First, we recommend an even greater emphasis on individually tailored messages. Such tailoring may range from the relatively simple (i.e., referencing the participant's name) to the more complex (i.e., basing the types of activities one is asked to do, or the type of feedback one receives, on their levels of perceived threat and efficacy, past behaviors, etc.). Second, such interventions might work best when used to complement, rather than to replace, more traditional school-based HIV prevention curricula. For example, traditional classroom-based interventions will clearly be able to do more if they also contain activities designed to be completed outside of class. The findings reported here suggest that knowledge, attitudes, and self-efficacy are prime targets for computer- and Internet-based interventions. Finally, though working with schools proved successful, partnerships with other organizations (e.g., other community organizations) might be just as effective.

## Acknowledgments

The project discussed in this chapter was funded by National Institute of Mental Health Grant R01 MH16876 awarded to the University of Kentucky, Rick S. Zimmerman, Principal Investigator. The authors would also like to acknowledge the important contributions of three additional research team members: Erin Abner, Pamela Cupp, and Gary Hansen.

## References

Barth, R. P. (1996). *Reducing the risk: Building skills to prevent pregnancy, STD, & HIV* (3rd ed.). Santa Cruz, CA: ETR Associates.

Campbell, D. T., & Stanley, J. C. (1963). *Experimental and quasi-experimental designs for research.* Boston: Houghton Mifflin.

Roberto, A. J., Zimmerman, R. S., Carlyle, K., & Abner, E. L. (2007). A computer-based approach to preventing pregnancy, STD, and HIV in rural adolescents. *Journal of Health Communication, 12,* 53–76.

Roberto, A. J., Zimmerman, R. S., Carlyle, K., Abner, E. L., Cupp, P. K., & Hansen, G. L. (2007). The effects of a computer-based HIV, STD, and pregnancy prevention intervention: A nine-school trial. *Health Communication, 21,* 115–124.

Witte, K., Meyer, G., & Martell, D. P. (2001). *Effective health risk messages: A step-by-step guide.* Newbury Park, CA: Sage.

# Author Index

# Subject Index

## A

activists
  prevention policy, 317
  public health policy, 317
ACT UP, 81
adolescent multimedia programs, 424
Advancing HIV Prevention (AHP), 297
  CDC, 312
  knowledge enthymeme, 304
  policy shifts, 318
  preventive actions, 304
  public health policy, 318
  SAFE, 300
  science *vs.* politics response, 309–314
adverse health effects, 335
African Americans, 195
  adolescents, 389–394
    females, 390
  AIDS information, 402
  community, 404
  families
    HIV infection percentages, 183
    sexual risk taking, 182
  fathers, 176
  heritage roles, 201
  HIV information, 402
  infected, 211
  mothers, 174, 177–178, 179
    adolescent daughters, 180
    religious beliefs, 179
  parent–child HIV/AIDS
      communications, 172, 179
  protests, 228
  rates of STDs, 196
  religious institutions, 208
  STDs, 269
  teens, 269
  women, 195, 389
    HIV, 268
    STD, 45
  youth, 199

agenda-setting process, 278
  components, 279, 289
  policy attention, 292
age- sex-based communication, 177
AHP. *see* Advancing HIV Prevention
      (AHP)
AIDS. *See* Autoimmune Deficiency
      Syndrome (AIDS)
AIDS Community Demonstration Projects,
      357
AIDS Project Los Angeles (APLA), 310
AIDS service organizations (ASOs), 102
American soap operas, 260
America Responds to AIDS (ARTA), 227
anger, 32
antiretrovirals, 67, 339
  dosing schedules, 338
APLA. *see* AIDS Project Los Angeles
      (APLA)
application-driven HIV test, 153
ARTA. *see* America Responds to AIDS
      (ARTA)
Asian Americans, 30
  campaigns, 293
  HIV/STD, 30
ASOs. *see* AIDS service organizations
assertion, 32
assertiveness
  definitions, 32
  negotiation, 37
  training approach, 33
audience segmentation HIV/AIDS media
      campaigns, 226–227
Autoimmune Deficiency Syndrome (AIDS).
      *see also* HIV/AIDS; specific
      topics e.g. prevention
  hotlines, 264
  specialist nurse, 340

Printed in the United States
201531BV00003BA/7-12/P